M000099290

Nearest-Neighbor Methods in Learning and Vision

Nearest-Neighbor Methods in Learning and Vision: Theory and Practice

edited by
Gregory Shakhnarovich
Trevor Darrell
Piotr Indyk

The MIT Press
Cambridge, Massachusetts
London, England

©2005 Massachusetts Institute of Technology

All rights reserved. No part of this book may be reproduced in any form by any electronic or mechanical means (including photocopying, recording, or information storage and retrieval) without permission in writing from the publisher.

This book was set in LaTeX by the authors and was printed and bound in the United States of America

Library of Congress Cataloging-in-Publication Data

Nearest-Neighbor Methods in Learning and Vision: Theory and Practice / edited by Gregory Shakhnarovich, Trevor Darrell and Piotr Indyk.
    p. cm. — (Neural information processing series)

Includes bibliographical references and index.
ISBN 0-262-19547-X (alk. paper)
1. Nearest neighbor analysis (Statistics)-Congresses. 2. Machine learning-Congresses. 3. Algorithms-Congresses. 4. Geometry-Data processing-Congresses. I. Shakhnarovich, Gregory. II. Darrell, Trevor. III. Indyk, Piotr. IV. Series.
QA278.2.N43 2006 00.6.3'1-dc22   2005053124

10 9 8 7 6 5 4 3 2 1

Contents

Series Foreword

The yearly Neural Information Processing Systems (NIPS) workshops bring together scientists with broadly varying backgrounds in statistics, mathematics, computer science, physics, electrical engineering, neuroscience, and cognitive science, unified by a common desire to develop novel computational and statistical strategies for information processing, and to understand the mechanisms for information processing in the brain. As opposed to conferences, these workshops maintain a flexible format that both allows and encourages the presentation and discussion of work in progress, and thus serve as an incubator for the development of important new ideas in this rapidly evolving field.

The Series Editors, in consultation with workshop organizers and members of the NIPS Foundation Board, select specific workshop topics on the basis of scientific excellence, intellectual breadth, and technical impact. Collections of papers chosen and edited by the organizers of specific workshops are built around pedagogical introductory chapters, while research monographs provide comprehensive descriptions of workshop-related topics, to create a series of books that provides a timely, authoritative account of the latest developments in the exciting field of neural computation.

Michael I. Jordan and Thomas Dietterich

Preface

Regression and classification methods based on similarity of the input to stored examples have been part of the arsenal in statistics and computer science for decades. Despite consistently good performance in a number of domains, these methods have not been employed as widely in applications where very large sets of high-dimensional data are involved. Two of the main reasons for this are the computational complexity of similarity search in high-dimensional spaces, often seen as prohibitive, and the sensitivity of the exemplar-based methods to the choice of distance measure. The main focus of this book is on advances in computational geometry and machine learning that may alleviate these problems, and on emerging applications in the field of computer vision in which the benefit of these advances is often dramatic.

The book contains contributions by participants in the workshop on nearest-neighbor methods in learning and vision, held in Whistler, British Columbia, as part of the annual conference on Neural Information Processing Systems (NIPS) in December 2003. The workshop brought together researchers from theory of computation, machine learning, and computer vision. Its goal was to bridge the ostensible gaps between these disciplines and explore the state of the art in nearest-neighbor search methods on the one hand, and the emerging applications of these methods in learning and vision on the other hand. The chapters, organized into three corresponding parts, are representative of the ideas presented and discussed at the workshop.

We hope that this book will be of interest to the students, researchers, and practitioners of machine learning and computer vision, to whom it may provide inspiration and ideas as well as useful solutions to specific problems. In addition, we expect that the book will be of interest to researchers in computational geometry and algorithms, for whom it presents intersting application domains in need of new efficient algorithms.

We would like to aknowledge Paul Viola, who co-organized the NIPS workshop with us. We would also like to thank all those who attended the workshop and participated in the discussions, and the authors of the chapters for their excellent contributions to the workshop and now to this book. Finally, we are grateful to the workshop chairs of NIPS 2003, to the editors of the series, and to the staff of MIT Press, in particular Bob Prior and Katherine Almeida, without all of whom this project would not have succeeded.

Gregory Shakhnarovich
Brown University

Trevor Darrell, Piotr Indyk
Massachusetts Institute of Technology, Cambridge

1 Introduction

Gregory Shakhnarovich, Piotr Indyk, and Trevor Darrell

The nearest-neighbor (NN) problem occurs in the literature under many names, including the *best match* or the *post office* problem. The problem is of significant importance to several areas of computer science, including pattern recognition, searching in multimedia data, vector compression, computational statistics, and data mining. For many of these applications, including some described in this book, large amounts of data are available. This makes nearest-neighbor approaches particularly appealing, but on the other hand it increases the concern regarding the computational complexity of NN search. Thus it is important to design algorithms for nearest-neighbor search, as well as for the related classification, regression, and retrieval tasks, which remain efficient even as the number of points or the dimensionality of the data grows large. This is a research area on the boundary of a number of disciplines: computational geometry, algorithmic theory, and the application fields such as machine learning. This area is the focus of this book, which contains contributions from researchers in all of those fields.

Below we define the exact and approximate nearest-neighbor search problems, and briefly survey a number of popular data structures and algorithms developed for these problems. We also discuss the relationship between the nearest-neighbor search and machine learning. Finally, we summarize the contents of the chapters that follow.

1.1 The Nearest-Neighbor Search Problem

The *exact* nearest-neighbor search problem in a Euclidean space is defined as follows:

Definition 1.1 (Nearest neighbor) *Given a set P of points in a d-dimensional space $\Re^d$, construct a data structure which given any* query *point q finds the point in P with the smallest distance to q.*

The problem is not fully specified without defining the distance between an arbitrary pair of points p and q. Typically, it is assumed that this distance is induced by an l_s norm. That is, the distance between p and q is defined as $\|p - q\|_s$, where $\|x\| = (\sum_{i=1}^{d} |x_i|^s)^{1/s}$. Other (more general) notions of distance are possible as well.

A naive algorithm for this problem is as follows: given a query q, compute the distance from q to each point in P, and report the point with the minimum distance. This *linear scan* approach has query time of $\Theta(dn)$. This is tolerable for small data sets, but is too inefficient for large ones. The "holy grail" of the research in the area is to design an algorithm for this problem that achieves *sublinear* (or even *logarithmic*) query time.

The nearest-neighbor problem has been extensively investigated in the field of computational geometry. As a result of this research effort, many efficient solutions have been discovered for the case when the points lie in a space of *constant* dimension. For example, if the points lie in the plane, the nearest-neighbor problem can be solved with $O(\log n)$ time per query, using only $O(n)$ storage [36, 27]. Similar results can be obtained for other problems as well. Unfortunately, as the dimension grows, the algorithms become less and less efficient. More specifically, their space or time requirements grow *exponentially* in the dimension. In particular, the nearest-neighbor problem has a solution with $O(d^{O(1)} \log n)$ query time, but using roughly $n^{O(d)}$ space [11, 29].

At the same time, many data structures that use the optimal $O(dn)$ space are known (e.g., see the survey [9] for a review of nearest-neighbor data structures from the database perspective). These data structures often provide significant speedups on many data sets. At the same time, they are known to suffer from linear query time for "high enough" dimension (e.g., see [9], p. 365).

The lack of success in removing the exponential dependence on the dimension led many researchers to conjecture that no efficient solutions exist for this problem when the dimension is sufficiently large (e.g., see [31]). At the same time, it raised the question: Is it possible to remove the exponential dependence on d, if we allow the answers to be *approximate*? The approximate nearest neighbor search problem is defined as follows.

Definition 1.2 (c-Approximate nearest neighbor) *Given a set P of points in a d-dimensional space $\Re^d$, construct a data structure which given any query point q, reports any point within distance at most c times the distance from q to p, where p is the point in P closest to q.*

During recent years, several researchers have shown that indeed in many cases approximation enables reduction of the dependence on dimension from exponential to polynomial. A survey of these results can be found in [23]. In addition, there are many approximate nearest-neighbor algorithms that are more efficient than the exact ones, even though their query time and/or space usage is still exponential in the dimension. This includes the algorithms given in [3, 5, 12, 26, 10, 20, 1]. The algorithm in [5] has an efficient implementation (ANN); see [2] for details.

In the following we present an brief overview of three data structures: kd-trees (and relatives), balltrees, and locality-sensitive hashing (LSH).

1.1.1 Kd-Trees

The kd-tree [8] is a data structure invented by Jon Bentley in 1975. Despite its fairly old age, kd-tree and its variants remain probably the most popular data structures used for searching in multidimensional spaces, at least in main memory. According to Google Scholar, the paper [8] that introduced this data structure is one of the most cited papers in computational geometry, with 734 citations as of June 2005.

Given a set of n points in a d-dimensional space, the kd-tree is constructed recursively as follows. First, one finds a median of the values of the ith coordinates of the points (initially, $i = 1$). That is, a value M is computed, so that at least 50% of the points have their ith coordinate greater-or-equal to M, while at least 50% of the points have their ith coordinate smaller than or equal to M. The value of x is stored, and the set P is partitioned into P_L and P_R, where P_L contains only the points with their ith coordinate smaller than or equal to M, and $|P_R| = |P_L| \pm 1$. The process is then repeated recursively on both P_L and P_R, with i replaced by $i + 1$ (or 1, if $i = d$). When the set of points at a node has size 1, the recursion stops.

The resulting data structure is a binary tree with n leaves, and depth $\lceil \log n \rceil$. In particular, for $d = 1$, we get a (standard) balanced binary search tree. Since a median of n coordinates can be found in $O(n)$ time, the whole data structure can be constructed in time $O(n \log n)$.

For the problem of finding the nearest neighbor in P of a given query q, several methods exist. The first one was suggested in the original paper. However, it was quickly superseded by a different procedure, introduced in [25] (the original procedure was deleted from the journal version of [8]). The latter search procedure is as follows. The search starts from the root of the tree, and is recursive. At any point in time, the algorithm maintains the distance R to the point closest to q encountered so far; initially, $R = \infty$. At a leaf node (containing, say, point p') the algorithm checks if $\|q - p'\| < R$. If so, R is set to $\|q - p'\|$, and p' is stored as the closest point candidate. In an internal node, the algorithm proceeds as follows. Let M be the median value stored at the node, computed with respect to the ith coordinates. The algorithm checks if the ith coordinate of q is smaller than or equal to M. If so, the algorithm recurses on the left node; otherwise it recurses on the right node. After returning from the recursion, the algorithm performs the "bounds overlap ball" test: it checks whether a ball of radius R around q contains any point in $\Re^d$ whose ith coordinate is on the opposite side of M with respect to q. If this is the case, the algorithm recurses on the yet-unexplored child of the current node. Otherwise, the recursive call is terminated. At the end, the algorithm reports the final closest-point candidate.

It was shown in [25] that if the data and the query point are chosen independently at random from a random distribution (say from a d-dimensional hypercube $[0,1]^d$), then the procedure terminates in time $G(d)\log n$, for some function G. However, $G(d)$ is exponential in d, at least for values of d that are "small" compared to $\log n$; note that the running time is always at most $O(dn)$. It is easy to construct data sets which achieve this worst-case running time.

A different search procedure is obtained by modifying the order in which the nodes are visited. Specifically, several authors [4, 5, 6, 21] proposed to examine the nodes in the order of their distance to the query point (the exact definition of this process depends on the implementation). This enables the algorithm to locate a "close enough" neighbor much faster. For example, experiments in [4] indicate that this "priority" approach enables finding very good approximate nearest neighbors up to ten times faster than the original kd-tree search procedure.

Another bonus of the priority search approach is that one can prove worst-case guarantees for the running times of the resulting algorithm (for a somewhat modified data structure, called box-decomposition tree, see [5]). Further results of this type are given in [17].

1.1.2 Balltrees and Metric Trees

Balltrees, introduced by Omohundro in [34], are complete binary trees, where the leaves correspond to the data points and each interior (non-leaf) node corresponds to a ball in the data space. The ball associated with a given node is required to be the smallest ball that contains the balls associated with that node's children. Closely related to balltrees are *metric trees* [38], in which a node is constructed by thresholding the distance between the points it contains and a pivot.

In contrast to kd-trees, the regions associated with sibling nodes in balltrees and metric trees may intersect and do not have to cover the entire space. This may allow a more flexible coverage of the space, reflecting the structure inherent in the data, and thus make the data structure more efficient for data embedded in high-dimensional spaces. A number of algorithms have been proposed for fast construction, updating, and searching of these data structures [34, 38, 32]. For a more detailed description, see section 4.2 in chapter 4.

1.1.3 Locality-Sensitive Hashing (LSH)

LSH, as well as several other algorithms discussed in [23], is *randomized*. The randomness is typically used in the construction of the data structure. Moreover, these algorithms often solve a *near*-neighbor problem, as opposed to the *nearest*-neighbor problem. The former can be viewed as a decision version of the latter. Formally, the problem definitions are as follows. A point p is an R-*near neighbor* of q if the distance from p to q is at most R.

Definition 1.3 (Randomized c-approximate near-neighbor) *Given a set P of points in a d-dimensional space $\Re^d$, and parameters $R > 0$, $\delta > 0$, construct a data structure which, given any* query *point q, does the following with probability $1 - \delta$: if there is an R-near neighbor of q in P, it reports a cR-near neighbor of q in P.*

Definition 1.4 (Randomized near-neighbor reporting) *Given a set P of points in a d-dimensional space $\Re^d$, and parameters $R > 0$, $\delta > 0$, construct a data structure which, given any* query *point q, reports each R-near neighbor of q in P with probability $1 - \delta$.*

Note that, in the second definition, the probabilities of reporting different R-near neighbors might *not* be independent. Also note that, in both problems, the value R is known during the preprocessing time. Therefore, by scaling the coordinates of all points, we can assume that $R = 1$.

Among the algorithms discussed in [23], the LSH algorithm is probably the one that has received most attention in the practical context. Its main idea is to hash the data points using several hash functions so as to ensure that, for each function, the probability of collision is much higher for points which are close to each other than for those which are far apart. Then, one can determine near neighbors by hashing the query point and retrieving elements stored in buckets containing that point.

The LSH algorithm can be used to solve either the approximate or the exact near-neighbor problem. It relies on the existence of *LSH functions*, defined in the following manner. Consider a family $\mathcal{H}$ of hash functions mapping $\Re^d$ to some universe U.

Definition 1.5 (Locality-sensitive hashing) *A family $\mathcal{H}$ is called (r, cr, P_1, P_2)-sensitive if for any $p, q \in \Re^d$*

- *if $\|p - q\| \leq R$ then $\mathrm{P}_{\mathcal{H}}[h(q) = h(p)] \geq P_1$,*
- *if $\|p - q\| \geq cR$ then $\mathrm{P}_{\mathcal{H}}[h(q) = h(p)] \leq P_2$.*

In order for a LSH family to be useful, it has to satisfy $P_1 > P_2$.

An LSH family can be utilized as follows. Given a family $\mathcal{H}$ of hash functions with parameters (r, cr, P_1, P_2) as in the above definition, we amplify the gap between the "high" probability P_1 and the "low" probability P_2 by concatenating several functions. In particular, for k and L specified later, we choose L functions $g_j(q) = (h_{1,j}(q), \ldots, h_{k,j}(q))$, where $h_{t,j}(1 \leq t \leq k, 1 \leq j \leq L)$ are chosen independently and uniformly at random from $\mathcal{H}$. During preprocessing, we store each $p \in P$ (input point set) in the bucket $g_j(p)$, for $j = 1, \ldots, L$. Since the total number of buckets may be large, we retain only the nonempty buckets by resorting to hashing the values $g_j(p)$.

To process a query q, we search through the buckets $g_1(q), \ldots, g_L(q)$. Two concrete strategies are possible:

1. Interrupt search after finding the first L' points (including duplicates).

2. Continue search until all points from the buckets are retrieved.

It is shown in [24] that the first strategy, with $L' = 3L$, enables solving the *randomized c-approximate near-neighbor problem*, with parameters R and δ, for some constant $\delta < 1$. To obtain that guarantee, it suffices to set L to $\Theta(n^\rho)$, where $\rho = \frac{\ln 1/P_1}{\ln 1/P_2}$. Note that this implies that the algorithm runs in time proportional to n^ρ, which is sublinear in n if $P_1 > P_2$.

On the other hand, in practice, the second strategy appears to be more popular, presumably since it avoids the need to specify the additional parameter L'. Also, there is no need to specify c, since the algorithm can solve the exact near neighbor problem, as described in the remainder of this paragraph. The analysis in [24] can be used to show that the second strategy enables solving the randomized *exact near-neighbor reporting problem* for a given parameter R. The value of δ depends on the choice of the parameters k and L; alternatively, for each δ one can provide parameters k and L so that the error probability is smaller than δ. The query time is also dependent on k and L: it could be as high as $\Theta(n)$ in the worst case, but for many data sets a proper choice of parameters results in a sublinear query time. See more details in chapter 3.

The quality of LSH functions is characterized by the parameter ρ. It was shown in [24, 19] that if the distance is measured according to the l_1 norm, then there exists a (R, cR, P_1, P_2)-sensitive family of functions with $\rho = 1/c$. In chapter 3 another family of functions is described which works if the distances are measured according to the l_s norm for $s \in (0, 2]$.

1.2 Nearest-Neighbor Methods in Learning and Vision

In the context of machine learning, nearest-neighbor methods are applied to supervised problems. Suppose one is given a *reference set*–a set of examples for which the target concept (a class label, function value, etc.) is known, and a *query*, for which such a value is unknown and is to be recovered. The nearest-neighbor approach consists of finding one or more examples most similar to the query, and using the labels of those examples to produce the desired estimate of the query's label.

This broad description leaves two important questions:

1. What are the criteria of similarity? The answer depends on the underlying distance measure as well as on the selection criteria, e.g., the k examples closest to the query for a fixed k, or the examples closer than a fixed threshold r. The choices of these criteria are known to have a very significant influence on the performance on the algorithm.

2. How are the labels from the neighbors to be combined? The simplest way is to take the majority vote, in classification setup, or the average,

in regression setup. However, more sophisticated methods, such as locally weighted regression, have been shown to produce sometimes dramatically better results.

The following fundamental property of nearest-neighbor classification has been shown by Cover and Hart in [15]. Let $R(n)$ be the expected probability of error of the M-category nearest-neighbor classifier for a training set of n examples. Then the limit $R = \lim_{n \to \infty} R(n)$ is bounded by $R^* \leq R \leq R^*(2 - MR^*/(M-1))$, where R^* stands for the *Bayes risk–* the probability of error of the optimal classifier given the distribution of the data. A similar result can be shown for the nearest-neighbor regression [13].

Unfortunately, these asymptotic results do not necessarily translate into similar bounds in practice when training sets of finite size are used. As has been shown by Cover in [14], the rate of convergence to this limit may be arbitrarily slow. A significant body of work has been devoted to analysis of nearest-neighbor performance on samples of finite size. Although no "distribution-free" bounds have been found, it is possible to characterize the finite sample risk of the nearest-neighbor classifier based on various properties of the input space and the data distribution (see [18, 35, 37] for some interesting results). Moreover, despite the lack of theoretical guarantees, it has often been observed that the nearest-neighbor classifiers perform very well in practice, and achieve accuracy equivalent to or even better than that of significantly more complicated methods; see, e.g., the extensive comparative study reported in [16].

Similar success has been seen in the application of nearest-neighbor methods to a variety of vision tasks, such as shape matching [22, 7] and object recognition [33, 30, 28]. However, in computer vision the limitations of some nearest-neighbor search methods have particularly high impact, since the data here is typically high-dimensional, and in many cases the databases required to sufficiently represent the visual phenomena are large. On the other hand, appropriate similarity measures in vision applications are often more expensive than the Euclidean distance. Furthermore, these measures may not even be metrics. All this poses a challenge for a practitioner interested in using an example-based technique in a computer vision problem. Possible solutions include randomized approximate algorithms, embedding techniques, and machine learning algorithms for adapting the data structures for the properties of the data in the given domain. The book describes some of the recent advances in these directions.

1.3   Contributions to this book

Theory

The book opens with two contributions from computational geometry. Chapter 2, by Clarkson, focuses on the formulation of exact nearest-neighbor search, and studies this problem in metric spaces. In particular, it investigates the various dimensionality properties that make the problem tractable in practice, and presents theoretical results. Chapter 3, by Andoni, Datar, Immorlica, Indyk, and Mirrokni, is devoted to a randomized algorithm that allows approximate as well as exact similarity search in very high dimensions in time sublinear in the size of the database. The algorithm is an extension of LSH, described in 1.1.3, to a family of distance metrics beyond the l_1 norm.

Learning

The unifying theme of the three chapters in the second part of the book is exploring the ways to make the nearest-neighbor approach practicable in machine learning application where the dimensionality of the data, and the size of the data sets, make the naive methods for nearest-neighbor search prohibitively expensive. In chapter 4, Liu, Moore, and Gray notice that in nearest-neighbor classification, what matters for the decision is the distribution of labels of the query's neighbors, rather than the neighbors themselves. They use this observation to develop new algorithms, using previously introduced balltree data structures, that afford a significant speedup while maintaining the accuracy of the exact k-nearest-neighbor classification.

Chapter 5, by Vijayakumar, D'Souza, and Schaal, is devoted to methods that build a local model of the target function in the vicinity of the query by finding its neighbors in the reference set. The chapter proposes an approach that extends such local learning methods to very high-dimensional spaces by exploiting the low intrinsic dimensionality within a neighborhood. Another contribution is a new Bayesian regression algorithm. The proposed framework has been shown to be fast and accurate in a number of applications, including real-time motor control tasks for robots.

Chapter 6, by Athitsos, Alon, Sclaroff, and Kollios addresses the issue that arises in the context of many applications of nearest-neighbor methods in learning, be they for classification, regression, or database retrieval. When computing the distance of interest is expensive, a significant reduction in search time may be gained if a cheap way exists to evaluate the relative distances from the query and eliminate the majority of the reference examples from contention, thus requiring the distance to be explicitly computed only on a small subset of the database. The approach proposed in this chapter is to learn an embedding of the original distance into a Euclidean space, in which the ranking with respect to the Manhattan metric reflects the ranking under the original distance. Connecting this chapter to the following ones, the approach is evaluated on two computer vision tasks: estimating the articulated pose of human hands and classifying sign language utterances.

Vision

The chapters in the third part of the book describe successful applications of LSH to vision tasks. Moreover, as some of the chapters show, the basic LSH framework may be adapted to better fit the properties of the data space and the task at hand.

In chapter 7, Shakhnarovich, Viola, and Darrell deal with a regression task: estimating articulated body pose from images of people. The basic idea here is to learn, using pairs of images with known poses, hash functions sensitive to the distance in the pose space. The resulting method, parameter-sensitive hashing, allows very fast example-based estimation of pose using a very large set of labeled examples. Chapter 8, by Grauman and Darrell, is concerned with database retrieval scenarios where the distance is known but very expensive to compute: the earth mover's distance (EMD) between contours. The authors propose a technique, based on multiresolution histograms, that embeds the contours into a Euclidean space of very high dimensions, and replaces EMD with the Manhattan distances between sparse points in that space, thus allowing application of very fast approximate search algorithms such as LSH. The experiments on data sets of handwritten digits and human body contours show that with this embedding, neighbor-based methods remain very accurate while gaining dramatic speedup.

In contrast to the previous chapters, the task of interest in chapter 9, by Shimshoni, Georgescu, and Meer, is an unsupervised one: clustering. Specifically, the authors show how LSH can be used to reduce the complexity of mean-shift clustering, and apply the resulting algorithm to the tasks of visual texture classification and image segmentation. They also propose significant modifications in the algorithms for constructing the data structure used to index the examples: the partitions in the hash tables are data driven.

Finally, in chapter 10 Frome and Malik present an application of LSH to another vision task: automatic classification of vehicles from their three-dimensional range scans. The approach proposed by the authors relies on LSH to perform fast search in a set of reference objects represented using shape context–a representation that has been shown to be useful but also to make distance calculations very costly. This chapter, too, presents a modification of the basic LSH algorithm: Associative LSH. In this algorithm, the results returned by LSH for a query are further refined by local search, improving the quality of the approximate nearest-neighbor and consequently affording a gain in classification accuracy.

References

1. S. Arya and T. Malamatos. Linear-size approximate Voronoi diagrams. *In Proceedings of the ACM-SIAM Symposium on Discrete Algorithms*, pages 147–155, 2002.

2. S. Arya and D. Mount. ANN: Library for approximate nearest neighbor searching. `http://www.cs.umd.edu/~mount/ANN/`.

3. S. Arya and D. Mount. Approximate nearest neighbor searching. *In Proceedings of the Fourth Annual ACM-SIAM Symposium on Discrete Algorithms*, pages 271–280, 1993.

4. S. Arya, D. Mount, J. Storer, and M. Cohn. Algorithms for fast vector quantization. *Data Compression Conference*, pages 381–390, 1993.

5. S. Arya, D.M. Mount, N.S. Netanyahu, R. Silverman, and A. Wu. An optimal algorithm for approximate nearest neighbor searching. *In Proceedings of the Fifth Annual ACM-SIAM Symposium on Discrete Algorithms*, pages 573–582, 1994.

6. J. Beis and D. Lowe. Shape indexing using approximate nearest neighbour search in high-dimensional spaces. *Proceedings of the IEEE Computer Society Conference on Computer Vision*, page 1000, 1997.

7. S Belongie, J. Malik, and J. Puzicha. Shape Matching and Object Recognition Using Shape Contexts. *IEEE Transactions on Pattern Analysis and Machine Intelligence*, April 2002.

8. J.L. Bentley. Multidimensional binary search trees used for associative searching. *Communications of the ACM*, 18:509–517, 1975.

9. C. Bohm, S. Berchtold, and D. A. Keim. Searching in high-dimensional spaces: Index structures for improving the performance of multimedia databases. *ACM Computing Surveys (CSUR)*, 33(3), 2001.

10. T.M. Chan. Approximate nearest neighbor queries revisited. *In Proceedings of the Thirteens Annual ACM Symposium on Computational Geometry*, pages 352–358, 1997.

11. K. Clarkson. A randomized algorithm for closest-point queries. *SIAM Journal on Computing*, 17:830–847, 1988.

12. K. Clarkson. An algorithm for approximate closest-point queries. *In Proceedings of the Tenth Annual ACM Symposium on Computational Geometry*, pages 160–164, 1994.

13. T. M. Cover. Estimation by the nearest neighbor rule. *IEEE Transactions on Information Theory*, 14:21–27, January 1968.

14. T. M. Cover. Rates of Convergence for Nearest Neighbor Procedures. In *Proc. 1st Ann. Hawaii Conf. Systems Theory*, pages 413–415, January 1968.

15. T. M. Cover and P. E. Hart. Nearest neighbor pattern classification. *IEEE Transactions on Information Theory*, 13:21–27, January 1967.

16. D. Michie, D.J. Spiegelhalter, and C.C. Taylor, editors. *Machine Learning, Neural and Statistical Classification.* Ellis Horwood, 1994.

17. C. Duncan, M. Goodrich, and S. Kobourov. Balanced aspect ratio trees: Combining the advantages of kd-trees and octrees. *Journal of Algorithms,* 38:303, 2001.

18. K. Fukunaga and D. M. Hummels. Bias of nearest neighbor error estimates. *IEEE Transactions on Pattern Analysis and Machine Intelligence,* PAMI-9(1):103–112, January 1987.

19. A. Gionis, P. Indyk, and R. Motwani. Similarity search in high dimensions via hashing. *In Proceedings of the 25th International Conference on Very Large Data Bases (VLDB),* 1999.

20. S. Har-Peled. A replacement for Voronoi diagrams of near linear size. *Annual Symposium on Foundations of Computer Science,* 2001.

21. G. Hjaltason and H. Samet. Ranking in spatial databases. *Proceedings of the 4th Symposium on Spatial Databases,* pages 83–95, 1995.

22. D. Huttenlocher, G. Klanderman, and W. Rucklidge. Comparing images using the hausdorff distance,. *IEEE Transactions on Pattern Analysis and Machine Intelligence,* 15, 1993.

23. P. Indyk. Nearest neighbors in high-dimensional spaces. *CRC Handbook of Discrete and Computational Geometry,* 2003.

24. P. Indyk and R. Motwani. Approximate nearest neighbor: towards removing the curse of dimensionality. *Proceedings of the Symposium on Theory of Computing,* 1998.

25. J.L. Bentley J.K. Friedman and R.A. Finkel. An algorithm for finding best matches in logarithmic expected time. *ACM Transactions on Mathematical Software,* 3:209–226, 1977.

26. J. Kleinberg. Two algorithms for nearest-neighbor search in high dimensions. *Proceedings of the Twenty-Ninth Annual ACM Symposium on Theory of Computing,* 1997.

27. R. Lipton and R. Tarjan. Applications of a planar separator theorem. *SIAM Journal on Computing,* 9:615–627, 1980.

28. S. Mahamud and M. Hebert. The optimal distance measure for object detection. In *IEEE Conf. on Computer Vision and Pattern Recognition,* Madison, WI, June 2003.

29. S. Meiser. Point location in arrangements of hyperplanes. *Information and Computation,* 106:286–303, 1993.

30. B. W. Mel. SEEMORE: Combining color, shape, and texture histogramming in a neurally inspired approach to visual object recognition. *Neural Computation,* 9(4):777–804, 1997.

31. M. Minsky and S. Papert. *Perceptrons.* MIT Press, Cambridge, MA, 1969.

32. Andrew Moore. The anchors hierarchy: Using the triangle inequality to survive high-dimensional data. In *Proceedings of the Twelfth Conference on Uncertainty in Artificial Intelligence,* pages 397–405. AAAI Press, 2000.

33. S. A. Nene and S. K. Nayar. A simple algorithm for nearest neighbor search in high dimensions. *IEEE Transactions on Pattern Analysis and Machine Intelligence*, 19(9):989–1003, September 1997.

34. S. M. Omohundro. Five balltree construction algorithms. Technical Report TR-89-063, International Computer Science Institute, Berkeley, CA, December 1989.

35. D. Psaltis, R. R. Snapp, and S. S. Venkatesh. On the Finite Sample Performance of the Nearest Neighbor Classifier. *IEEE Transactions on Information Theory*, 40(3):820–837, May 1994.

36. M. I. Shamos and D. Hoey. Closest point problems. *Proceedings of the Sixteen IEEE Symposium of Foundations of Computer Science*, pages 152–162, 1975.

37. R. R. Snapp and S. S. Venkatesh. Asymptotic derivation of the finite-sample risk of the k nearest neighbor classifier. Technical Report UVM-CS-1998-0101, University of Vermont, Burlingotn, Burlington, VT, October 1997.

38. J.K. Uhlmann. Satisfying general proximity/similarity queries with metric trees. *Information Processing Letters*, 40:175–179, 1991.

I THEORY

2   Nearest-Neighbor Searching and Metric Space Dimensions

Kenneth L. Clarkson

Given a set S of points in a metric space with distance function D, the *nearest-neighbor searching* problem is to build a data structure for S so that for an input query point q, the point $s \in S$ that minimizes $D(s,q)$ can be found quickly. We survey approaches to this problem, and its relation to concepts of metric space dimension. Several measures of dimension can be estimated using nearest-neighbor searching, while others can be used to estimate the cost of that searching. In recent years, several data structures have been proposed that are provably good for low-dimensional spaces, for some particular measures of dimension. These and other data structures for nearest-neighbor searching are surveyed.

2.1   Introduction

The problem of *nearest-neighbor search* is to build a data structure for a set of objects so that, given a query object q, the nearest object in the set to q can be found quickly.

That is, suppose $\mathbb{U}$ is a set and D is a *distance measure* on $\mathbb{U}$, a function that takes pairs of elements of $\mathbb{U}$ and returns a nonnegative real number. Then given a set $S \subset \mathbb{U}$ of size n, the *nearest-neighbor searching* problem is to build a data structure so that, for an input query point $q \in \mathbb{U}$, an element $a \in S$ is found with $D(q,a) \leq D(q,x)$ for all $x \in S$. We will call the members of S *sites*, to distinguish them from other members of $\mathbb{U}$, and say that the answer a is *nearest* in S to q. Put another way, if we define $D(x,S)$ as $\min\{D(x,s) \mid s \in S\}$, then we seek the site s such that $D(q,s) = D(q,S)$.

This problem has been studied for a long time, and has many names in a large and diverse literature. In an early proposal for a solution, due to McNutt (as discussed by Knuth[60]), it was called the *post office problem*. In another early proposal, it was called *best-match file searching* [15]. In the database or information-retrieval literature, it might be called the problem of *building an index for similarity search* [50]. In the information theory literature, it arises as the problem of *building a vector quantization encoder* [69, 42]. In the pattern recognition (or statistics or learning theory) literature, it might be called the problem of building a *fast nearest-neighbor classifier* [34, 26].

This chapter surveys the problem of nearest neighbor searching in the general metric space setting, together with additional dimensionality properties that make instances of the problem tractable. The meaning of "tractable" here is vague, but mainly refers to data structures that are not too big, but allow queries that are fast, where "not too big" means roughly $O(n)$, and "fast" means $o(n)$, as $n \to \infty$.

Some basic constructions of metric spaces are also reviewed, as are some ways of "repairing" a distance measure that does not quite satisfy all the properties needed for a metric space.

Some concepts of dimension we consider include the *Assouad* dimension, the *box* dimension, and a dimension based on *doubling measures*. These concepts have been studied in measure theory and harmonic analysis. As discussed in Subsection 2.5.2, the theoretical computer science community has in recent years begun to study spaces of bounded Assouad dimension, and some of their results include provably efficient data structures for nearest-neighbor searching [21, 64, 44]. Some stronger efficiency results have also been given for spaces satisfying a stronger condition based on *doubling measure* [58, 11, 48]. Some of these algorithms, or related ones, have been implemented, with promising results [22, 11]. Also, some experimental results have been obtained regarding the correlation dimension of a space and the cost of some nearest-neighbor searching problems [10].

These results are described here in the context of the large variety of algorithms and data structures that have been proposed for nearest-neighbor searching. It is remarkable that there are so many such algorithms, especially considering that the distance measure is used simply as a "black box" function that takes two objects and returns a nonnegative real number.

To put these applications of dimensional properties in perspective, we survey a variety of dimensional concepts for metric spaces and for metric measure spaces, and relate them to nearest neighbors. In addition to the box and Assouad dimensions, we consider also for metric spaces the Hausdorff and packing dimensions. For metric measure spaces, the pointwise, energy, and quantization dimensions are discussed, as well as doubling measures, and also the general Rènyi dimensions, which include the information and correlation dimensions. Nearest-neighbor searching is a key component of several estimators of these dimensions, while some estimates of dimension allow bounds for costs related to nearest-neighbor queries. These relations are discussed in Section 2.5.

As an example of the interplay of dimensions and nearest neighbors, suppose a metric space has a measure. Here we will assume that the measure is a probability distribution. The *pointwise dimension* at point x tells how quickly the measure of a ball $B(x, \epsilon)$ centered at x goes to zero, as its radius ϵ goes to zero. The pointwise dimensions of points in the space are closely related to the Hausdorff, information, and energy dimensions of the measure. Now suppose a set of n sites S comprises random points that are independently distributed according to the given measure. It turns out that the pointwise dimension at x can be estimated as the ratio of $\log n$ to the distance of x to its nearest neighbor in S. That is, the pointwise dimension is related to how fast the nearest-neighbor distance goes to zero as n goes to infinity. This is discussed in Subsection 2.4.2. The pointwise dimension has been proposed in the database literature as a way to determine how large the answer to a fixed-radius neighbor query is likely to be. (Such a query asks for all sites inside a given ball.) It is a basic concept of *multifractal* analysis, as used in studying dynamical systems [79].

As another example: ϵ-nets are a kind of well-distributed subset of a metric space, such that every point in the space is within distance ϵ of the net. The box dimension of the space determines the rate at which the size of such nets increases, as a function of $1/\epsilon$. There is a greedy algorithm for finding ϵ-nets that has been applied to building data structures for nearest-neighbor searching,[13, 97, 22, 45] as well as other optimization problems [39]. These relations are discussed in Section 2.4 and Subsection 2.5.2.4.

2.1.1 Scope, and Survey of Surveys

There are many important aspects of nearest-neighbor searching that are not covered here, but have been surveyed elsewhere.

Several surveys of nearest-neighbor searching in $\Re^d$ have been done: one focuses on high-dimensional spaces[53]; another on closest-pair problems, including insertions and deletions of sites [86]; and another [1] on data structures to allow *moving* sites to be handled efficiently [6, 56, 7]. A recent survey [12] and book [78] describe nearest-neighbor searching from a database perspective.

There are at least two prior surveys of searching in general metric spaces [17, 50]. These surveys discuss in detail many algorithms that have arisen in practice.

The primary concern here is with reducing the number of distance evaluations needed to answer a query. There is a substantial body of work on increasing the efficiency of search by speeding up distance evaluations. Some of these techniques are simple and practical, such as avoiding the evaluation of square roots, or stopping distance evaluations when the distance value is known accurately enough. Other techniques show that distances can be estimated quickly using randomization. Related techniques involve the "embedding" of the metric space in a low-dimensional space, a very active area of research [54].

The basic conditions for provably fast search that we consider relate to various concepts of dimension, many of which include the possibility of non-integral, or *fractal* dimension [31, 29]. A rigorous, thorough, and accessible introduction to fractal dimension, including statistical considerations for estimators of dimension, is given by Cutler[24].

2.1.2   Caveat Lector

The algorithms described in Section 2.3 are given only the most cursory overview. The discussion of dimension in Section 2.4 may well neglect some basic conditions needed for mathematical rigor, while the discussion of algorithms in Section 2.5 may not accurately reflect the data structures that are being abstracted and simplified. The bibliography should be helpful, however.

2.1.3   Related Problems and Applications

Nearest-neighbor problems arise in many application areas, including information retrieval, classification, data compression, databases, and dynamical systems. The tasks of vector quantization and nearest-neighbor classification are illustrative.

The *vector quantization* problem is the following: let X denote a random variable in $\mathbb{U}$, with distribution μ. An *n-quantizer* for μ is a function f on $\mathbb{U}$ that takes a point X to one of a set of at most n points in $\mathbb{U}$. That set is called the *codebook*. Let $\mathcal{F}_n$ be the set of all n-quantizer functions. Then the nth quantization error for $\mathbb{U}$ is

$$V_n(\mu) := \inf_{f \in \mathcal{F}_n} E\rho(D(X, f(X))), \qquad (2.1)$$

the cheapest expected cost of representing X by $f(X)$, where the cost is a function $\rho()$ of the distance of X to $f(X)$, and the expectation is with respect to the distribution μ. If the value X was information to transmit over a channel, then an identifying number for $f(X)$ from 1 to n could be transmitted instead, and $f(X)$ recovered from that number on the other end of the channel. The quantization error is the expectation for how badly the received value $f(X)$ distorts the true value X.

Often $\mathbb{U}$ is $\Re^d$, the distance is Euclidean, and $\rho(a) = a^v$ for some value $v > 0$, in which case the nth quantization error is of *order v*.

Nearest-neighbor searching arises in vector quantization as the task of implementing f, after the codebook set has been chosen. Sometimes the codebook is *structured* in a way that allows fast and easy search, as for example when it comprises points on a regular grid. However, for a given distribution, the optimal codebook may be *unstructured*, and look like nothing but an arbitrary point set. (For such unstructured codebooks, the need for fast encoding has led to the use of *tree* encoders, which are not guaranteed to answer a query with the nearest site, or even a near one. However, such encoders work well in practice.) Vector quantization, and the *quantization dimension*, are discussed further in §2.4.3.

As noted above, the problem of classification has long been approached using nearest-neighbor searching [26]. Points in the space (typically $\Re^d$) correspond to sets of objects, and the point coordinates encode various properties of the objects. Each object also has a "color," say red or blue, corresponding to some additional important property. The sites S are a "training set," each of known color. A nearest-neighbor classifier takes as input a query point of unknown color, and returns the color of the nearest site in the training set, or the color of the majority of the nearest k sites. That returned value is a prediction of the true color of the query point.

Thus the nearest-neighbor searching problem arises in finding the closest sites in the training set. Note that, however, it is not necessary to find the nearest sites, but only their colors. It is sometimes possible to use this simplification of the problem to obtain a faster algorithm [74, 70].

We turn now to other computational problems, closely related to nearest-neighbor searching, that arise in applications. One mentioned for classification is *k-nearest neighbors* (*k*-NN): given an integer k and query point q, find the k sites that are closest to q. That is, nearest-neighbor searching is the special case of k-NN searching with $k = 1$. Another related problem is distance *range searching*: build a data structure so that given distance value r and query point q, all sites $p \in S$ with $D(q,p) \leq r$ can be found quickly. If we were given the nearest-neighbor distance $D(q,S)$ by an oracle, then answering the range query with parameter $r = D(q,S)$ would answer the nearest neighbor query.

Approximate Queries. Sometimes it may not be necessary to find the nearest neighbor, but only a (δ)-*near* neighbor, that is, one whose distance is within a δ factor of the nearest distance, for some $\delta > 1$. (Note the distinction between "k-nearest" and "(δ)-near.") Such *approximate* nearest neighbor queries are of interest in their own right, and may have much faster algorithms than those for nearest neighbor queries. Moreover, near neighbors can sometimes be used to find nearest neighbors, as discussed in Subsection 2.5.2.

Reverse Queries. Another related problem is that of building a data structure for *reverse* or *inverse* nearest neighbor queries, where the input is similar, but the answer is not the site nearest to query point q, but rather the sites that have q as their (second) nearest neighbor in $S \cup \{q\}$, that is, the answer is the set of sites

$$\{s \in S \mid D(s,q) \leq D(s, S \setminus \{s\})\}.$$

As with (forward) nearest-neighbor searching, this problem also can be generalized with k and ϵ: given k and site q, find all sites that have q as kth nearest neighbor, or given $\epsilon > 0$, find all sites such that q is within

$1 + \epsilon$ of closest. This problem has arisen as a computational bottleneck in event-driven astrophysical simulations [3], and as a notion of "influence" in decision support and referral systems[62, 85]. It also arises as a subproblem in building data structures for nearest-neighbor queries, as mentioned in Subsection 2.5.2.4.

A key property for reverse queries is that in some circumstances, such as those given for Lemma 2.3, the answer size is bounded by a value independent of $|S|$, the number of elements of S. The intuition, considering points in the plane, is that as more and more sites have q as a nearest neighbor, at some point two of the sites must be closer to each other than to q.

Batched Queries. There are several general problems that might be solved using a data structure for nearest-neighbor searching, or k-NN searching. For example, the *closest-pair* problem is to find the two sites s and s' such that $D(s, s') = \min\{D(p, p') \mid p, p' \in S, p \neq p'\}$. This could be solved by applying a data structure for 2-nearest-neighbors to each site in turn. (Here we must have 2-nearest-neighbors because the closest site to a site s is s itself.) Similarly, the *all-k-nearest-neighbor* (all-k-NN) problem is to find, for each site s, the k sites closest to s. Solving this problem is a common preprocessing step for "manifold reconstruction" in the computational geometry[36], learning theory[83], and computer graphics[52] literatures. Note that the answer to the closest-pair problem can easily be found using the answer to the all-k-NN problem. Similarly, the max-min distance

$$\max_i \min_j D(s_i, s_j),$$

which has been proposed as a diversity measure [2], can be found among the all-k-NN output. The *correlation integral* problem is a range query analog of all-nearest neighbors: given a value $r > 0$, find all pairs of sites within distance r of each other. This problem arises in computing the *correlation dimension* of S, discussed in Subsection 2.4.2.

Bichromatic Problems In addition to the "chromatic" problem of nearest-neighbor classification mentioned above, another class of problems is *bichromatic*. The input is two sets S and S', and the closest pair of sites, one from each set, is desired. (That is, sites in S are "red," and those in S' are "blue," and the closest two-color pair is wanted, hence the problem is bichromatic.) Another bichromatic problem is called a kind of *spatial join* in the database literature: given distance value D, find for each site $s \in S$, the sites in S' that are within distance D of s [10].

2.2 Metric Space Properties, Construction, and Repair

So far, we have only described nearest-neighbor searching problems in great generality, and have not even given any properties of the distance measure

D, except that it maps from pairs of points to real numbers. In instances of these problems, $\mathbb{U}$ and D have many properties that can be used to obtain solutions to the nearest-neighbor problem. The main property that often holds is that $(\mathbb{U}, D)$ is a *metric space*, described next. An additional condition that often applies is that $(\mathbb{U}, D)$ has bounded dimension, for some concept of dimension, as discussed in Section 2.4.

2.2.1 Metric Spaces

The distance function D of a metric space $(\mathbb{U}, D)$ satisfies the following conditions, for all $x, y, z \in \mathbb{U}$:

1. nonnegativity: $D(x, y) \geq 0$;
2. small self-distance: $D(x, x) = 0$;
3. isolation: $x \neq y$ implies $D(x, y) > 0$;
4. symmetry: $D(x, y) = D(y, x)$;
5. the triangle inequality: $D(x, z) \leq D(x, y) + D(y, z)$.

2.2.2 Distance Measure Repairs

A great many instances of nearest-neighbor searching naturally have an associated metric space. Moreover, it is worth noting that if any one of the conditions 3 to 5 fails, while the others hold, there is a natural associated function that is a metric, described next.

Condition 3, isolation, fails: here $(\mathbb{U}, D)$ is a called a *pseudometric*. Partition $\mathbb{U}$ into equivalence classes based on D, where x and y are equivalent if and only if $D(x, y) = 0$. With the natural distance $D([x], [y]) = D(x, y)$ on the classes, the result is a metric space.

Condition 4, symmetry, fails: $(\mathbb{U}, D)$ is a *quasi-metric*. The related measure $\hat{D}(x, y) := (D(x, y) + D(y, x))/2$ will satisfy symmetry, and so yield a metric space.

Condition 5, the triangle inequality, fails: a *semimetric*, or *positively-weighted undirected graph*. A related metric can be found using *shortest paths*: let

$$\hat{D}(x, y) := \inf \sum_i D(z_i, z_{i+1}),$$

where the infimum is taken over all sequences in $\mathbb{U}$ of the form

$$x = z_1, z_2, \ldots, z_N = y,$$

for all $N > 1$. Note that $\hat{D}$ satisfies the triangle inequality, and is a metric, possibly after patching up the "small self-distance" condition. This is the shortest path distance in the graph whose vertices are the points, a *graph metric*.

This repair of the triangle inequality is often used in the other direction: given a finite metric space $(\mathbb{U}, D)$, a graph with vertex set $\mathbb{U}$ and with few edges is found, such that the resulting graph metric is a good approximation to the original metric D. Such graphs are called *spanners*; these have been the focus of considerable research and application.

Another conceivable repair for the triangle inequality is to use $\hat{D}(x,y) := D(x,y)^{1/w}$; for sufficiently large w, $\hat{D}$ satisfies the triangle inequality. If only $w = \infty$ will suffice, then the uniform metric ($D(x,y) = 1$ if $x \neq y$) is the resulting $\hat{D}$. Otherwise, with $w < \infty$, this approach might be of interest, since it preserves inequalities among distances, so the nearest neighbor in D is also the nearest in $\hat{D}$. For finite spaces, $\max_{x,y,z \in \mathbb{U}, x \neq y} \log_2(D(x,z)/D(x,y))$ would be large enough, for example; this quantity is bounded by the *spread*, which is discussed in Subsection 2.5.2. Note that this transformation preserves distance rank: if y is farther from x than z, it will also be under the repaired version. So distance measures that do not obey the triangle inequality might be transformed into metrics, with the answers to nearest-neighbor queries preserved. On the other hand, this transformation flattens the distance, and so may make clusters less distinct, and degrade some searching algorithms.

The repair of quasi-metrics given above is computationally trivial. Pseudometrics do not really need "repair" for nearest-neighbor searching: it is only necessary to keep in mind that the answer is a representative of an equivalence class, and the possibility that distinct sites have distance zero. The repair of the triangle inequality may be difficult to apply in the context of nearest-neighbor searching (although see the string edit distance below). However, graph metrics are a concept of considerable interest and importance in optimization [54]. Given an arbitrary distance function (mapping from ordered pairs to the nonnegative reals) that has $D(x,x) = 0$, an associated metric could be found by using shortest paths to obtain a function that satisfies the triangle inequality, then averaging to enforce symmetry, and finally grouping into equivalence classes to achieve isolation.

2.2.3   Metric Space Constructions

One very basic metric space for any given set $\mathbb{U}$ is, as noted, the uniform metric, where for all $x, y \in \mathbb{U}$, $D(x,y) = 1$ if $x \neq y$, and $D(x,x) = 0$. Another basic space is the set of real numbers $\Re$, with distance $|x - y|$ for $x, y \in \Re$. Moreover, metric spaces can be constructed from other spaces. In the following, suppose $(\mathbb{U}, D)$ is a metric space, as are some $(\mathbb{U}_1, D_1) \ldots (\mathbb{U}_d, D_d)$.

– Submetrics. Plainly, any $(\mathbb{U}', D')$, where $\mathbb{U}' \subset \mathbb{U}$ and D' is D restricted to $\mathbb{U}' \times \mathbb{U}'$, is a metric space.

– Products. Let $\hat{\mathbb{U}}$ be the cross-product $\mathbb{U}_1 \times \mathbb{U}_2 \times \ldots \mathbb{U}_d$, that is, the d-tuples over the $\mathbb{U}_i$. For some value p with $1 \leq p \leq \infty$, define $\hat{D}$ as follows: for $x, y \in \hat{\mathbb{U}}$, let

$$\hat{D}(x, y) := \left(\sum_i D_i(x_i, y_i)^p \right)^{1/p},$$

the product metric. When all $\mathbb{U}_i = \Re$ and $D_i(x, y) = |x - y|$, this yields $\Re^d$ with the ℓ_p distance measures, so $\hat{D}(x, y) = \|x - y\|_p$. When $p = d = 2$, this is simply the Euclidean plane. When $p = 1$ and all the D_i are the uniform metric, the result is the Hamming distance.

– Strings. Let $\mathbb{U}^*$ denote the strings over $\mathbb{U}$. Suppose $\hat{D}$ is a distance measure on $\mathbb{U}^*$ defined as follows: when deletion or addition of one character from x yields y, then $\hat{D}(x, y) = 1$; when replacement of a character a in x by a character b yields y, then $\hat{D}(x, y) = D(a, b)$. Then $(\mathbb{U}^*, \hat{D})$ is a semimetric, and its shortest path "repair," as discussed above, is called the string edit, or Levenshtein distance. In other words, the string edit distance between $x, y \in \mathbb{U}^*$ is the minimum cost sequence of deletion, insertion, or replacement operations to obtain y from x. If deletion and insertion have infinite cost, then this is a kind of Hamming distance on strings. This measure might be used for spelling correction, and for comparing genetic sequences.

– Subsets. The Hausdorff distance between subsets of $\mathbb{U}$ is

$$\hat{D}(S, T) := \min\{D'(S, T), D'(T, S)\},$$

where

$$D'(S, T) := \sup_{s \in S} \inf_{t \in T} D(s, t).$$

Such a distance might be used for geometric shapes. (Technically, this is only a pseudometric, but it is a metric for all closed bounded subsets.) Another commonly used distance between subsets is

$$D(S, T) := \inf_{s \in S, t \in T} D(s, t).$$

Note that this is not a metric.

When $\mathbb{U}$ has a measure μ, the distance $\mu(A \Delta B)$ has been studied, where $A \Delta B$ is the symmetric difference of A and B; this metric generalizes the Hamming distance.

– Nonnegative combinations. Suppose the $\mathbb{U}_i$ are all equal, a set $\mathbb{U}$, but the D_i are different. Given $\alpha_1 \ldots \alpha_d$ with $\alpha_i \geq 0$, define $\hat{D}$ by $\hat{D}(x, y) := \sum_i \alpha_i D_i(x, y)$. Then $(\mathbb{U}, \hat{D})$ is a metric, a nonnegative combination of the originals. (In particular, scaling a single metric by a positive constant also gives a metric.) In other words, the set of metrics on $\mathbb{U}$ is closed under nonnegative combination, and forms a cone; such cones are well studied [27].

– Metric Transforms. If f is a real-valued function of the nonnegative reals, and $f(0) = 0$, and $f(z)$ is monotone increasing and concave for $z \geq 0$, then $\hat{D}(x, y) := f(D(x, y))$ is a metric [27]. For example, if f is twice differentiable, $f'(z) \geq 0$, and $f''(z) \leq 0$ for $z \geq 0$, then f is monotone increasing and concave. One such function is $f(z) := z^\epsilon$, for any given ϵ with $0 < \epsilon < 1$. The new metric $D(x, y)^\epsilon$ is sometimes called the *snowflake* or *power transform* of the original. The function with $f(z) = z/(1 + z)$ also satisfies the given conditions, and yields a bounded distance measure.

– Steinhaus Transform. If (U, D) is a metric space and $a \in U$, then $(U, \hat{D})$ is also a metric space, where

$$\hat{D}(x, y) := \frac{2D(x, y)}{D(x, a) + D(y, a) + D(x, y)}.$$

This is sometimes called the *Steinhaus transform*[27].
When this transform is applied to the distance $D(A, B) = \mu(A \Delta B)$, and with a being the null set Φ, the result is

$$\begin{aligned}
\hat{D}(A, B) &= \frac{2\mu(A \Delta B)}{\mu(A \Delta \Phi) + \mu(B \Delta \Phi) + \mu(A \Delta B)} \\
&= \frac{2\mu(A \Delta B)}{\mu(A) + \mu(B) + \mu(A \Delta B)} = \frac{2\mu(A \Delta B)}{2\mu(A \cup B)} \\
&= \frac{\mu(A \Delta B)}{\mu(A \cup B)},
\end{aligned}$$

which is called the *Steinhaus distance* [27]. The special case for finite sets $|A \Delta B|/|A \cup B|$ is called the *Tanimoto distance* [82], *resemblance* [14], *set similarity distance* [16], *Jaccard distance* [55, 87], or *Marczewski-Steinhaus distance* [71]. It has been proven a metric in several ways [27, 87, 98, 16].

The above follows in part Deza and Laurent [27], and also Indyk and Matoušek [54]; the latter describe other metric constructions, including the *earth-mover* (or *Mallows*[68]), *Fréchet*, and *block-edit* distances.

The above hardly exhausts the distances and metrics that have been considered, even by applying the constructions repeatedly. For example, for two probability distributions on $\mathbb{U}$ with density functions f and g, the α-divergence of f and g is

$$\frac{1}{\alpha - 1} \ln \int f^\alpha g^{1-\alpha},$$

which has the Kullback-Leibler ($\alpha \to 1$) and Hellinger ($\alpha = 1/2$) divergences as special cases. This is not a metric, however.

There is even a distance measure between metric spaces, which can be defined for spaces Z and Z' as the Hausdorff distance between $\kappa(Z)$ and $\kappa(Z')$, where these are Kuratowski embeddings of Z and Z', as mentioned in

Subsection 2.3.1, and the embeddings are chosen to minimize the Hausdorff distance, among all such embeddings [47].

The Pearson Correlation Distance. A distance measure on $\Re^d$ commonly used for biological sequences is derived from the *Pearson correlation*: For point $x = (x_1, \ldots, x_d) \in \Re^d$, let $\eta := \sum_i x_i / d$, and $x' := (x_1 - \eta, x_2 - \eta, \ldots, x_d - \eta)$, and finally $\hat{x} := x'/\|x'\|_2$. That is, the coordinates of x are normalized to have mean zero, and to have $\|\hat{x}\|_2 = 1$, a unit vector in the Euclidean norm. The Pearson correlation of $x, y \in \Re^d$ is then the dot product $\hat{x} \cdot \hat{y}$. The commonly-used derived distance measure is $1 - \hat{x} \cdot \hat{y}$. While this measure does not satisfy the small self-distance or triangle inequality conditions for a metric, note that

$$\|\hat{x} - \hat{y}\|_2^2 = \hat{x} \cdot \hat{x} + \hat{y} \cdot \hat{y} - 2\hat{x} \cdot \hat{y} = 2(1 - \hat{x} \cdot \hat{y}).$$

That is, the square root of the commonly used measure is proportional to the ordinary Euclidean distance between $\hat{x}$ and $\hat{y}$. Therefore, only the small self-distance condition fails for this variant, and metric space (even Euclidean space) methods can be used.

2.3 Using Triangle Inequalities

2.3.1 Triangle Inequality Bounds

The properties of metric spaces allow some basic observations that can yield significantly faster algorithms for nearest-neighbor searching. These follow from the triangle inequality, which allows bounds on a distance we may not have computed, say $D(q, s)$, to be derived from two distances we may already know, say $D(q, p)$ and $D(p, s)$. The following simple properties hold.

Lemma 2.1 *For $q, s, p \in \mathbb{U}$, any value r, and any $P \subset \mathbb{U}$,*

1. $|D(p, q) - D(p, s)| \leq D(q, s) \leq D(q, p) + D(p, s)$;
2. $D(q, s) \geq D_P(q, s) := \max_{p \in P} |D(p, q) - D(p, s)|$;
3. *if $D(p, s) > D(p, q) + r$ or $D(p, s) < D(p, q) - r$, then $D(q, s) > r$;*
4. *if $D(p, s) \geq 2D(p, q)$, then $D(q, s) \geq D(q, p)$.*

Proof Applying the triangle inequality in the three possible ways,

$$D(q, s) \leq D(q, p) + D(p, s)$$
$$D(p, s) \leq D(p, q) + D(q, s)$$
$$D(q, p) \leq D(q, s) + D(s, p)$$

The first of these is the upper bound for $D(q, s)$ in (1), and the other two imply the lower bound of (1). Claim (2) follows from (1), the two parts of Claim (3) follow from the last two inequalities, respectively, and Claim (4) follows from Claim (3) with $r = D(p, q)$. ∎

The value $D_P(q, s)$, that is a lower bound for $D(q, s)$, is used in the AESA algorithm, as discussed below(§2.3.2.2).

If sites in $\mathbb{U}$ are represented by the vector of their distances to P, then $D_P(q, s)$ is the ℓ_∞ (coordinate-wise maximum) distance between the representatives of q and s. Because $D_P(q, s) \leq D(q, s)$, the mapping from the original $(\mathbb{U}, D)$ to $(\Re^{|P|}, D_\infty)$ is said to be *contractive*; such contractive mappings can be helpful in distance range searching: if the problem is mapped to the vector representation, then the answer to a query corresponds to a superset of the answer in the original space [49].

Moreover, $D_P(q, s) \leq D(q, s)$ is an equality if both q and s are in P. That is, the sites $s \in P$ can be represented by the vector of their distances to P, and the ℓ_∞ (coordinate-wise maximum) distance between those vectors is the original distance. This shows that any finite space of m sites can be embedded in the ℓ_∞ space of dimension m. This embedding is due to Kuratowski [47, 54].

2.3.2   Orchard's Algorithm, AESA, Metric Trees

The above bounds from the triangle inequality give a way to avoid computing the distance from a query point q to many of the sites, by giving bounds on their distance that allow the sites to be ruled out as nearest.

2.3.2.1   *Orchard's Algorithm*

For example, consider the following simple scheme. For each site p, create a list of sites in increasing order of distance to p.

To find the closest site to a query point q, pick some site c as an initial candidate for the nearest site. Compute $D(c, q)$, and walk along the list for c, computing distances to the sites on the list. If some site s is closer to q than c, set $c := s$. Now repeat the same procedure, using the new c and its list, and so on. Suppose some such list is traversed to a site s with $D(c, s) > 2D(c, q)$. Then by Lemma 2.1(4), c is the closest site: any remaining site on the list for c must be farther from q than c is. (Here c takes the role of p in the lemma.)

This algorithm, due to Orchard[77], is simple and fast[101], particularly in high dimension ($\mathbb{U}$ is $\Re^{64}$, for example). However, it needs $\Omega(n^2)$ preprocessing, making it inappropriate for large databases. Even worse, it needs $\Omega(n^2)$ storage. For many applications this is fatal. However, for the target application of vector quantization, the preprocessing and storage costs can be acceptable.

Orchard's algorithm is an instance of a "traversal" method, and so can be accelerated using the *skip list* technique, as discussed in Subsection 2.5.2.3.

One refinement for Orchard's algorithm is to ensure that the distance from q to any given site is computed only once per query; one way to do this is to keep a mark bit for each site, which is initially zero for all sites. When the distance to a site is computed, the mark bit is set to one, and the site is entered in a linked list. When a site is considered for distance computation, if the mark bit is set to one, the site can be ignored: it cannot be closer than the current site. After a query, the linked list is walked, and the mark bits are set to zero for sites on the list. Such a scheme allows the mark bits to be maintained in a time proportional to the number of distance evaluations.

The Annulus Method. To ease the storage burden, a different scheme is to keep only one of the sorted lists for Orchard's algorithm, proceeding as follows. For some site p^*, build a list of the other sites and their distances to p^*, sorted by increasing distance. As in Orchard's algorithm, maintain a candidate closest site c. To find sites closer to q than c, walk on the list for p^* from the position of c, alternately in each direction, and compute distances. As in Orchard's algorithm, if a site s is found that is closer to q than c, set $c := s$ and continue. If a site s on the lower side has $D(p^*, s) < D(p^*, q) - D(c, q)$, then no further sites on the lower side need be considered, by Lemma 2.1(3). (Here the r of the lemma is $D(c, q)$, and the p of the lemma is p^*.) Similarly, if a site on the higher side has $D(p^*, s) > D(p^*, q) + D(c, q)$, then no further sites on the higher side need be considered. If both conditions hold, then the current candidate c is closest.

Orchard's method, the annulus method, and other methods are discussed and tested in [101].

2.3.2.2 AESA

The Approximating and Eliminating Search Algorithm, or AESA [94, 95], applies the bounds of Lemma 2.1 in a more thorough way than Orchard's algorithm or the annulus method, and like Orchard's method, uses $\Omega(n^2)$ preprocessing and storage. The AESA algorithm precomputes and stores distances $D(x, y)$ for all $x, y \in S$, and uses the lower bound function D_P defined in Lemma 2.1. When AESA answers a query for point q, every site $x \in S$ is in one of three states:

– *Known*, so that $D(x, q)$ has been computed; the Known sites form a set P;
– *Unknown*, so that only a lower bound $D_P(x, q)$ is available;
– *Rejected*, so that $D_P(x, q)$ is larger than the distance of the closest Known site.

The algorithm starts with all sites x Unknown, with $D_P(x, q) = \infty$, and repeats the following steps until all sites are Rejected or Known:

1. pick the Unknown site x with the smallest $D_P(x, q)$;
2. compute $D(x, q)$, so that x becomes Known;
3. update the smallest distance r known to q;
4. set $P := P \cup \{x\}$, and for all Unknown x', update $D_P(x', q)$; make x' Rejected if $D_P(x', q) > r$.

Based on its definition,

$$D_{P\cup\{x\}}(x', q) = \max\{D_P(x', q), |D(x, q) - D(x, x')|\},$$

so it is easy to maintain its value as sites are added to P.

There will be a need to break ties in the picking step 1, as at the beginning, when all sites have $D_P(x, q) = \infty$. This might be done at random.

While this scheme is simple and answers queries quickly, the quadratic preprocessing and storage limit its applicability. The *Linear* Approximating and Eliminating Search Algorithm, or LAESA [73], reduces these needs by precomputing and storing the distances from all sites to only a subset V of the sites, called *pivots*. The algorithm proceeds as in AESA, but only applies the update step 4 when $x \in V$. The algorithm therefore picks the pivots preferentially in step 1.

The LAESA algorithm works best when the pivots are well separated [73]; similar observations motivate many algorithms, as discussed in Subsection 2.5.2.2, to use ϵ-nets (defined in the next section) in a way similar to pivot sets.

While AESA makes very thorough use of bounds that are implied by the triangle inequality, perhaps the ultimate in that direction is the work of Shasha and Wang[84], whose algorithm considers a matrix of upper and lower bounds on the distances among points in $S \cup \{q\}$, and finds the closure of the bounds implied by the distance evaluations. The set of evaluated distances gives a semimetric, or nonnegatively weighted undirected graph. The triangle inequality gives an upper bound on the distance between two sites by way of the shortest path in the graph, and a lower bound by way of such upper bounds and evaluated distances.

2.3.2.3   Metric Trees

While the storage needs of the data structures of the last section are considerable, those of *metric trees* are quite modest. A metric tree $T(S)$ can be built as follows: if $|S| = 1$, the tree has one node; otherwise,

1. pick a ball B, with a site as center;
2. recursively construct $T(S \cap B)$ and $T(S \setminus B)$;
3. make these two trees the children of the root;
4. store a description of B at the root, including its center site.

Each node of a metric tree thus corresponds to the intersection of the balls and ball-complements stored at its ancestors in the tree. When answering a query for point q, the tree is traversed and distances to the ball centers of nodes are computed. As the traversal progresses, the minimum of the computed distances gives an upper bound on the nearest-neighbor distance, and thus the radius of a ball B_q centered at q. When a node in the tree is visited, the regions of the two children of the node are considered; if B_q can be proven not to meet the region of a child, based on the ball data in the path to the root, then the child need not be visited. Otherwise, the child is visited. (Here Lemma 2.1(3) gives a means for such a proof, using the current upper bound on the nearest-neighbor distance as r.) The cost of answering a query is proportional to the number of nodes explored.

In the seventies, McNutt(as discussed by Knuth [60]) proposed a data structure similar to metric trees, where children of a node are $T(S \cap B)$ and $T(S \setminus B')$, and B' is a ball with the same center, but slightly smaller radius than B. Thus some sites might be stored in both subtrees. This overlap makes for a data structure that needs more space, but allows some queries to be answered with less backtracking, that is, without needing to explore both children.

Burkhard and Keller [15] proposed a multibranch version for discrete-valued metrics. Metric trees, in many variations, were also invented by Omohundro [76], by Uhlmann[91], and by Yianilos[99], and they have a large literature. For further discussion of them, prior surveys can be consulted [50, 17].

2.4 Dimensions

While it is easy to construct or encounter metric spaces for which brute-force search is the fastest possible, it is still useful to consider situations in which something faster can be done. Moreover, it may be that the properties of the space that make it desirable to do nearest-neighbor search also make it possible to do the search quickly.

One such property is that of bounded dimension of the metric space, for a wide variety of definitions of the term *dimension*. Such a definition gives a way of assigning a real number to a metric space; all the definitions we consider coincide (assign the same number) for "simple" sets. So the dimension of $\Re^d$, or an open subset of it, is d for any of these definitions, and the dimension of a d-manifold in $\Re^{d'}$ will always be d, regardless of how big d' is. That is, the dimensions are generally "intrinsic," and rely on properties of the given metric space itself, not on any space in which the given space happens to reside.

In physics and statistics, there has long been interest in the use of nearest-neighbor searching for the purpose of estimating the dimension of a space. The correlation integral and correlation dimension were mentioned in Subsection 2.1.3 above. The k-NN problem is intimately related to the information dimension, as discussed below. The correlation and information dimensions are both instances of the generalized, or Rènyi, dimension spectrum; here there is a numerical parameter v so that $\dim_v Z$ is a measure of dimension, where the information dimension corresponds to $v = 1$, and the correlation dimension corresponds to $v = 2$. The Rènyi spectrum is much-studied in the area of chaotic, multifractal systems, such as turbulence, the web, network traffic [33], and Bayesian belief networks [43].

Another dimension value on the Rènyi spectrum can be computed by way of minimum spanning trees, or other extremal geometric graphs, as discussed in Section 2.5.

This section will survey some of these concepts of dimension, and the relations among them. Only a glimpse will really be given here; as mentioned earlier, for a more thorough understanding the survey by Cutler is helpful [24].

2.4.1   Dimensions of Metric Spaces

To discuss the many concepts of dimension, the notions of coverings and packings are crucial. These concepts will also appear in algorithms, as discussed in §2.5.2 below.

Coverings and packings. We will consider bounded metric spaces $Z = (\mathbb{U}, D)$, so that there is some r with $D(x, y) < r$ for all $x, y \in \mathbb{U}$. Given $\epsilon > 0$, an ϵ-*cover* (by balls) of Z is a set $Y \subset \mathbb{U}$ with the property that for every $x \in \mathbb{U}$, there is some $y \in Y$ with $D(x, y) < \epsilon$. Put another way, let

$$B(y, \epsilon) := \{x \in \mathbb{U} \mid D(x, y) < \epsilon\}.$$

Then Y is an ϵ-cover if and only if $\mathbb{U} = \cup_{y \in Y} B(y, \epsilon)$. Put still another way, Y is an ϵ-cover of $\mathbb{U}$ if and only if the Hausdorff distance (cf. §2.2.1) of $\mathbb{U}$ to Y is less than ϵ.

The *covering number* $\mathcal{C}(\mathbb{U}, \epsilon)$ is the size of the smallest ϵ-covering of $\mathbb{U}$. (Here the dependence of the covering number on the distance function D is implicit.) For example, if $\mathbb{U}$ is the unit square in the plane, the covering number is $\Theta(1/\epsilon^2)$ as $\epsilon \to 0$, since a disk of radius ϵ can cover only an area proportional to ϵ^2. In general, the covering number of a unit hypercube in $\Re^d$ is $\Theta(1/\epsilon^d)$, for similar reasons.

The quantity $\log_2 \mathcal{C}(\mathbb{U}, \epsilon)$ is called the ϵ-*entropy* or *metric entropy*, a function of ϵ. This measures the number of bits needed to identify an element of the space, up to distortion ϵ. Referring to Subsection 2.1.3, the elements of the cover could constitute a codebook for an n-quantizer with $n = \mathcal{C}(\mathbb{U}, \epsilon)$. Such a quantizer would need $\log_2 n$ bits to transmit an approximation to a member $x \in \mathbb{U}$, such that the worst-case (not expected) distortion $D(x, f(x))$ is no more than ϵ.

A subset $Y \subset \mathbb{U}$ is an ϵ-*packing* if and only if $D(x, y) > 2\epsilon$ for every $x, y \in Y$. That is, the set of balls $\{B(y, \epsilon) \mid y \in Y\}$ are disjoint.

The *packing number* $\mathcal{P}(\mathbb{U}, \epsilon)$ is the size of the largest ϵ-packing. The packing number is closely related to the covering number, as shown in the following lemma.

Lemma 2.2 *[61] For given $\epsilon > 0$ and metric space $(\mathbb{U}, D)$, if $\mathcal{P}(\mathbb{U}, \epsilon)$ and $\mathcal{C}(\mathbb{U}, \epsilon)$ are finite, then*

$$\mathcal{P}(\mathbb{U}, \epsilon) \leq \mathcal{C}(\mathbb{U}, \epsilon) \leq \mathcal{P}(\mathbb{U}, \epsilon/2).$$

Proof A maximal $(\epsilon/2)$-packing P has the property that no point $s \in \mathbb{U}$ has $D(s, P) > \epsilon$; otherwise such a site could be added to P. That is, a maximal $(\epsilon/2)$-packing P is an ϵ-cover, and so the smallest ϵ-cover can be no larger.

On the other hand, for a given ϵ-cover Y, and ϵ-packing P, every point in P must be in $B(y, \epsilon)$ for some $y \in Y$. However, no two $p, p' \in P$ can be in the same such ball: then $D(p, p') < 2\epsilon$ by the triangle inequality, contradicting the assumption that P is an ϵ-packing. So every ϵ-packing is no larger than any ϵ-cover. ∎

Nets and the Greedy Algorithm. The close relation of packing and covering is illuminated by the fundamental concept of ϵ-*nets*. A set $Y \subset \mathbb{U}$ is an ϵ-*net* of $(\mathbb{U}, D)$ if it is both an ϵ-cover and an $(\epsilon/2)$-packing.

An ϵ-net can be constructed by the following greedy algorithm, whose input is $\epsilon \geq 0$ and maximum allowed size k, as well as the metric space $(\mathbb{U}, D)$. The algorithm: pick $s \in \mathbb{U}$ arbitrarily, and set $Y := \{s\}$. Repeat the following: pick an $s \in \mathbb{U}$ that maximizes $D(s, Y) = \min\{D(s, y) \mid y \in Y\}$. If $D(s, Y) < \epsilon$ or $|Y| \geq k$, stop. Otherwise, set $Y := Y \cup \{s\}$, and continue.

The returned Y is an ϵ'-cover for some ϵ', with $\epsilon' < \epsilon$ if k is large enough. Let the ith site added to Y be denoted s_i, and let Y_i denote the set Y before s_i is added. Since the sequence $D(s_i, Y_i)$, for $i = 2 \ldots, |Y|$, is nonincreasing, every member of Y is at least ϵ' from every other member, and so Y is an $(\epsilon'/2)$-packing, and hence an ϵ'-net. Since Y is an $(\epsilon'/2)$-packing, by the Lemma above, any $(\epsilon'/2)$-cover must have at least $|Y|$ members. If this greedy algorithm is run with input $\epsilon = 0$, then the output Y will have size k, and any $(\epsilon'/2)$-cover must have at least k members; that is, the algorithm gives a cover distance ϵ' no more than twice the best possible for k sites: it is an approximation algorithm for the *k-center problem*, of finding the k points whose maximum distance to any point in $\mathbb{U}$ is minimized. Gonzalez [39], and, independently, Hochbaum and Shmoys [51], showed that this is the best possible approximation factor for a polynomial-time algorithm on a general metric space, unless $P = NP$.

As mentioned, this algorithm has been used in building nearest-neighbor data structures [13, 97, 22, 44]. It has also been used in computational chemistry[96], where it is one version of the *Bawden-Lajiness algorithm*.

Box Dimension. The *box dimension* $\dim_B(Z)$ of $Z = (\mathbb{U}, D)$ can be defined as follows: it is the d such that the covering number satisfies

$$\mathcal{C}(\mathbb{U}, \epsilon) = 1/\epsilon^{d + o(1)} \tag{2.2}$$

as $\epsilon \to 0$, if such a d exists. That is, the covering (and packing) numbers depend roughly polynomially on the scale of measurement ϵ, and $\dim_B(Z)$

is the limiting degree of that polynomial. The above condition on d is often expressed as

$$d = \lim_{\epsilon \to 0} \frac{\log \mathcal{C}(\mathbb{U}, \epsilon)}{\log(1/\epsilon)}.$$

The box dimension need not be an integer; sets with nonintegral dimension are often called *fractals*. A set can also have zero measure but be fully dimensioned; for example, space-filling curves in the plane have box dimension two, but area zero. The rational numbers have box dimension one, but length zero. (This last property is generally viewed, mathematically, as "bad" in that for other dimensions, the dimension of a countable union $\cup_i U_i$ is no more than $\sup_i \dim U_i$, so the rationals "should" have dimension zero. This can be patched up, resulting in the *modified box dimension*, which turns out to be equal to the *packing dimension*.)

Another view of the box dimension is that it is the critical value for the box *t-content* $\mathcal{C}(\mathbb{U}, \epsilon)\epsilon^t$. That is, suppose each ball in the cover has volume proportional to at most ϵ^t, as would be true in $\Re^t$. Then the box t-content is a rough overestimate of the volume of $\mathbb{U}$, since it is the sum of volumes of a small collection of sets whose union contains $\mathbb{U}$. Suppose the covering number is $1/\epsilon^{d+o(1)}$; then the t-content is $\epsilon^{t-d+o(1)}$, as $\epsilon \to 0$, which goes to 0 for $t > d$, and ∞ for $t < d$. That is, d is the supremum of the t for which the t-content is infinite, or the infinum of the t for which the t-content is zero.

Hausdorff and Packing Dimensions. A similar relationship holds for some other concepts of dimension: the dimension is the critical value for a t-content function. For example, generalizing on ϵ-covers slightly, suppose we call a collection $\mathcal{E}$ of balls an ϵ-cover when $\mathbb{U} \subset \cup_{B \in \mathcal{E}} B$, and $\mathrm{diam}(B) \leq \epsilon$ for all $B \in E$, where $\mathrm{diam}(B) := \sup_{x,y \in B} D(x,y)$. Now consider the t-content

$$\inf\{\sum_{B \in \mathcal{E}} \mathrm{diam}(B)^t \mid \mathcal{E} \text{ an } \epsilon\text{-cover of } \mathbb{U}\}.$$

This is a *Hausdorff t-measure*, and the corresponding critical value is the *Hausdorff dimension* $\dim_H Z$. (Really, this is the Hausdorff *ball t-measure*, as discussed below.) Note that a cover $\mathcal{E}$ could contain many more balls than $\mathcal{C}(Z, \epsilon)$, but balls smaller than ϵ count less in the sum.

A similar construction as for Hausdorff measure, but with covers $\mathcal{E}$ replaced with packings, and the infimum replaced with a supremum, leads to the *packing t-measure*, and the *packing dimension*[90, 88]. (The Hausdorff and packing t-measures are better behaved mathematically than the box t-content, since they are *outer measures*, hence the different names.)

Variations. There are many variations of these constructions; for example, the limit may not always exist, so $\limsup$ or $\liminf$ are used instead, leading to *upper* or *lower* versions of these dimensions, respectively. These are denoted as $\overline{\dim}_H(Z)$ for the upper Hausdorff dimension, and $\underline{\dim}_H(Z)$ for the lower Hausdorff dimension, and similarly for other dimensions. The

Hausdorff dimension, and other dimensions, exist if and only if the upper and lower versions are equal.

The Hausdorff measure is usually defined with the covers $\mathcal{E}$ allowed to include arbitrary subsets; this changes the t-measure by some factor, but not the basic dependence on ϵ, and so the dimension is the same. In $\Re^d$, the covering or packing can be done with, for example, boxes for all three versions of dimension, and similarly the measures change by a factor but the dimension remains the same.

Furthermore, it is not necessary to consider boxes of all possible sizes and shapes. For $Z = (\mathbb{U}, D)$ with $\mathbb{U} \subset \Re^d$, and D an ℓ_p distance, an equivalent definition of box dimension can be made using *quadtrees* (also known as hyperoctrees, dyadic cubes, or Besicovitch nets), as follows: put the set $\mathbb{U}$ in a cube; divide the cube into 2^d equal-sized subcubes, divide those into equal sized cubes, and so on, so that at the kth step, there are 2^{kd} equal-sized cubes. Let $\mathcal{B}_{2^{-k}}(\mathbb{U})$ denote the minimum number of such cubes at step k needed to contain $\mathbb{U}$. Then the upper box dimension $\overline{\dim}\,Z$ is the d' such that $\mathcal{B}_{2^{-k}}(\mathbb{U}) = 2^{kd'+o(k)}$ as $k \to \infty$. The occupied cubes in this description correspond to the nodes of a quadtree data structure for $\mathbb{U}$.

Assouad dimension, a.k.a. Uniform Metric Dimension, Doubling Constant. The *Assouad dimension* $\dim_A(Z)$, for space $Z = (\mathbb{U}, D)$ is related to the box dimension, but satisfies a stronger, more uniform condition: it is the value d, if it exists, such that

$$\sup_{x \in \mathbb{U}, r>0} \mathcal{C}(B(x,r), \epsilon r) = 1/\epsilon^{d+o(1)} \tag{2.3}$$

as $\epsilon \to 0$ [66, 5].

So $\dim_A(Z)$ is at least as large as the box dimension of any ball from the space. This dimension is bounded if and only if $Z = (\mathbb{U}, D)$ is a *doubling space*, meaning that there is a constant C so that that any ball $B(x, 2r)$ is contained in the union of at most 2^C balls of radius r; that is, any $2r$-ball has an r-cover. Sometimes C itself is termed the *doubling dimension*, and 2^C the *doubling constant*. Let $\text{doub}_A(Z)$ denote this version of the doubling dimension. The numbers are related by $\dim_A(Z) \le \text{doub}_A(Z)$; in fact we can say that the cover size in (2.3) above is bounded by $O(1/\epsilon^{\text{doub}_A(Z)})$.

From the close relation of packings and coverings, another way to express the doubling condition is that no ball $B(x, r)$ contains an $(r/2)$-packing with more than 2^C members.

Coping with Finiteness. If $\mathbb{U}$ is finite, then $(\mathbb{U}, D)$ has dimension zero for any of these dimensions except $\text{doub}_A Z$, since $\mathcal{C}(Z, \epsilon) \le n$ for any ϵ. However, the box dimension can be estimated by considering the covering number as a function of ϵ, over some range of ϵ values, and fitting $\log \mathcal{C}(Z, \epsilon)$ to $\log \epsilon$ within that range. Moreover, if $S \subset \mathbb{U}$, then $\dim S \le \dim \mathbb{U}$ for any of these dimensions, and $\text{doub}_A S \le \text{doub}_A \mathbb{U}$, that is, a bound on the dimension of $\mathbb{U}$ gives a bound on the dimension of its subsets.

2.4.2   Dimensions of Metric Measure Spaces

Another category of dimensions applies to metric measure spaces $(\mathbb{U}, d, \mu)$, where a set $\mathbb{U}$ is equipped with both a metric D and a measure μ. (We will assume that $\mu(\mathbb{U}) = 1$, so μ defines a probability distribution, and the measure of a set is the probability mass that it contains.)

Recall that a measure μ is a nonnegatively valued function on subsets of $\mathbb{U}$, with at least the following properties: the empty set ϕ has $\mu(\phi) = 0$; if $A \subset B$, then $\mu(A) \leq \mu(B)$; and $\mu(\cup_i A_i) \leq \sum_i \mu(A_i)$, for $A_1, A_2, \cdots \subset \mathbb{U}$.

The metric spaces that are input for nearest-neighbors problems are of course finite, and a given finite set has measure zero for many measures of interest. However, the counting measure μ_c can be used, for which $\mu_c(A) = |A|$, the number of elements of A. A common input of interest is a random sample from μ, with the sites independently generated with distribution μ. Moreover, often we consider such sets of independently identically distributed sites $S = \{x_1, x_2, \ldots, x_n\}$ as $n \to \infty$. Since the *empirical measure* $\mu_S(A) := \mu_c(A \cap S)/n$ satisfies

$$\lim_{n \to \infty} \mu_S(A) = \mu(A)$$

with probability one, for any given $A \subset \mathbb{U}$, various properties of μ can be estimated using S. Also, some properties of metric measure spaces can be defined also for finite spaces, for example, the *doubling measure* property.

Doubling Measure. A metric measure space $Z = (\mathbb{U}, D, \mu)$ with a doubling measure[47] is one for which there is a number $\text{doub}_M(Z)$ such that $\mu(B(x, 2r)) \leq \mu(B(x, r))2^{\text{doub}_M(Z)}$ for all x and r. Such a space is also called a *growth-restricted metric*[58] or *Federer measure* or a *diametrically regular* measure [32]. The definition is sometimes relaxed, so that only balls $B(x, r)$ with $\mu(B(x, r))$ sufficiently large need satisfy the doubling condition.

For such a space there is a smallest number $\dim_D(Z)$ such that

$$\sup_{x \in \mathbb{U}, r > 0} \mu(B(x, r))/\mu(B(x, \epsilon r)) = 1/\epsilon^{\dim_D(Z) + o(1)},$$

as $\epsilon \to 0$. (cf. (2.3).) It is not hard to show that $\text{doub}_A(Z) \leq 4 \, \text{doub}_M(Z)$[64] and that $\dim_A(Z) \leq \dim_D(Z)$.

If the inputs to a nearest-neighbor searching problem are such that $(S \cup \{q\}, D, \mu_c)$ is a doubling measure, then several provably good data structures exist for searching S, as discussed below (§2.5.2). Note that it is *not* the case that any subset of a growth-restricted space is growth-restricted. However, this relation can hold approximately for *random* subsets.

Rènyi Spectrum and Dimensions. For a metric measure space $(\mathbb{U}, D, \mu)$, and a value $\epsilon \geq 0$, define μ_ϵ by $\mu_\epsilon(x) = \mu(B(x, \epsilon))$, and for a value v, let

$$\|\mu_\epsilon\|_v := \left[\int_{\mathbb{U}} \mu_\epsilon^v d\mu \right]^{1/v} = \left[\int_{\mathbb{U}} \mu(B(y, \epsilon))^v d\mu(y) \right]^{1/v}.$$

That is, μ_ϵ is a "smoothed" version of μ, and $\|\mu_\epsilon\|_v$ is its L_v norm with respect to μ. For integral $v \geq 1$, it is not too hard to see that for random points $X_1 \ldots X_{v+1}$ with distribution μ, $\|\mu_\epsilon\|_v^v$ is the probability that $X_2 \ldots X_{v+1}$ are all within distance ϵ of X_1. So $\|\mu_\epsilon\|_v^v$ is the probability distribution (as a function of ϵ) for the vth nearest-neighbor distance of $v + 1$ points.

In particular, $\|\mu_\epsilon\|_1$ is the probability that X_1 and X_2 are within distance ϵ of each other. Since this is a kind of spatial correlation, $\|\mu_\epsilon\|_1$ is also known as the *correlation* integral. For S a random sample with distribution μ, the correlation integral can be estimated by the number of pairs of sites in S at distance less than ϵ, divided by $\binom{n}{2}$. The expectation of this estimate is $\|\mu_\epsilon\|_1$.

The *generalized Rènyi dimension* $\dim_v(\mu)$ is the value d, if it exists, such that

$$\|\mu_\epsilon\|_{v-1} = \epsilon^{d+o(1)},$$

as $\epsilon \to 0$. The Rènyi entropy of order v is $\log\|\mu_\epsilon\|_{v-1}$, and so the Rènyi dimension is the limit of the ratio of the Rènyi entropy to $\log \epsilon$, as $\epsilon \to 0$ [81, 24].

The Rènyi dimension can be defined even for $v = 1$, by considering the limiting value of $\|\mu_\epsilon\|_v$ as $v \to 0$. If the limit exists, the result is equal to the *information dimension* of μ, which will be denoted as $\dim_1(\mu)$, and equal to the d such that

$$\int_{\mathbb{U}} \mu_\epsilon(y) \log(\mu_\epsilon(y)) d\mu(y) = \epsilon^{d+o(1)}, \tag{2.4}$$

as $\epsilon \to 0$.

The family of values $\dim_v(\mu)$, for $v \in \Re$, is called the *Rènyi spectrum*.

Pointwise Dimension, $f_\mu(\alpha)$. The information dimension is closely related to the *pointwise dimension* $\alpha_\mu(x)$ for $x \in \mathbb{U}$, also known as the *local dimension* or *Hölder exponent*. It is defined as the d, if it exists, such that

$$\mu(B(x, \epsilon)) = \epsilon^{d+o(1)},$$

as $\epsilon \to 0$. That is,

$$\alpha_\mu(x) = \lim_{\epsilon \to 0} \frac{\log \mu(B(x, \epsilon))}{\log \epsilon}, \tag{2.5}$$

with a lower version $\underline{\alpha}_\mu(x)$ defined using lim inf instead of lim, and similarly an upper version. The definition of information dimension suggests that $\dim_1(\mu) = E[\alpha_\mu(x))]$, taking the expectation with respect to μ, and indeed for bounded measures the equality holds, under some general conditions [24].

The pointwise dimension is also related to the Hausdorff and packing dimensions of μ: the upper Hausdorff dimension $\overline{\dim}_H(\mu)$ is the infinum of the Hausdorff dimensions of all subsets of $\mathbb{U}$ with measure 1, that is,

$$\overline{\dim}_H(\mu) := \inf\{\dim_H A \mid A \subset \mathbb{U}, \mu(A) = 1\}.$$

(Recalling here our assumption that μ is a probability distribution, so $\mu(\mathbb{U}) = 1$.) The packing dimension of a measure can be defined analogously. The upper Hausdorff dimension can also be expressed in terms of the pointwise dimension:

$$\overline{\dim}_H(\mu) = \inf\{\beta \mid \underline{\alpha}_\mu(x) \le \beta, \text{almost all } x\}$$

So the upper Hausdorff dimension is an upper bound for the pointwise dimension of all points, except for a set of measure zero. (See Edgar [29],3.3.14.) The lower Hausdorff dimension, and upper and lower packing dimensions, also can be expressed as bounds for the pointwise dimension.

Some spaces are *exact-dimensional*, meaning that all points have the same pointwise dimension, except for a set of measure zero. For $(\mathbb{U}, D, \mu)$, let $f_\mu(\alpha)$ denote the Hausdorff dimension of the subset of $\mathbb{U}$ comprising those points with pointwise dimension α. (Sometimes the box dimension is used instead here.) For exact-dimensional spaces, $f_\mu(\alpha)$ is zero for all but one value of α, but other spaces have a more elaborate structure under this *multifractal* analysis. Moreover, the values of $f_\mu(\alpha)$ can be computed from the Rènyi spectrum, using the Legendre transform.

Box-Counting Versions. Just as with the dimensions of metric spaces, for subsets of $\Re^d$ these dimensions are also readily defined in a box-counting, or "quadtree" form: the level i cubes of the quadtree are those cubes of size 2^{-i} that have nonzero measure. Then the value $\sum_{c \text{ level } i} \mu(c)^v$ is within a constant factor of $\|\mu_{2^{-i}}\|_{v-1}^{v-1}$, and yields the same dimension value. (The difference in exponents, that is, v vs. $v-1$, is due to the implicit additional factor of $\mu(x)$ in the integral defining $\|\mu_\epsilon\|_v$.)

In this formulation, the set function for the information dimension becomes

$$\sum_{c \text{ at level } i} \mu(c) \log \mu(c),$$

an estimate of the Shannon information, while the set function for the correlation dimension is

$$\sum_{c \text{ at level } i} \mu(c)^2,$$

and $\dim_0(Z)$ is seen to equal the box dimension of the support of μ.

Again, a given finite or countable metric space (S, D, μ) will have dimension zero, according to the above definitions, but under the assumption that S is i.i.d. with distribution μ, the empirical measure using S gives a way of estimating the dimension of μ. The quadtree cells of interest for estimating the information dimension are those that contain at least one site, and the estimator for the information dimension set function becomes

$$\sum_{c \text{ at level } i} \mu_S(c) \log \mu_S(c).$$

We would like to use the limit, as $\epsilon \to 0$, of the limit of this function as $n \to \infty$, but instead the value for given $\epsilon = 2^{-i}$ is estimated using "sufficiently large" n. (Using such estimates for a range of ϵ scales leads to a dimension estimate via line-fitting, as mentioned for metric space dimension.) It is the complication of relating ϵ and n that has led to consideration of nearest-neighbor-based estimators, where the scale of measurement is set by the sample size n itself.

Relations Among the Dimensions. As noted above, there are some basic inequalities among these notions of dimension. If $\dim_T(Z)$ denotes the topological dimension, we have

$$\dim_T(Z) \leq \dim_H(Z) \leq \dim_0(Z) = \dim_B(Z) \leq \dim_A(Z) \leq \dim_D(Z),$$

when the given values exist. The inequalities can be strict. Also for metric measure space Z, $\dim_q(Z) < \dim_{q'}(Z)$ if $q > q'$, so in particular $\dim_2(Z) \leq \dim_1(Z) \leq \dim_0(Z)$.

Some of these inequalities are clear intuitively. The Assouad dimension is roughly a uniform, homogeneous, worst-case version of the box dimension, so it is not surprising that $\dim_B(Z) \leq \dim_A(Z)$. The box dimension is based on a t-content that is a restricted form of that for the Hausdorff measure, so $\dim_H(Z) \leq \dim_B(Z)$ is intuitively clear. The existence of a doubling measure implies the existence of a doubling constant, implying $\dim_A(Z) \leq \dim_D(Z)$.

2.4.3 Quantization and Energy Dimensions

For completeness, we note yet two more concepts of dimension for measures. Each is equal to the box dimension in a limiting case. The *quantization* dimension is related to the ability to apply the procedure of vector quantization. Let X denote a random variable in $\mathbb{U}$, with distribution μ. As discussed in §2.1.3, an *n-quantizer* for μ is a function f on $\mathbb{U}$ that takes a point X to one of at most n points in $\mathbb{U}$. Also $\mathcal{F}_n$ is the set of all such n-quantizer functions, and the nth quantization error for $\mathbb{U}$ of order v is

$$V_{n,v}(\mu) := \inf_{f \in \mathcal{F}_n} ED(X, f(X))^v, \qquad (2.6)$$

the cheapest expected cost of representing X by $f(X)$, where the cost is the vth power of the distance of X to $f(X)$. The *quantization dimension of order v* of $Z = (\mathbb{U}, D, \mu)$ is

$$\dim_Q(Z) := \lim_{n \to \infty} -v \frac{\log n}{\log V_{n,v}(\mu)},$$

that is,

$$V_{n,v}(\mu) = n^{-v/\dim_Q(Z) + o(1)} \qquad (2.7)$$

as $n \to \infty$.

The quantization dimension can also be defined for $v = \infty$, and with "upper" and "lower" versions, and these are equal to the upper and lower box dimension of the support of μ.

Graf and Luschgy [40] discuss the quantization dimension in detail.

The *energy* dimension is defined as follows. The *Riesz t-energy* of a measure is

$$I_t(\mu) := \int \int \frac{1}{D(x,y)^t} d\mu(x) d\mu(y),$$

and the energy dimension is $\sup\{t \mid I_t(\mu) < \infty\}$.

This energy is related to the pointwise dimension: for given x, it can be shown [72] that

$$\int \frac{1}{D(x,y)^t} d\mu(y) = t \int_0^\infty r^{-t-1} \mu(B(x,r)) dr.$$

If $\mu(\mathbb{U})$ is bounded, and the upper pointwise dimension is bounded everywhere by some $v > t$, that is, for all $x \in \mathbb{U}$, $\mu(B(x,r)) = O(r^v)$, then $I_t(\mu)$ is bounded.

A discrete version of the energy is, for $S = \{x_1 \ldots x_n\}$ with distribution μ,

$$I_t(S) = \frac{1}{n^2} \sum_{i \neq j} \frac{1}{D(x_i, x_j)^t}.$$

Minimizing this energy is a way to produce "well-distributed" points [46]. Note that for large t, the small distances will dominate, and a minimizer will be approximately a packing. The results of Hardin and Saff [46] imply that the minimum energy $I_t(S)$ for n points in a d-manifold contained in $\Re^{d'}$ is

$$n^{t/d-1+o(1)} \tag{2.8}$$

as $n \to \infty$, for $t > d$.

2.5   Dimensions and Nearest-Neighbor Searching

2.5.1   Dimension Estimation

Dimension measures and nearest-neighbor searching are related in both directions: the computation of some dimensional measures can be done using nearest-neighbor searching, and spaces with bounded dimension can have faster nearest-neighbor searching data structures, both theoretically and empirically.

Nearest-neighbor Searching for Dimension Estimation. In the former direction, we have already seen that the correlation integral can be estimated using a fixed-radius all-sites query. Historically, the quadtree-based view was proposed first, and the distance-based version was proposed as a more accurate empirical estimator [41].

For a given set of sample points, the quadtree estimate is easier to compute than the correlation integral, and so Belussi and Faloutsos[10] use the quadtree estimator in the context of database *spatial joins*. One kind of spatial join is the set of pairs of sites within distance ϵ of each other, for some given ϵ. That is, its size is exactly the distance-based estimate of the correlation integral, times $\binom{n}{2}$. Belussi and Faloutsos propose the quadtree estimator (together with a line fit) to help estimate the answer size for spatial joins.

Pointwise Dimension. So far, estimators based on quadtrees and fixed-radius queries have been considered; a class of estimators even more directly related to nearest-neighbor search are those based on k-NN search. For example, Cutler and Dawson [25] showed that the pointwise dimension (2.5), related to the information dimension, has the kth nearest-neighbor distance as an estimator:

$$\alpha_\mu(x) = \lim_{n \to \infty} \frac{\log(k/n)}{\log \delta_{k:n}(x)}, \tag{2.9}$$

with probability 1, where n is the sample size and $\delta_{k:n}(x)$ is the distance of x to its kth nearest neighbor in the sample. In other words,

$$\delta_{1:n}(x) = n^{-1/\alpha_\mu(x)+o(1)} \tag{2.10}$$

as $n \to \infty$. Similar observations were made by Pettis et al. [65], Verveer and Duin [93], and van de Water and Schram [92]. A derivation of a similar estimator via maximum likelihood was given by Levina and Bickel [67].

Heuristically, (2.9) can be understood by considering ϵ_k such that the ball $B(x, \epsilon_k)$ has probability mass $\mu(B(x, \epsilon_k)) = k/n$. The expected number of points in the sample falling in $B(x, \epsilon_k)$ is k, and so $\delta_{k:n}(x) \approx \epsilon_k$, and therefore

$$k/n = \mu(B(x, \epsilon_k)) \approx \epsilon_k^{\alpha_\mu(x)} \approx \delta_{k:n}(x)^{\alpha_\mu(x)},$$

using the definition of pointwise dimension, and (2.9) follows after taking logarithms and dividing. This relation to pointwise dimension suggests that nearest-neighbor distances might be helpful in estimating other related dimensional measures, such as the information, energy, and even Hausdorff dimension.

A paper of Tao et al. [89], related to that of Belussi and Faloutsos [10], uses estimates of the pointwise dimension for nearest-neighbor query cost and size estimation; given (S, D), the pointwise dimension for each site in a sample $P \subset S$ is estimated, and then for a given query point, the pointwise dimension estimate for a nearby sample site is used. The pointwise dimension estimate is done with the counting measure, and is called a *local power law*.

A worst-case bound on the pointwise dimension of a graph metric is used by Gao and Zhang [38] in the context of routing. In view of the relation of the Hausdorff and pointwise dimensions, perhaps their bound is a kind of graph Hausdorff dimension.

Extremal Graphs as Dimensional Estimators. In the setting of Euclidean manifolds, Costa and Hero [23] propose the use as dimension estimators of the minimum spanning tree, matching, k-NN graph, or other extremal graphs. Suppose G is such a graph for a set of n sites independently, identically distributed on a d-manifold. For v with $0 < v < d$, let

$$L(G, v) := \sum_{e \text{ an edge of } G} \ell(e)^v,$$

an edge length power sum of G. Costa and Hero use the fact, going back to the celebrated results of Beardwood et al. [9], that

$$L(G, v)/n = n^{-v/d + o(1)}$$

as $n \to \infty$, for the extremal graphs just mentioned, and others. (cf. (2.7), (2.8), (2.10)) Yukich's monograph [100] surveys results in this setting.) This allows the topological dimension d of a manifold to be estimated as a function of $L(G, v)$ and n, so for example,

$$d = \lim_{n \to \infty} \frac{\log(1/n)}{\log(L(G, 1)/n)}$$

with probability one.

This expression matches (2.9) for the case of the 1-nearest-neighbor graph in a d-manifold, since $L(G, 1)/n$ is the mean nearest-neighbor distance in the graph, and all points in the manifold have pointwise dimension d. Moreover, algorithms to find the extremal graphs involve nearest-neighbor queries. These estimators also provide their own scaling: there is no ϵ to go to zero, as in the definitions of the dimensions, but rather the scale of measurement $1/n$ is a consequence of the nearest-neighbor relations involved.

Kozma et al.[63] have shown a somewhat similar relation between the minimum spanning tree and the upper box dimension: for a bounded metric space $(\mathbb{U}, D)$, let the *minimum spanning tree dimension* be the infimum of the values t such that there is some δ with $L(T(S), t) \leq \delta$ for all $S \subset \mathbb{U}$, where $T(S)$ is the minimum spanning tree of S. That is, $\sup_{S \subset \mathbb{U}} L(T(S), t)$ is a t-content of $\mathbb{U}$, and this minimum spanning tree dimension is its critical value. Kozma et al. show that this dimension is equal to the upper box dimension of $(\mathbb{U}, D)$. They do this by way of a series of packings implicitly constructed in the course of building a minimum spanning tree.

A further, heuristic, relation with box dimension: if we change the greedy ϵ-net algorithm of Subsection 2.4.1 only "slightly," to take at each step the point whose minimum distance is smallest, instead of largest, then the minimum spanning tree results by connecting each newly added point to its nearest neighbor in the current set.

Kégl[59] proposes using an upper bound on the packing number and a simple form of line-fitting as an estimate of the box dimension, although not using the greedy ϵ-net algorithm discussed in Subsection 2.4.1.

2.5.2   Constant Dimension and Nearest-Neighbors Search

2.5.2.1   *Basic Properties, Spread*

Some basic properties of metric spaces $Z = (S, D)$ with bounded Assouad dimension, that is, constant doubling dimension, are useful in nearest neighbor searching. Recall that for Z with constant doubling dimension, there is a value $d = \text{doub}_A(Z)$ so that any ball of radius r has an $(r\epsilon)$-cover of size at most $O(1/\epsilon^d)$, as $\epsilon \to 0$. As shown below, this implies a reverse nearest-neighbor condition: every site $s \in S$ is nearest neighbor to $O(2^{O(d)} \log \Delta(S))$ sites, where $\Delta(S)$ is the ratio of the distance between the farthest pair of sites to the distance between the closest pair of sites.

Before that nearest-neighbor condition is shown, a brief digression on the ratio $\Delta(S)$: it is known variously as the *distance ratio*, *aspect ratio*, and *spread*, where the last seems to be most common. Algorithms for nearest-neighbor searching problems that depend on the spread have been known for some time: for example, algorithms for the all-nearest-neighbors or all-k-NN in $\Re^d$ that take $O(n \log \Delta(S))$ time[18, 37]. Less anciently, combinatorial properties of point sets in $\Re^d$ with very low spread have also been described[28, 30], and bounds have been given for classical clustering algorithms in terms of the spread [45]. Note also that the spread gives a bound to the exponent of Subsection 2.2.1 related to the "repair" of a distance measure for the triangle inequality.

Although it is not as elegant to include a dependence on the spread in a bound, often that dependence is only on the logarithm of the spread. Making an algorithm more complicated to remove such dependence is unlikely to be worth the trouble in practice.

Here is the reverse nearest-neighbor condition mentioned. It holds not just for nearest neighbors, but in the more general setting of "kth (γ)-nearest" neighbors. A site a is *kth (γ)-nearest to a site b*, with respect to S, if there are at most $k-1$ sites in S whose distance to b is within a factor of γ of the distance of the nearest to b in $S \setminus \{b\}$.

Lemma 2.3 *For a metric space $Z = (S, D)$ with doubling dimension $d = \dim_A(Z)$, and any site $s \in S$, the number of sites $s' \in S$ for which s is k-th (γ)-near in S to s' is $O((2\gamma)^d k \log \Delta(S))$, as $1/\gamma \to 0$.*

Proof   First consider $k = 1$, that is, (γ)-near neighbors, and a ball $B(s, 2r)$ for some $r > 0$. As discussed in §2.4.1, there is an (r/γ)-cover of $B(s, 2r)$ of size $O((2r/(r/\gamma))^d) = O((2\gamma)^d)$. Therefore any site s' with $r < D(s, s') \leq 2r$ has some site in the (r/γ)-cover that is closer to s' than $D(s, s')$ by a factor of at least $r/(r/\gamma) = \gamma$, and the number of sites s' with $r < D(s, s') \leq 2r$ that have s (γ)-near is $O((2\gamma)^d)$.

If p is the closest point in S to s, at distance r', then consideration of $r = 2r', 4r', 8r', \ldots$, shows that at most $\log \Delta(S)$ values of r need be considered, each contributing at most $O((2\gamma)^d)$ sites with s (γ)-near in S.

For $k = 2$, all sites of the covers in the above construction are removed from S; this leaves a metric space with fewer sites but the same doubling constant. New covers can be constructed using the remaining sites, showing that there two sites that are closer to a given site s' than $D(s, s')/\gamma$.

For $k > 2$, build such nets k times.   ∎

Doubling Constant Spaces vs. Euclidean. For Euclidean spaces, there is a sharper form of the above bound, as applied to kth nearest neighbors: for $S \subset \Re^d$, a site is kth nearest to at most $k2^{O(d)}$ other sites. It is not clear if this condition alone makes searching in Euclidean spaces much easier.

Another condition satisfied by subsets of Euclidean spaces is that for any site s and query q, if s is nearest neighbor to q, then it is possible to prove this using the Delaunay neighbors of s. (Sites a and b are Delaunay neighbors if there is some ball with a and b on its boundary sphere, and no sites in its interior.) If s is closer to q than any Delaunay neighbor of s is to q, then s is closest to q in S. A site may have many Delaunay neighbors, even in the plane, but for random sites under many probability distributions, a site may have $O(1)$ expected Delaunay neighbors. If the nearest neighbor to the query can be "guessed," then in such cases its status can be proven in constant expected time. Any similar condition for metric spaces seems to include a dependence on the spread.

Note that conversely, if s is not nearest to q, then one of its Delaunay neighbors is closer, suggesting a walk from Delaunay neighbor to Delaunay neighbor toward q; analogs of such an approach are discussed in Subsection 2.5.2.3.

2.5.2.2 *Divide and Conquer*

We next consider applying a *divide-and-conquer* approach to building a data structure and answering a query. Under some conditions, it is possible to split the searching problem into subproblems: the set of sites S is expressed as the union of sets $S_1, S_2, \ldots$, so that for any query point q, the nearest in S to q is in one of the sets S_i, and there is an efficient test to verify that condition. A natural tree data structure $\mathcal{T}(S)$ could be found in this setting by recursively finding $\mathcal{T}(S_i)$ for all S_i, and making each of these a child of the root of the tree. The search algorithm is then: apply this "effective test" to choose S_i, and then recursively search $\mathcal{T}(S_i)$.

Such a data structure is appealing, in that it requires no "back-tracking," that is, it is a tree structure for which the search proceeds from the root, along a single path, to a leaf.

Key properties of such an approach are a bound on $\max_i |S_i|$, and on the total $\sum_i |S_i|$. The former determines the number of levels in the data structure, and the latter is needed to determine the size of the data structure.

One example of such a scheme is an algorithm by Clarkson for the Euclidean case [19].

In the examples below, the divide-and-conquer scheme is based on finding the nearest neighbor to q in a subset $P \subset S$. To motivate such approaches, we return to some basic considerations regarding nearest-neighbor search.

Bounds Using the Nearest in a Subset. The task of nearest-neighbor searching can be viewed as having two parts: finding the nearest neighbor, and proving that all other sites are *not* the nearest neighbor. Moreover, any nearest-neighbor algorithm, at any given time while processing a query, has computed the distance from the query point q to some subset P of the sites. So the algorithm needs to use the distance evaluations from q to P to prove that some sites cannot be the answer to the query. What is the most effective way to do this?

Looking at Lemma 2.1(1), to show that $s \in S \setminus P$ is far from q, given that the distance from some $p \in P$ to q is known, the lower bound of

$$|D(p,q) - D(p,s)|$$

for $D(q,s)$ can be used. It is hard to tell, considering different members p of P, which p would maximize this expression. However, to maximize the difference of the two distances in the expression, one might try to make one distance or the other as small as possible. The $p \in P$ that minimizes $D(p,q)$ is of course the nearest in P to q, while the $p \in P$ that minimizes $D(p,s)$ is the nearest in P to s. So if some $p \in P$ is close to q and far from s, or close to s and far from q, then it gives a proof that s cannot be close to q.

These considerations suggest that one major piece of information for a query point q is the closest site in P. Next we will consider how such information can be used, together with the doubling constant and doubling measure conditions, to suggest some data structures for nearest-neighbor searching that have provable properties. These data structures will be inefficient in their resource bounds, but will illustrate the relations involved.

In each of the three examples below, a subset P of S of size m will be found, together with a ball B_p for each $p \in P$. (B_p is typically, but not always, centered at p.) These will have the property that for query point q, if p is nearest to q in P, then up to some conditions, the nearest neighbor to q in S is contained in B_p. Moreover, some progress will be made by this, either because B_p is small, or there are not too many sites in it. The three cases considered are:

– The space has a doubling constant, P is an ϵ-net, and either q is far enough away from p that p itself is approximately nearest, or B_p contains the nearest to q in S. Each ball B_p is smaller by a constant factor than a ball containing S.

– The space is an (empirical) doubling measure, P is a random subset, and B_p contains the nearest to q in S with very high probability. Moreover, B_p contains $O(n(\log n)/m)$ sites.

– The space has a doubling constant and the queries are *exchangeable* with the sites. Here P is a random subset, and B_p contains the nearest to q in S with controllably high probability $1 - 1/K$, for given K. Moreover, B_p is expected to contain $O((Kn/m)\log^2 \Delta(S))$ sites.

A direct approach for using these constructions is, again, to apply them recursively: to build $\mathcal{T}(S)$, find the subset P and balls B_p for each $p \in P$, then recursively build $\mathcal{T}(S \cap B_p)$ for each $p \in P$. To search for the nearest neighbor in S to query point q, find $p \in P$ closest to q, then recursively search $\mathcal{T}(S \cap B_p)$.

The first approach we consider uses ϵ-nets, which were defined in Subsection 2.4.1.

Divide and Conquer: Doubling Constant Spaces. Consider a metric space $Z = (\mathbb{U}, D)$ with bounded doubling dimension $d = \mathrm{doub}_A(Z)$, input sites $S \subset \mathbb{U}$, and the problem of building a data structure for approximate nearest-neighbor search. Suppose we scale the distance measure so that the sites fit in a ball of radius one, and suppose the subset P is a δ^2-net, for a parameter $\delta > 0$. That means, in particular, that any site in S is within δ^2 of a site in P. Moreover, the doubling dimension condition means that there is a limit on how many sites are in a δ^2-net, namely, $O(1/\delta^{2d})$. Now suppose a query point q has p as nearest neighbor in P, and a as nearest neighbor in S, and also the nearest neighbor of a in P is $p_a \in P$. Then $D(a, p_a) \leq \delta^2$, and so

$$D(q,p) \leq D(q,p_a) \leq D(q,a) + D(a,p_a) \leq D(q,a) + \delta^2.$$

That is, if $D(q,a) > \delta$, then p is $(1 + \delta)$-near to q in S. Otherwise, with $D(q,a) \leq \delta$, we have

$$D(p,a) \leq D(p,q) + D(q,a) \leq 2\delta + \delta^2 \leq 3\delta, \tag{2.11}$$

for $\delta < 1$. At the cost of searching the sites of P, we have confined the answer to the query to a ball $B_p := B(p, 3\delta)$, unless p itself is an acceptable answer. Suppose we recursively build a data structure, for each $p \in P$, for $S \cap B(p, 3\delta)$, with $\delta < 1/6$. Then at depth t in such a data structure, the sites are in a ball of radius $1/2^t$.

The building of such a data structure must stop when there is only one site in the current set S. Thus the depth of this data structure, and the cost of searching it for a nearest neighbor, is proportional to $\log \Delta(S)$. The data structure sketched above can answer an approximate nearest neighbor query in time $O(2^{O(d)} \log \Delta(S))$, if δ and so $m = |P| = O(1/\delta^{2d})$ are constants.

Divide and Conquer: Doubling Measure Spaces. Consider now a metric space $(\mathbb{U}, D)$ for which the empirical measure μ_C is doubling for $S \subset \mathbb{U}$ and

$q \in \mathbb{U}$. Recall from Subsection 2.4.2 that such a space has the property that $|S \cap B(x,r)| \geq |S \cap B(x,2r)|/2^C$ for a value C, for all $x \in S \cup \{q\}$ and $r > 0$.

Hereafter, we may abbreviate $|S \cap B(x,r)|$ as $|B(x,r)|$.

Fix a query point q, and let P be a random subset of S, obtained by choosing each site of S independently, with probability m/n, for a parameter m. The expected size of P is m. For $p \in P$, consider ϵ_p chosen so that $|B(p,\epsilon_p)| = Kn(\log n)/m$, where $n := |S|$ and the values of K and m are to be determined. For $p \in P$, suppose $D(q,p) \leq \epsilon_p/2$, and p is nearest to q in P. Then the nearest site to q in S is contained in $B(p,\epsilon_p)$, by Lemma 2.1(4). On the other hand, if $\beta := D(q,p) > \epsilon_p/2$, then

$$|B(q,\beta)| \geq |B(q,3\beta)|/4^C \geq |B(p,\epsilon_p)|/4^C \geq Kn(\log n)/m4^C.$$

where the second inequality follows from $B(p,\epsilon_p) \subset B(q,3\beta)$, which follows, for $x \in B(p,\epsilon_p)$, from

$$D(q,x) \leq D(q,p) + D(p,x) \leq \beta + \epsilon_p \leq 3\beta.$$

The probability that p is nearest to q in P is no more than the probability that $B(q,\beta)$ has no points of P, which is no more than

$$(1 - m/n)^{Kn(\log n)/m4^C} \leq e^{-K(\log n)/4^C} = 1/n^{K/4^C}.$$

If $K/4^C > 10$, for example, then q will have p nearest in P with probability no more than $1/n^{10}$.

We have the following lemma.

Lemma 2.4 *Suppose $(\mathbb{U}, D)$ is a metric space, $S \subset \mathbb{U}$, and $q \in \mathbb{U}$, such that there is some constant C for which*

$$|S \cap B(x,r)| \geq |S \cap B(x,2r)|/2^C$$

for all $x \in S \cup \{q\}$ and r. Suppose P is a random subset of S, where $p \in S$ is chosen independently for P with probability m/n. Then with probability at least $1 - 1/n^{K/4^C}$, the nearest neighbor to q in S will be contained in a subset of S of size $Kn(\log n)/m$.

If $m := 10K \log n$, that size is $n/10$, so if a data structure is built for each subset recursively, the depth will be $\log n$. Choosing $K := 10(\log n)4^C$ then means that the probability that any step in a search for a given q will fail is no more than about $1/n^9$.

Divide and Conquer: Exchangeable Queries. We have seen that for metric spaces with a doubling constant, it is possible to build a data structure for approximate nearest-neighbor searching, and for doubling measure spaces, it is possible to build a data structure for exact searching. While the schemes given above are crude, the best data structures known for metric spaces under these conditions have a similar behavior: approximate for doubling constant, exact for doubling measure. This is dissatisfying, because the doubling measure condition seems very fragile. The doubling constant condition is more robust, but approximation algorithms have the difficulty that for some metric spaces, and some applications, they may have poor precision: for points uniformly distributed in high dimension, *every* site is not much more distant, relatively speaking, than the nearest site. An approximation algorithm might return any site at all.

A better goal, then, would be a data structure for exact queries that is provably good for doubling constant spaces. Unfortunately, no such data structure is known, so it is worth asking for additional conditions under which provably good data structures can be built.

One such condition is known: when the queries have the same distribution as the sites, that is, they are *exchangeable*. The assumption here is of some random generator of sites and queries, such that the following is true: for a presented query point q, the sets $P \cup \{q\}$ and P' have the same distribution, when P and P' are random subsets of S, and P has one less site than P'. This would hold, for example, when the sites and queries are independently, identically distributed random variables, or if the sites and queries were chosen at random from some large discrete set. Such conditions roughly hold, for example, for vector quantization, where the sites are specifically chosen to be representative of the distribution of the queries.

This condition, together with constant doubling dimension, imply some useful bounds. In particular, a divide-and-conquer construction analogous to those previously given is as follows: pick a random subset $P \subset S$ of size m, then pick a random subset $\hat{P} \subset S$ of size Km, where K and m will be determined. For each $p \in P$, consider the site $q_p \in \hat{P}$ that has p nearest in P, but is farthest away among all such sites in $\hat{P}$. We will show that the ball $B_p := B(q_p, 3D(p, q_p))$ is likely to contain the answer site, for exchangeable query points q with p nearest in P. We will also show that there are not too many sites expected in B_p.

Lemma 2.5 *Under the conditions just above, for $s \in \hat{P}$ with p nearest to s in P and a nearest to s in S, it holds that $D(a, q_p) \le 3D(p, q_p)$.*

Proof Since q_p is farther from p than s, $D(s, a) \le D(s, p) \le D(q_p, p)$, and so

$$D(q_p, a) \le D(q_p, p) + D(p, s) + D(s, a) \le 3D(p, q_p),$$

using the triangle inequality and assumptions.   ∎

Lemma 2.6 *Under the conditions of the previous lemma, if q is an exchangeable query point with p nearest in P, then with probability $1 - 1/K$, the nearest neighbor to q in S is contained in $B(q_p, 3D(p, q_p))$.*

Proof If $D(q, p) \leq D(q_p, p)$, the previous lemma shows that the nearest neighbor of q in S is contained in $B(q_p, 3D(p, q_p))$, as desired. So the construction fails only if $D(q, p) > D(q_p, p)$, that is, if q is the point in $P_q := \{q\} \cup \hat{P}$ that is farthest from p, among all points in P_q that have p nearest in P; that is q is the "q_p" of P_q. There are m such points in P_q, and since q is exchangeable, the probability that it is chosen to be one of those m points is $m/(Km + 1) < 1/K$. The lemma follows. ∎

So the probability is at least $1 - 1/K$ that the nearest neighbor to q is in $B_p := B(q_p, 3D(q_p, p))$, that is, is a (3)-near neighbor of q_p. The next lemma bounds the expected number of such (3)-near neighbors.

Lemma 2.7 *For $P \subset S$ a random subset of size m, $\hat{P} \subset S$ a random subset of size Km, and q an exchangeable query, there are an expected*

$$2^{O(d)} O(Kn/m) \log^2 \Delta(S)$$

sites x such that: there is some q' in $\hat{P}$ with x a (3)-near site with respect to P, and some $p \in P$ that is nearest in P to q and q'.

We really only need to bound the expected number of sites x in such a configuration with $q' = q_p$. It seems easier, however, to bound the number with a weaker condition on q'. The set of such sites x, for a given $p \in P$, contains $B(q_p, 3D(q_p, p)) \cap S$.

Proof Let P' be any subset of S with $m + 2$ sites. Consider any $x \in S \setminus P'$. The number of sites $\hat{q}' \in P'$ with x (3)-near in P' is at most $2^{O(d)} \log \Delta(S)$, from Lemma 2.3. (Here we apply the lemma to $P' \cup \{x\}$ with $\gamma = 3$, and use the fact that the spread of that set is no more than $\Delta(S)$.) Let $p \in P'$ be the nearest to $\hat{q}'$ in P'. The number of sites $\hat{q} \in P'$ with p as nearest or second nearest is $2^{O(d)} \log \Delta(S)$. (It is possible that $\hat{q}'$ is nearest to $\hat{q}$ in P', and we want to be able to discount that, so second nearest p is considered.)

That is, at most $2^{O(d)} \log^2 \Delta(S)$ configurations of sites $\hat{q}'$, p, and $\hat{q}$ in P' satisfy the conditions:

1. $\hat{q}'$ has x (3)-nearest in P',

2. $\hat{q}'$ has p nearest in P', and

3. $\hat{q}$ has p nearest or second nearest in P'.

Consider now an exchangeable query q, and q' a random member of $\hat{P}$. We have that q and q' are random members of $P \cup \{q, q'\}$. Therefore the probability there are also $p \in P'$ and $x \in S \setminus P'$ such that q, q', p, and x satisfy conditions 1-3, with q in the role of $\hat{q}$ and q' in the role of $\hat{q}'$, is the number of such configurations divided by $(m + 1)(m + 2)$, namely $(2^{O(d)} \log^2 \Delta(S))/(m + 2)(m + 1)$. The result follows by multiplying by Km, to account for averaging over the members of $\hat{P}$ by picking random $q' \in \hat{P}$, and also multiplying by $n - m$, to account for all choices of x. ∎

Nearly-Linear Data Structures. The above claims were not proposed in the literature exactly as given, since their direct application to divide and conquer does not result in the most efficient data structures. However, the ϵ-net scheme roughly follows the ideas of Krauthgamer and Lee[64], while the empirical doubling measure (growth-restricted) scheme follows ideas of an earlier paper by Karger and Ruhl[58]. Finally, the "exchangeable queries" model follows a still earlier paper [21].

The problem with applying the direct approach, as described in Subsection 2.5.2.2, is that the sizes of the subproblems are too big: ideally, the sum of the subproblem sizes $|B_p \cap S|$, over $p \in P$, would be n, but it can be much larger than that. As a result, the resulting data structures, if built with small P, use superlinear storage.

However, for the two approaches described above that employ a random subset, it is possible to use a sample size αn, where α is a fixed fraction; applying this approach recursively to P, the resulting data structure needs storage close to linear in n, although exponential in the doubling dimension. The $M(S, Q)$ algorithm of [21] uses a scheme like this.

Applying this approach to the divide-and-conquer scheme for doubling measure would yield, in the course of construction, a sequence of nested random subsets,

$$S = P_0 \supset P_1 \supset P_2 \supset \ldots \supset P_h, \tag{2.12}$$

where $|P_i| \approx \alpha^i n$, and $h \approx \log_{1/\alpha} n$. Each P_i is a random subset of P_{i-1}, for $i > 0$, and a random subset of S.

Another way to build nested random subsets is via random permutations: if $p_1, p_2, \ldots, p_n$ is a random permutation of S, then any prefix $\{p_1, p_2, \ldots, p_m\}$ is a random subset. Random permutations, and subsets, can be built one site at a time, picking p_{m+1} as a random element of $S \setminus \{p_1, p_2, \ldots, p_m\}$.

A roughly analogous idea for the ϵ-net scheme would be to use the ϵ-net P to divide and conquer, not the searching problem in S, but instead the searching problem for a larger ϵ-net P' (that is, one with smaller ϵ). There is a nested sequence of subsets as in (2.12) above, but (assuming S is in a ball of radius $1/2$), each P_i is $(1/2^{h-i})$-net, and $h \approx \Delta(S)$. This is roughly the approach taken by Krauthgamer and Lee[64], with additional refinements; they obtain also dynamic data structures that support insertion and deletion of sites.

The ϵ-net divide-and-conquer approach can also use a permutation: the one that arises from the greedy ϵ-net construction procedure described in Subsection 2.4.1. This permutation is used in [22] and [44].

2.5.2.3 *Traversal Data Structures and Skip Lists*

Four ways of generating a nested sequence of subsets of the sites were just described, two for the random approaches, and two for the ϵ-net approaches.

The first way could also be described as follows: each site is given a level number $i \geq 0$, and the level is chosen independently for each site, where the probability that level i is assigned is $1/2^{i+1}$. Starting at the highest level, the search algorithm finds the closest site at level i, and then must consider a small number of sites to determine the closest site at level $i - 1$ or higher, repeating until the closest site at level 0 is found.

This description shows that the data structure is similar to a *skip list*[80], which is a way to accelerate searching in a linear list of ordered values; such searching is the one-dimensional version of nearest-neighbor searching.

The skip list approach can be applied to a broader set of methods for nearest-neighbor searching, which could be characterized as graph-searching or *traversal* methods.

Orchard's method (see Subsection 2.3.2.1) is an example: recall that for Orchard's method, each site s has a corresponding list L_s, sorted by increasing distance from s. The search algorithm maintains a candidate closest site c, and repeats the following steps:

1. walk down L_c, until a site c' closer to q than c is found, or the distance of the list entry to c exceeds $2d(c, q)$;

2. if no such site is found, return c as nearest; otherwise $c := c'$.

In Subsection 2.5.2, a way of searching in Euclidean spaces was described, using Delaunay neighbors: each site s has a list N_s of its Delaunay neighbors. For every point q and site s, recall that either some Delaunay neighbor site $s' \in N_s$ is closer to q than s, or else s is the closest site. That is, the same traversal procedure as in Orchard's algorithm can be applied to the Delaunay neighbor lists, in the Euclidean case.

While the Delaunay method can be very expensive, because the total number of Delaunay neighbors can be large, in the Euclidean case there are some traversal approximation algorithms. Given $\epsilon > 0$, Arya and Mount[4] found an easily computed list L_s of size independent of the number of sites, such that for any q, if s is closer to q than any member of L_s, then s is $(1 + \epsilon)$-near to q in s. This yields a traversal approximation algorithm. In this setting, it is possible to find a list with the same properties as described for Arya and Mount, and whose size is within a provably small factor of the smallest possible for such a list[20].

In the metric-space setting, Navarro [75] proposed a heuristic data structure with a similar but somewhat more complicated searching method. His construction is very similar to one of those of Arya and Mount.

Even when the sizes of the lists L_s are small, it may be that the query time is large, because the path from the starting site to the answer must hop over many sites. However, the skip list technique can be applied to accelerate any traversal method; it was first applied in the nearest-neighbor setting by Arya and Mount. It was expressed above in terms of a nested sequence of random subsets, but it could also be described as follows: assign the sites to levels probabilistically, as above, and for a site s at level i, build the search lists $L_{s,j}$ with respect to P_j, for each $j \leq i$. (As before, P_j is the set of sites at level j or lower.) Starting at some site at the highest level h, perform the traversal procedure using lists $L_{s,h}$, until the nearest site at level h is found, then use the level $h-1$ lists, and so on, until the nearest at level 0 is found. In some cases the same effect can be achieved as follows: for s at level i, concatenate its lists $L_{s,i}, L_{s,i-1}, \ldots, L_{s,0}$, and search this grand concatenated list using the basic traversal method. This might be called a skip-list-accelerated traversal method.

Although it was not derived in the same way, the $M(S, Q)$ data structure of [21] behaves something like such a data structure: the data structure comprises, for each site, a list of sites, the searching method is the traversal above, and the search is provably fast. However, the nested sequence of subsets was generated using a random permutation.

Note that Orchard's algorithm might be accelerated in this way, and in the doubling measure setting, each list L_s for Orchard's method need not include all the sites, by an analysis similar to that for the divide-and-conquer construction.

2.5.2.4 *Voronoi Grouping*

The storage requirements of data structures are often their critical limitation, and for nearest-neighbor searching that limitation is particularly acute. Even with storage that is $O(n)$, as in some of the data structures cited above, a dependence in the storage on the doubling constant, or other large constant, makes the data structures unsuitable for many applications.

One way to make a data structure that uses less space is to give up on pure divide and conquer. In the examples above, the condition that p is nearest to the query q in P constitutes a certificate that the nearest site a to q in S is contained in B_p, up to the various additional caveats given. One less "greedy" approach is the following: view each $p \in P$ as the "leader" of a "group" of sites, those sites in S for which p is nearest in P. The set of points that has a given site closest is called its *Voronoi region*, and so this approach might be called Voronoi grouping.

A key value associated with a leader $p \in P$ is its *covering radius* r_p, the distance to the farthest site in its group. Thus each leader $p \in P$ has an associated ball $B(p, r_p)$ that contains all the sites in its group, although not all sites in $B(p, r_p)$ are in the group led by p. However, if at some point the nearest distance to a query q is bounded above by some δ, and $D(q, p) > \delta + r_p$, then none of the sites led by p can be nearest. So the covering radius gives a way of ruling out groups, even if it does not give a way to "rule them in," as in divide and conquer.

An early proposal for Voronoi grouping, called "bisector trees" [57] had $|P| = 2$; that is, the sites would be split according to which of two sites was closer, and child subtrees built for each set. To search the tree, the closest site currently known is maintained, and a subtree need not be searched if its sites can be ruled out using the covering radius, as above.

(A very early proposal by Fukunaga and Narendra [35] for nearest-neighbor searching uses Voronoi grouping with a large branching factor, that is, $|P|$ is large. Their method does not apply to general metric spaces.)

Another data structure that uses Voronoi grouping is GNAT[13], where $|P|$ is typically a large constant, and one proposed way to choose P is find an ϵ-net of a random sample. There are no proven results about its performance, however.

We turn now to sketching data structures related to those for which provable bounds have been found. Here the approach is generally something like that for divide and conquer: when answering a query, a sequence of larger and larger subsets is considered, and for each subset, the sites that cannot be ruled out as the leaders of the answer a are maintained.

To apply this idea to the ϵ-net approach, consider the nested sequence of ϵ_i-nets P_i described above, with $\epsilon_i := 1/2^{h-i}$, for ϵ-net divide and conquer. (Recall that D has been scaled to have maximum value 1.) For each $p \in P_i$, suppose its leader in P_{i+1}, the closest $p' \in P_{i+1}$, has been found in preprocessing, and stored. A way to answer a query is to find, for $i = h, h-1, \ldots, 0$, the set Q_i containing all sites in P_i that are at a distance from the query point q no more than $D(q, P_i) + 2\epsilon_i$. Let $Q_h := P_h$, the coarsest net. Suppose inductively that $Q_i \subset P_i$ satisfies the distance condition. Then Q_{i-1} can be found from Q_i, because if $p' \in P_i$ is the leader of a site $p \in P_{i-1}$ with

$$D(q,p) \le D(q, P_{i-1}) + 2\epsilon_{i-1} \le D(q, P_i) + \epsilon_i,$$

then the distance of q to p' is at most

$$D(q, p') \le D(q,p) + D(p', p) \le D(q, P_i) + 2\epsilon_i,$$

and so $p' \in Q_i$.

This is roughly the technique of Beygelzimer et al. [11], who prove resource bounds for it in the doubling measure model.

The following lemma gives a slightly different way of applying this idea.

Lemma 2.8 *For query point q, and $P \subset S$, suppose $p' \in P$ is nearest to q in P, and $a \in S \setminus P$ is nearest to q in S. If $p \in P$ is nearest to a in P, then*

$$D(a,p) \le D(a, p') \le 2D(q, p'),$$

and

$$D(q,p) \le 3D(q, p'),$$

and

$$D(p, p') \le 4D(q, p').$$

So any leader in P of a is a (3)-near neighbor of q in P.

Proof We have

$$D(a, p) \le D(a, p') \le D(a, q) + D(q, p') \le 2D(q, p'),$$

using the triangle inequality and the assumptions. So

$$D(q, p) \le D(q, a) + D(a, p) \le D(q, p') + 2D(q, p') = 3D(q, p').$$

Finally, $D(p, p') \le D(q, p') + D(q, p) \le 4D(q, p')$. ∎

This lemma was used by Hildrum et al. [48] to prove bounds for a randomized data structure along generally similar lines: an increasing nested sequence of random subsets $P_h \subset P_{h-1} \subset \dots \subset P_0 = S$ is considered, generated with the skip-list technique; each $p \in P_i$ has a link to its leader in P_{i+1}; to answer a query, a subset Q_i is maintained such that Q_i contains the (3)-near neighbors of q in P_i.

The same lemma was used in a previous paper for doubling constant spaces in the exchangeable queries model[21], to obtain a provably efficient data structure, and it also figures in an algorithm for *approximate distance oracles* [8].

Recently Har-Peled and Mendel [44] have shown, among many other things, that the greedy permutation can be computed using the Voronoi grouping approach, with a near-linear time bound for constant doubling dimension spaces. Clarkson [22] proposed and implemented a roughly similar algorithm, but without analysis. These algorithms proceed site by site, for $j = 1 \dots n$, processing a site p_j and making it a leader. Each leader, that is, each site in $P_j := \{p_1, \dots, p_j\}$, has maintained for it the set of sites in S for which it is nearest in P_j. Such a set for each p_i is maintained in a heap, ordered by distance to p_i, with the largest distance on top. The top of each such heap is itself kept in a heap, so that the site $p \in S \setminus P_j$ for which $D(p, P_j)$ is largest can found, and chosen to be p_{j+1}. When p_{j+1} is processed, a key operation is to find the set of sites that it leads, those for which it is closest in P_{j+1}. In other words, a reverse nearest-neighbor query is done for p_{j+1}. Such queries can be answered quickly, using some information acquired while building P_j.

2.6 Concluding Remarks

The problem of nearest-neighbor searching and various concepts of metric space dimension have been seen to be related in a variety of interesting ways.

A few obvious questions arise: Does constant doubling dimension allow a data structure for exact queries, without the exchangeability condition?

Can efficiency be proven for algorithms under weaker dimensional conditions than doubling measure or doubling constant? Can extremal graphs be used to estimate metric measure space dimensions in a broader setting than Euclidean d-manifolds?

References

1. P. K. Agarwal, L. J. Guibas, H. Edelsbrunner, J. Erickson, M. Isard, S. Har-Peled, J. Hershberger, C. Jensen, L. Kavraki, P. Koehl, M. Lin, D. Manocha, D. Metaxas, B. Mirtich, D.. Mount, S. Muthukrishnan, D. Pai, E. Sacks, J. Snoeyink, S. Suri, and O. Wolefson. Algorithmic issues in modeling motion. *ACM Computing Surveys*, 34(4):550–572, 2002.

2. D. K. Agrafiotis and V. S. Lobanov. An efficient implementation of distance-based diversity measures based on k-d trees. *J. Chem. Inf. Comput. Sci.*, 39:51–58, 1999.

3. R. Anderson and B. Tjaden. The inverse nearest neighbor problem with astrophysical applications. In *SODA '01: Proceedings of the Twelfth Annual ACM-SIAM Symposium on Discrete Algorithms*, pages 767–768. Society for Industrial and Applied Mathematics, 2001.

4. S. Arya and D. M. Mount. Approximate nearest neighbor queries in fixed dimensions. In *SODA '93: Proceedings of the Fourth Annual ACM-SIAM Symposium on Discrete Algorithms*, pages 271–280. Society for Industrial and Applied Mathematics, 1993.

5. P. Assouad. Plongements lipschitziens dans R^n. *Bulletin de la Societe Mathematique de France*, 111:429–448, 1983.

6. M. J. Atallah. Some dynamic computational geometry problems. *Comput. Math. Appl.*, 11:1171–1181, 1985.

7. J. Basch, L. J. Guibas, and J. Hershberger. Data structures for mobile data. In *SODA '97: Proceedings of the Eighth Annual ACM-SIAM Symposium on Discrete Algorithms*, pages 747–756. Society for Industrial and Applied Mathematics, 1997.

8. S. Baswana and S. Sen. Randomized graph data-structures for approximate shortest paths. In D. P. Mehta and S. Sahni, editors, *Handbook on Data Structures*. Chapman & Hall, London, 2004.

9. J. Beardwood, J. Halton, and J. Hammersley. The shortest path through many points. *Proceedings of the Cambridge Philosophical Society*, 55:299–327, 1959.

10. A. Belussi and C. Faloutsos. Self-spatial join selectivity estimation using fractal concepts. *ACM Trans. Inf. Syst.*, 16(2):161–201, 1998.

11. A. Beygelzimer, S. Kakade, and J. Langford. Cover trees for nearest neighbor. `http://hunch.net/~jl/projects/cover_tree/paper/paper.ps`, 2004.

12. C. Böhm, S. Berchtold, and D. A. Keim. Searching in high-dimensional spaces: Index structures for improving the performance of multimedia databases. *ACM Computing Surveys*, 33(3):322–373, 2001.

13. S. Brin. Near neighbor search in large metric spaces. In *VLDB '95: Proceedings of the Twenty-First International Conference on Very Large Data Bases*, pages 574–584. Morgan Kaufmann Publishers Inc., 1995.

14. A. Broder. On the resemblance and containment of documents. In *SEQUENCES '97: Proc. Compression and Complexity of Sequences 1997*, page 21. IEEE Computer Society, 1997.

15. W. A. Burkhard and R. M. Keller. Some approaches to best-match file searching. *Commun. ACM*, 16:230–236, 1973.

16. M. S. Charikar. Similarity estimation techniques from rounding algorithms. In *STOC '02: Proceedings of the Thirty-Fourth Annual ACM Symposium on Theory of Computing*, pages 380–388. ACM Press, 2002.

17. E. Chávez, G. Navarro, R. Baeza-Yates, and J. L. Marroquín. Searching in metric spaces. *ACM Computing Surveys*, 33(3):273–321, 2001.

18. K. L. Clarkson. Fast algorithms for the all nearest neighbors problem. In *FOCS '83: Proceedings of the 24th Symp. on Foundations of Computer Science*, 1983.

19. K. L. Clarkson. A randomized algorithm for closest-point queries. *SIAM J. Comp.*, pages 830–847, 1988.

20. K. L. Clarkson. An algorithm for approximate closest-point queries. In *SOCG '94:Proceedings of the Tenth Annual ACM Symposium on Computational Geometry*, pages 160–164, 1994.

21. K. L. Clarkson. Nearest neighbor queries in metric spaces. *Discrete & Computational Geometry*, 22:63–93, 1999.

22. K. L. Clarkson. Nearest neighbor searching in metric spaces: Experimental results for $sb(S)$. http://cm.bell-labs.com/who/clarkson/Msb/readme.html, 2003.

23. J. Costa and A. O. Hero. Geodesic entropic graphs for dimension and entropy estimation in manifold learning. *IEEE Trans. Signal Proc.*, 2004.

24. C. D. Cutler. A review of the theory and estimation of fractal dimension. In H. Tong, editor, *Dimension Estimation and Models*. World Scientific, 1993.

25. C. D. Cutler and D. A. Dawson. Estimation of dimension for spatially-distributed data and related theorems. *Journal of Multivariate Analysis*, 28:115–148, 1989.

26. L. Devroye, L. Györfi, and G. Lugosi. *A Probabilistic Theory of Pattern Recognition*. Springer-Verlag, New York, 1996.

27. M. Deza and M. Laurent. *Geometry of Cuts and Metrics*. Springer-Verlag, New York, 1997.

28. H. Edelsbrunner, P. Valtr, and E. Welzl. Cutting dense point sets in half. *Discrete & Computational Geometry*, 17:243–255, 1997.

29. G. A. Edgar. *Integral, Probability, and Fractal Measures*. Springer-Verlag, New York, 1998.

30. J. Erickson. Dense point sets have sparse Delaunay triangulations: or "–but not too nasty". In *SODA '02: Proceedings of the Thirteenth Annual ACM-SIAM Symposium on Discrete Algorithms*, pages 125–134. Society for Industrial and Applied Mathematics, 2002.

31. K. J. Falconer. *Fractal Geometry - Mathematical Foundations and Applications*. J. Wiley & Sons, Hoboken, NJ, 1990.

32. H. Federer. *Geometric Measure Theory*. Springer-Verlag, New York, 1969.

33. A. Feldmann, A. C. Gilbert, and W. Willinger. Data networks as cascades: investigating the multifractal nature of internet WAN traffic. In *SIGCOMM '98: Proceedings of the ACM SIGCOMM '98 Conference on Applications, Technologies, Architectures, and Protocols for Computer Communication*, pages 42–55. ACM Press, 1998.

34. E. Fix and J. L. Hodges Jr. Discriminatory analysis, non-parametric discrimination. Technical Report 4, USAF School of Aviation Medicine, 1951. Project 21-49-004.

35. K. Fukunaga and P. M. Narendra. A branch and bound algorithm for computing k-nearest neighbors. *IEEE Trans. on Computers*, C-24:750–753, 1975.

36. S. Funke and E. A. Ramos. Smooth-surface reconstruction in near-linear time. In *SODA '02: Proceedings of the Thirteenth Annual ACM-SIAM Symposium on Discrete Algorithms*, pages 781–790. Society for Industrial and Applied Mathematics, 2002.

37. H. N. Gabow, J. L. Bentley, and R. E. Tarjan. Scaling and related techniques for geometry problems. In *STOC '84: Proceedings of the Sixteenth Annual ACM Symposium on Theory of Computing*, pages 135–143. ACM Press, 1984.

38. J. Gao and L. Zhang. Tradeoffs between stretch factor and load balancing ratio in routing on growth restricted graphs. In *PODC '04: Proceedings of the Twenty-Third Annual ACM Symposium on Principles of Distributed Computing*, pages 189–196. ACM Press, 2004.

39. T. Gonzalez. Clustering to minimize the maximum intercluster distance. *Theoretical Computer Science*, 38:293–306, 1985.

40. S. Graf and H. Luschgy. *Foundations of Quantization for Probability Distributions*. Springer-Verlag, New York, 2000.

41. P. Grassberger and I. Procaccia. Measuring the strangeness of strange attractors. *Physica*, D9:189–208, 1983.

42. R.M. Gray and D. L. Neuhoff. Quantization. *IEEE Trans. Inform. Theory*, 44:2325–2383, 1993.

43. H. Guo and W. Hsu. On multifractal property of the joint probability distributions and its application to Bayesian network inference. In *The 7th Asia-Pacific Conference on Complex Systems*, 2004.

44. S. Har-Peled and M. Mendel. Fast construction of nets in low dimensional metrics, and their applications. In *SOCG '05: Proceedings of the Twenty-First Annual ACM Symposium on Computational Geometry*, 2005.

45. S. Har-Peled and B. Sadri. How fast is the k-means method? *Algorithmica*, 41(3):185–202, 2005.

46. D. P. Hardin and E. B. Saff. Discretizing manifolds via minimum energy points. *Notices of the AMS*, 51(10):1186–1194, 2004.

47. J. Heinonen. Geometric embeddings of metric spaces. Technical report, University of Jyväskylä, Finland, 2003. `http://www.math.jyu.fi/tutkimus/ber.html`.

48. K. Hildrum, J. Kubiatowicz, S. Ma, and S. Rao. A note on the nearest neighbor in growth-restricted metrics. In *SODA '04: Proceedings of the Fifteenth Annual ACM-SIAM Symposium on Discrete Algorithms*, pages 560–561. Society for Industrial and Applied Mathematics, 2004.

49. G. R. Hjaltason and H. Samet. Contractive embedding methods for similarity searching in metric spaces. Technical Report 4102, University of Maryland, 2000.

50. G. R. Hjaltason and H. Samet. Index-driven similarity search in metric spaces. *ACM Trans. Database Syst.*, 28(4):517–580, 2003.

51. D. S. Hochbaum and D. B. Shmoys. A best possible heuristic for the k-center problem. *Mathematics of Operations Research*, 10:180–184, 1985.

52. K. Hormann. From scattered samples to smooth surfaces. In *Proc. of Geometric Modeling and Computer Graphics*, 2003.

53. P. Indyk. Nearest neighbors in high dimensional spaces. In J. E. Goodman and J. O'Rourke, editors, *Handbook of Discrete and Computational Geometry*. CRC Press, second edition, 2004.

54. P. Indyk and J. Matoušek. Low distortion embeddings of finite metric spaces. In J. E. Goodman and J. O'Rourke, editors, *Handbook of Discrete and Computational Geometry*. CRC Press, second edition, 2004.

55. P. Jaccard. Etude comparative de la distribution florale dans une portion des Alpes et des Jura. *Bull. Soc. Vaudoise Sci. Nat*, 37:547–579, 1901.

56. S. Kahan. A model for data in motion. In *STOC '91: Proceedings of the Twenty-Third Annual ACM Symposium on Theory of Computing*, pages 265–277. ACM Press, 1991.

57. I. Kalantari and G. McDonald. A data structure and an algorithm for the nearest point problem. *IEEE Transactions on Software Engineering*, 9(5), 1983.

58. D. R. Karger and M. Ruhl. Finding nearest neighbors in growth-restricted metrics. In *STOC '02: Proceedings of the Thirty-Fourth Annual ACM Symposium on Theory of Computing*, pages 741–750. ACM Press, 2002.

59. B. Kégl. Intrinsic dimension estimation using packing numbers. In S. Becker, S. Thrun, and K. Obermayer, editors, *Advances in Neural Information Processing Systems 15*, pages 681–688. MIT Press, Cambridge, MA, 2003.

60. Donald Ervin Knuth. *The Art of Computer Programming, Volume 3: Sorting and Searching*. Addison-Wesley, Boston, 1998.

61. A. Kolmogorov and V. Tikhomirov. ϵ-entropy and ϵ-capacity of sets of functions. *Translations of the AMS*, 17:277–364, 1961.

62. F. Korn and S. Muthukrishnan. Influence sets based on reverse nearest neighbor queries. In *SIGMOD 2000: Proceedings of the ACM International Conference on Management of Data*, pages 201–212. ACM Press, 2000.

63. G. Kozma, Z. Lotker, and G. Stupp. The minimal spanning tree and the upper box dimension. arXiv:math.CO/0311481.

64. R. Krauthgamer and J. R. Lee. Navigating nets: simple algorithms for proximity search. In *SODA '04: Proceedings of the Fifteenth Annual ACM-SIAM Symposium on Discrete Algorithms*, pages 798–807. Society for Industrial and Applied Mathematics, 2004.

65. K.W.Pettis, T.A.Bailey, A.K.Jain, and R.C. Dubes. An intrinsic dimensionality estimator from near-neighbor information. *IEEE Transactions on Pattern Analysis and Machine Intelligence*, 1:25–37, 1979.

66. D.G. Larman. A new theory of dimension. *Proc. London Math. Soc. (3rd Series)*, pages 178–192, 1967.

67. E. Levina and P. J. Bickel. Maximum likelihood estimation of intrinsic dimension. In L. K. Saul, Y. Weiss, and L. Bottou, editors, *Advances in Neural Information Processing Systems 17*, pages 777–784. MIT Press, Cambridge, MA, 2005.

68. E. Levina and P.J. Bickel. The earth mover's distance is the Mallows distance: Some insights from statistics. In *Proc. ICCV '01*, pages 251–256, 2001.

69. Y. Linde, A. Buzo, and R. M. Gray. An algorithm for vector quantizer design. *IEEE Transactions on Communications*, 28:84–95, 1980.

70. T. Liu, A. W. Moore, and A. Gray. Efficient exact k-NN and nonparametric classification in high dimensions. In S. Thrun, L. Saul, and B. Schölkopf, editors, *Advances in Neural Information Processing Systems 16*. MIT Press, Cambridge, MA, 2004.

71. F. Marczewski and H. Steinhaus. On a certain distance of sets and the corresponding distance of functions. *Colloquium Mathematicum*, 6:319–327, 1958.

72. P. Mattila. *Geometry of Sets and Measures in Euclidean Spaces*. Cambridge University Press, Cambridge, 1995.

73. M. L. Micó, J. Oncina, and E. Vidal. A new version of the nearest-neighbour approximating and eliminating search algorithm (AESA) with linear preprocessing time and memory requirements. *Pattern Recognition Letters*, 15(1):9–17, 1994.

74. D. M. Mount, N. Netanyahu, R. Silverman, and A. Y. Wu. Chromatic nearest neighbor searching: A query sensitive approach. *Computational Geometry: Theory and Applications*, 17:97–119, 2000.

75. G. Navarro. Searching in metric spaces by spatial approximation. *VLDB Journal*, 11(1):28–46, 2002.

76. S. Omohundro. Five balltree construction algorithms. Technical report, International Computer Science Institute, 1989.

77. M. T. Orchard. A fast nearest-neighbor search algorithm. In *ICASSP '91: 1991 International Conference on Acoustics, Speech and Signal Processing*, volume 4, pages 2297–3000, 1991.

78. A. N. Papadopoulos and Y. Manolopoulos. *Nearest Neighbor Search: A Database Perspective*. Springer-Verlag, New York, 2005.

79. Y. B. Pesin. *Dimension Theory in Dynamical Systems. Contemporary views and applications*. University of Chicago Press, 1997.

80. W. Pugh. Skip lists: A probabilistic alternative to balanced trees. *Comm. ACM*, 33(6):668–676, 1990.

81. A. Rènyi. *Probability Theory*. North-Holland, New York, 1970.

82. D. Rogers and T. Tanimoto. A computer program for classifying plants. *Science*, 132(3434):1115–1118, 1960.

83. L. K. Saul and S. T. Roweis. Think globally, fit locally: unsupervised learning of low dimensional manifolds. *J. Mach. Learn. Res.*, 4:119–155, 2003.

84. D. Shasha and T.-L. Wang. New techniques for best-match retrieval. *ACM Trans. Inf. Syst.*, 8(2):140–158, 1990.

85. A. Singh, H. Ferhatosmanoglu, and A. Ş. Tosun. High dimensional reverse nearest neighbor queries. In *CIKM '03: Proceedings of the Twelfth International Conference on Information and Knowledge Management*, pages 91–98. ACM Press, 2003.

86. M. Smid. Closest-point problems in computational geometry. In J.-R. Sack and J. Urrutia, editors, *Handbook of Computational Geometry*. North-Holland, 2000.

87. H. Spaeth. *Cluster Analysis Algorithms for Data Reduction and Classification of Objects*. J. Wiley & Sons, Hoboken, NJ, 1980.

88. D. Sullivan. Entropy, Hausdorff measures old and new, and limit sets of geometrically finite Kleinian groups. *Acta Mathematica*, 153:259–277, 1984.

89. Y. Tao, C. Faloutsos, and D. Papadias. The power-method: a comprehensive estimation technique for multi-dimensional queries. In *CIKM '03: Proceedings of the Twelfth International Conference on Information and Knowledge Management*, pages 83–90. ACM Press, 2003.

90. C. Tricot. Two definitions of fractional dimension. *Math. Proceedings of the Cambridge Philosophical Society*, 91:57–74, 1982.

91. J. K. Uhlmann. Satisfying general proximity/similarity queries with metric trees. *Inform. Proc. Letters*, 40:175–179, 1991.

92. W. van de Water and P. Schram. Generalized dimensions from near-neighbor information. *Phys. Rev. A*, 37:3118–3125, 1988.

93. P. Verveer and R. Duin. An evaluation of intrinsic dimensionality estimators. *IEEE Transactions on Pattern Analysis and Machine Intelligence*, 17:81–86, 1995.

94. E. Vidal. An algorithm for finding nearest neighbours in (approximately) constant average time. *Pattern Recognition Letters*, 4:145–157, 1986.

95. E. Vidal. New formulation and improvements of the nearest neighbours in approximating and eliminating search algorithm (AESA). *Pattern Recognition Letters*, 15(1), 1994.

96. P. Willett. Molecular diversity techniques for chemical databases. *Information Research*, 2(3), 1996.

97. A. Wojna. Center-based indexing in vector and metric spaces. *Fundam. Inf.*, 56(3):285–310, 2003.

98. H. Xu and D. K. Agrafiotis. Nearest neighbor search in general metric spaces using a tree data structure with a simple heuristic. *J. Chem. Inf. Comput. Sci.*, 43:1933–1941, 2003.

99. P. N. Yianilos. Data structures and algorithms for nearest neighbor search in general metric spaces. In *SODA '93: Proceedings of the Fourth Annual ACM-SIAM Symposium on Discrete Algorithms*, pages 311–321. Society for Industrial and Applied Mathematics, 1993.

100. J. E. Yukich. *Probability theory of classical Euclidean optimization*, volume 1675 of *Lecture Notes in Mathematics*. Springer-Verlag, New York, 1998.

101. K. Zatloukal, M. H. Johnson, and R. Ladner. Nearest neighbor search for data compression. In M. Goldwasser, D. Johnson, and C. McGeoch, editors, *Data Structures, Nearest Neighbor Searches, and Methodology: Fifth and Sixth DIMACS Implementation Challenges*. AMS, 2002.

3   Locality-Sensitive Hashing Using Stable Distributions

Alexandr Andoni, Mayur Datar, Nicole Immorlica,
Piotr Indyk, and Vahab Mirrokni

In this chapter, we introduce and analyze a novel locality-sensitive hashing family. The family is defined for the case where the distances are measured according to the l_s norm, for any $s \in [0, 2]$. The hash functions are particularly simple for the case $s = 2$, i.e., the Euclidean norm. The new family provides an efficient solution to the (approximate or exact) randomized near-neighbor problem. Part of this work appeared earlier in [5].

3.1   The Locality-Sensitive Hashing Scheme Based on s-Stable Distributions

3.1.1 s-Stable Distributions

Stable distributions [10] are defined as limits of normalized sums of independent identically distributed variables (an alternative definition follows). The best-known example of a stable distribution is the Gaussian (or normal) distribution. However, the class is much wider; for example, it includes heavy-tailed distributions.

Definition 3.1 *A distribution $\mathcal{D}$ over $\Re$ is called s-stable if there exists $p \geq 0$ such that for any n real numbers $v_1 \ldots v_n$ and i.i.d. variables $X_1 \ldots X_n$ with distribution $\mathcal{D}$, the random variable $\sum_i v_i X_i$ has the same distribution as the variable $(\sum_i |v_i|^p)^{1/p} X$, where X is a random variable with distribution $\mathcal{D}$.*

It is known [10] that stable distributions exist for any $p \in (0, 2]$. In particular:

– a *Cauchy distribution* $\mathcal{D}_C$, defined by the density function $c(x) = \frac{1}{\pi}\frac{1}{1+x^2}$, is 1-stable;

– a *Gaussian (normal) distribution* $\mathcal{D}_G$, defined by the density function $g(x) = \frac{1}{\sqrt{2\pi}}e^{-x^2/2}$, is 2-stable.

We note from a practical point of view, despite the lack of closed form density and distribution functions, it is known [4] that one can generate s-stable random variables essentially from two independent variables distributed uniformly over $[0,1]$.

Stable distributions have found numerous applications in various fields (see the survey [8] for more details). In computer science, stable distributions were used for "sketching" of high-dimensional vectors by Indyk ([6]) and since have found use in various applications. The main property of s-stable distributions mentioned in the definition above directly translates into a sketching technique for high-dimensional vectors. The idea is to generate a random vector a of dimension d whose each entry is chosen independently from an s-stable distribution. Given a vector v of dimension d, the dot product $a \cdot v$ is a random variable which is distributed as $(\sum_i |v_i|^s)^{1/s} X$ (i.e., $||v||_s X$), where X is a random variable with s-stable distribution. A small collection of such dot products $(a.v)$, corresponding to different a's, is termed the sketch of the vector v and can be used to estimate $||v||_s$ (see [6] for details). It is easy to see that such a sketch is linearly composable, i.e., for any $p, q \in \Re^d$, $a \cdot (p - q) = a \cdot p - a \cdot q$.

3.1.2 Hash Family Based on s-Stable Distributions

We use s-stable distributions in the following manner. Instead of using the dot products $(a \cdot v)$ to estimate the l_s norm we use them to assign a hash value to each vector v. Intuitively, the hash function family should be locality sensitive; i.e., if two points (p, q) are close (small $||p-q||_s$), then they should collide (hash to the same value) with high probability and if they are far they should collide with small probability. The dot product $a \cdot v$ projects each vector to the real line. It follows from s-stability that for two vectors (p, q) the distance between their projections $(a \cdot p - a \cdot q)$ is distributed as $||p-q||_s X$ where X is an s-stable distribution. If we "chop" the real line into equiwidth segments of appropriate size w and assign hash values to vectors based on which segment they project onto, then it is intuitively clear that this hash function will be locality-sensitive in the sense described above.

Formally, each hash function $h_{a,b}(v) : \mathcal{R}^d \to \mathcal{N}$ maps a d-dimensional vector v onto the set of integers. Each hash function in the family is indexed by a choice of random a and b where a is, as before, a d-dimensional vector with entries chosen independently from an s-stable distribution and b is a real number chosen uniformly from the range $[0, w]$. For a fixed a, b the hash function $h_{a,b}$ is given by $h_{a,b}(v) = \lfloor \frac{a \cdot v + b}{w} \rfloor$

3.1.2.1 *Collision Probability*

We compute the probability that two vectors p, q collide under a hash function drawn uniformly at random from this family. Let $f_s(t)$ denote the probability density function of the **absolute value** of the s-stable distribution. We may drop the subscript s whenever it is clear from the context.

For the two vectors p, q, let $u = ||p-q||_s$ and let $p(u)$ denote the probability (as a function of u) that p, q collide for a hash function uniformly chosen from the family $\mathcal{H}$ described above. For a random vector a whose entries are drawn from an s-stable distribution, $a \cdot p - a \cdot q$ is distributed as cX where X is a random variable drawn from an s-stable distribution. Since b is drawn uniformly from $[0, w]$ it is easy to see that

$$p(u) = Pr_{a,b}[h_{a,b}(p) = h_{a,b}(q)] = \int_0^w \frac{1}{u} f_s(\frac{t}{u})(1 - \frac{t}{w})dt$$

For a fixed parameter w the probability of collision decreases monotonically with $u = ||p - q||_s$. Thus, as per the definition, the family of hash functions above is (R, cR, P_1, P_2)-sensitive for $P_1 = p(1)$ and $P_2 = p(c)$.

3.2   Approximate Near Neighbor

In what follows we will bound the ratio $\rho = \frac{\ln 1/P_1}{\ln 1/P_2}$, which as discussed earlier is critical to the performance when this hash family is used to solve the c-approximate near-neighbor problem.

Note that we have not specified the parameter w, for it depends on the value of c and s. For every c we would like to choose a finite w that makes ρ as small as possible.

We focus on the cases of $s = 1, 2$. In these cases the ratio ρ can be explicitly evaluated. We compute and plot this ratio and compare it with $1/c$. Note that $1/c$ is the best (smallest) known exponent for n in the space requirement and query time that is achieved in [7] for these cases.

For $s = 1, 2$ we can compute the probabilities P_1, P_2, using the density functions mentioned before. A simple calculation shows that $P_2 = 2\frac{tan^{-1}(w/c)}{\pi} - \frac{1}{\pi(w/c)} \ln(1 + (w/c)^2)$ for $s = 1$ (Cauchy) and $P_2 = 1 - 2norm(-w/c) - \frac{2}{\sqrt{2\pi}w/c}(1 - e^{-(w^2/2c^2)})$ for $s = 2$ (Gaussian), where $norm(\cdot)$ is the cumulative distribution function (cdf) for a random variable that is distributed as $N(0, 1)$. The value of P_1 can be obtained by substituting $c = 1$ in the formulas above.

For c values in the range $[1, 10]$ (in increments of 0.05) we compute the minimum value of ρ, $\rho(c) = min_w \log(1/P_1)/\log(1/P_2)$, using *Matlab*. The plot of c vs. $\rho(c)$ is shown in fig. 3.1. The crucial observation for the case $s = 2$ is that the curve corresponding to optimal ratio ρ ($\rho(c)$) lies strictly below the curve $1/c$. As mentioned earlier, this is a strict improvement over the previous best known exponent $1/c$ from [7]. While we have computed here $\rho(c)$ for c in the range $[1, 10]$, we believe that $\rho(c)$ is strictly less than $1/c$ for all values of c.

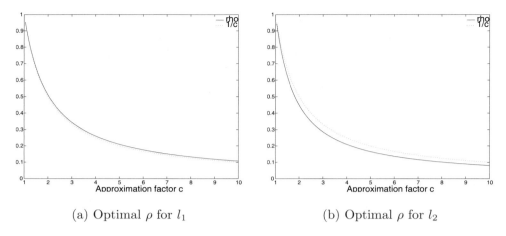

(a) Optimal ρ for l_1 (b) Optimal ρ for l_2

Figure 3.1   Optimal ρ vs. c.

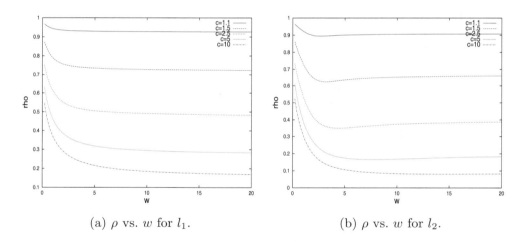

(a) ρ vs. w for l_1.   (b) ρ vs. w for l_2.

Figure 3.2 ρ vs. w.

For the case $s = 1$, we observe that the $\rho(c)$ curve is very close to $1/c$, although it lies above it. The optimal $\rho(c)$ was computed using *Matlab* as mentioned before. The *Matlab* program has a limit on the number of iterations it performs to compute the minimum of a function. We reached this limit during the computations. If we compute the true minimum, then we suspect that it will be very close to $1/c$, possibly equal to $1/c$, and that this minimum might be reached at $w = \infty$.

If one were to implement our locality-sensitive hashing scheme, ideally they would want to know the optimal value of w for every c. For $s = 2$, for a given value of c, we can compute the value of w that gives the optimal value of $\rho(c)$. This can be done using programs like *Matlab*. However, we

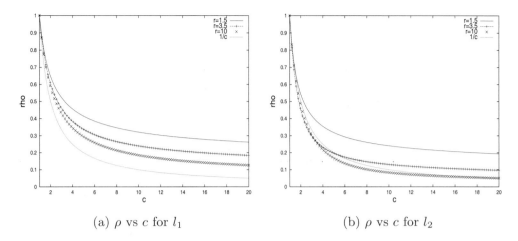

(a) ρ vs c for l_1 (b) ρ vs c for l_2

Figure 3.3 ρ vs c

observe that for a fixed c the value of ρ as a function of w is more or less stable after a certain point (see fig. 3.2). Thus, we observe that ρ is not very sensitive to w beyond a certain point and as long we choose w "sufficiently" away from 0, the ρ value will be close to optimal. Note, however that we should not choose w that is too large. As w increases, both P_1 and P_2 get closer to 1. This increases the query time, since k increases as $\log_{1/P_2} n$.

We mention that for the l_2 norm, the optimal value of w appears to be a (finite) function of c.

We also plot ρ as a function of c for a few fixed w values (see fig. 3.3). For $s = 2$, we observe that for moderate w values the ρ curve "beats" the $1/c$ curve over a large range of c that is of practical interest. For $s = 1$, we observe that as w increases the ρ curve drops lower and gets closer and closer to the $1/c$ curve.

3.3   Exact Near Neighbor

LSH can also be used to solve the randomized version of the exact near-neighbor problem. To use it for the exact near neighbor, we use the "strategy 2" of the basic LSH scheme, and keep only the R-near neighbors of q. Thus, the running time depends on the data set $\mathcal{P}$. In particular, the running time is slower for "bad" data sets, e.g., when for a query q, there are many points from $\mathcal{P}$ clustered right outside the ball of radius R centered at q (i.e., when there are many approximate near neighbors).

3.3.1   Parameters k and L of the LSH Scheme

There are two steps for choosing the parameters k and L that are optimal for a data set. First, we need to determine the bounds on k and L that guarantee the correctness of the algorithm. Second, within those bounds, we choose the values k and L that would achieve the best expected query running time.

Next, we derive the bounds that need to be satisfied by k and L to guarantee the correctness of the algorithm. We need to ensure that our data structure reports an R-near neighbor with a probability of at least $1 - \delta$. To analyze what condition this implies, consider a query point q and an R-near neighbor p of q. Let $P_1 = p(R)$. Then, $Pr_{g \in \mathcal{G}}[g(q) = g(p)] \geq P_1^k$. Thus, q and p fail to collide for all L functions g_i with probability at most $(1 - P_1^k)^L$. Requiring that the point q collides with p on some function g_i is equivalent to saying $1 - (1 - P_1^k)^L \geq 1 - \delta$, which implies that

$$L \geq \frac{\log 1/\delta}{-\log(1 - P_1^k)}. \tag{3.1}$$

Since we want to choose L as small as possible (for a fixed k), the best value for L is $L = \left\lceil \frac{\log 1/\delta}{-\log(1-P_1^k)} \right\rceil$.

Thus, one is free to choose only k since it is the only remaining degree of freedom in choosing parameters k and L.

To understand better how the choice of k affects the query running time, we decompose the running time into two terms, T_g and T_c. T_g is the time necessary for computing L functions g_i for the query point q as well as for retrieving the buckets $g_i(q)$ from hash tables; the expression for T_g is $T_g = O(dkL)$.

The second term, T_c, represents the time for computing the distance to all points encountered in the retrieved buckets; T_c is equal to $O(d \cdot \#collisions)$, where $\#collisions$ is the number of points encountered in the buckets $g_1(q), \dots g_L(q)$ for a query point q. The expected value of T_c is

$$E[T_c] = O(d \cdot E[\#collisions]) = O\left(dL \cdot \sum_{p \in \mathcal{P}} p^k(\|q - p\|)\right). \tag{3.2}$$

Intuitively, T_g increases as a function of k, while T_c decreases as a function of k. The latter is due to the fact that higher values of k magnify the gap between the collision probabilities of "close" and "far" points, which (for proper values of L) decreases the probability of collision of far points. Thus, typically there exists an optimal value of k that minimizes the sum $T_g + T_c$ (for a given query point q). Note that there might be different optimal k's for different query points, therefore the goal would be optimize the mean query time for all query points.

3.4   LSH in Practice: E²LSH

In this section we present a practitioner's view on how to implement the LSH scheme for solving the R-near-neighbor reporting problem in practice. Specifically, we describe a concrete method for choosing the algorithm's parameters, as well as present some implementation details that both clarify steps of the scheme and demonstrate how to optimize the scheme in practice.

The section is based on the package E²LSH (*Exact Euclidean LSH*), version 0.1, which is our current implementation of the LSH scheme [1]. E²LSH solves the exact near-neighbor reporting problem.

Note that E²LSH uses a few addition optimizations to improve the search performance, in addition to what is described below. Please refer to the manual [1] for more information.

3.4.1   Data Structure Construction

Before constructing the data structure, E2LSH first computes the parameters k, L as a function of the data set $\mathcal{P}$, the radius R, and the probability $1 - \delta$ as outlined in earlier sections. In what follows, we consider L as a function of k, and the question remains only of how to choose k.

For choosing the value k, the algorithm experimentally estimates the times T_g and T_c as a function of k. Remember that the time T_c is dependent on the query point q, and, therefore, for estimating T_c we need to use a set S of sample query points (the estimation of T_c is then the mean of the times T_c for points from S). The sample set S is a set of several points chosen at random from the query set. (The package also provides the option of choosing S to be a subset of the data set $\mathcal{P}$.)

Note that to estimate T_g and T_c precisely, we need to know the constants hidden by the $O(\cdot)$ notation in the expressions for T_g and T_c. To compute these constants, the implementation constructs a sample data structure and runs several queries on that sample data structure, measuring the actual times T_g and T_c. Note that T_g and T_c depend on k. Thus, k is chosen such that $T_g + \tilde{T}_c$ is minimal (while the data structure space requirement is within the memory bounds), where $\tilde{T}_c$ is the mean of the times T_c for all points in the sample query set S: $\tilde{T}_c = \frac{\sum_{q \in S} T_c(q)}{|S|}$.

Once the parameters k, m, L are computed, the algorithm constructs the data structure containing the points from $\mathcal{P}$.

3.4.2   Bucket Hashing

Recall that the domain of each function g_i is too large to store all possible buckets explicitly, and only nonempty buckets are stored. To this end, for each point p, the buckets $g_1(p), \ldots g_L(p)$ are hashed using the universal hash functions. For each function g_i, $i = 1 \ldots L$, there is a hash table H_i

containing the buckets $\{g_i(p) \mid v \in \mathcal{P}\}$. For this purpose, there are two associated hash functions $t_1 : \mathbb{Z}^k \to \{0, \dots, tableSize - 1\}$ and $t_2 : \mathbb{Z}^k \to \{0, \dots, C\}$. The function t_1 determines for an LSH bucket the index of the point in the hash table. The second hash function identifies the buckets in chains.

The collisions within each index in the hash table are resolved by chaining. When storing a bucket $g_i(p) = (x_1, \dots x_k)$ in its chain, instead of storing the entire vector $(x_1, \dots x_k)$ for bucket identification, we store only $t_2(x_1, \dots x_k)$. Thus, a bucket $g_i(p) = (x_1, \dots x_k)$ has only the following associated information stored in its chain: the identifier $t_2(x_1, \dots, x_k)$, and the points in the bucket, which are $g_i^{-1}(x_1, \dots x_k) \cap \mathcal{P}$.

The reasons for using the second hash function t_2 instead of storing the value $g_i(p) = (x_1, \dots x_k)$ are twofold. First, by using a fingerprint $t_2(x_1, \dots x_k)$, we decrease the amount of memory for bucket identification from $O(k)$ to $O(1)$. Second, with the fingerprint it is faster to look up an LSH bucket in the chain containing it. The domain of the function t_2 is chosen big enough to ensure with a high probability that any two different buckets in the same chain have different t_2 values.

All L hash tables use the same primary hash function t_1 (used to dermine the index in the hash table) and the same secondary hash function t_2. These two hash functions have the form

$$t_1(a_1, a_2, \dots, a_k) = \left(\left(\sum_{i=1}^{k} r'_i a_i \right) \mod P \right) \mod tableSize,$$
$$t_2(a_1, a_2, \dots, a_k) = \left(\sum_{i=1}^{k} r''_i a_i \right) \mod P,$$

where r'_i and r''_i are random integers, $tableSize$ is the size of the hash tables, and P is a prime.

In the current implementation, $tableSize = |\mathcal{P}|$, a_i are represented by 32-bit integers, and the prime P is equal to $2^{32} - 5$. This value of the prime allows fast hash function computation without using modulo operations. Specifically, without loss of generality, consider computing $t_2(a_1)$ for $k = 1$. We have that

$$t_2(a_1) = (r''_1 a_1) \mod (2^{32} - 5) = (low[r''_1 a_1] + 5 \cdot high[r''_1 a_1]) \mod (2^{32} - 5),$$

where $low[r''_1 a_1]$ are the low-order 32 bits of $r''_1 a_1$ (a 64-bit number), and $high[r''_1 a_1]$ are the high-order 32 bits of $r''_1 a_1$. If we choose r''_i from the range $\{1, \dots 2^{29}\}$, we will always have that $\alpha = low[r''_1 a_1] + 5 \cdot high[r''_1 a_1] < 2 \cdot (2^{32} - 5)$. This means that

$$t_2(a_1) = \begin{cases} \alpha & \text{, if } \alpha < 2^{32} - 5 \\ \alpha - (2^{32} - 5) & \text{, if } \alpha \geq 2^{32} - 5 \end{cases}$$

For $k > 1$, we compute progressively the sum $\left(\sum_{i=1}^{k} r_i'' a_i \right) \bmod P$ keeping always the partial sum modulo $(2^{32} - 5)$ using the same principle as the one above. Note that the range of the function t_2 thus is $\{1, \ldots 2^{32} - 6\}$.

3.4.3 Memory Requirement for LSH

The data structure described above requires $O(nL)$ memory (for each function g_i, we store the n points from $\mathcal{P}$). Since L increases as k increases, the memory requirement could be large for a large data set, or for a moderate data set for which optimal time is achieved with higher values of k. Therefore, an upper limit on memory imposes an upper limit on k.

Because the memory requirement is big, the constant in front of $O(nL)$ is very important. In E^2LSH, with the best variant of the hash tables, this constant is 12 bytes. Note that it is the structure and layout of the L hash tables that dictate memory usage.

Below we show two variants of the layout of the hash tables that we deployed. We assume that

- the number of points is $n \leq 2^{20}$;
- each pointer is 4 bytes long;
- *tableSize* $= n$ for each hash table.

One of the most straightforward layouts of a hash table H_i is the following. For each index l of the hash table, we store a pointer to a singly linked list of buckets in the chain l. For each bucket, we store its value $h_2(\cdot)$, and a pointer to a singly linked list of points in the bucket. The memory requirement per hash table is $4 \cdot tableSize + 8 \cdot \#buckets + 8 \cdot n \leq 20n$, yielding a constant of 20.

To reduce this constant to 12 bytes, we do the following. First, we index all points in $\mathcal{P}$, such that we can refer to points by index (this index is constant across all hash tables). Referring to a point thus takes only 20 bits (and not 32 as in the case of a pointer). Consider now a hash table H_i. For this hash table, we deploy a table Y of 32-bit unsigned integers that store all buckets (with values $h_2(\cdot)$) and points in the buckets (thus, Y is a hybrid storage table since it stores both buckets' and points' description). The table has a length of $\#buckets + n$ and is used as follows. In the hash table H_i, at index l, we store the pointer to some index e_l of Y; e_l is the start of the description of the chain l. A chain is stored as follows: $h_2(\cdot)$ value of the first bucket in chain (at position e_l in Y) followed by the indices of the points in this bucket (positions $e_l + 1, \ldots e_l + n_1$); $h_2(\cdot)$ value of the second bucket in the chain (position $e_l + n_1 + 1$) followed by the indices of the points in this second bucket (positions $e_l + n_1 + 2, \ldots e_l + n_1 + 1 + n_2$); and so forth.

Note that we need also to store the number of buckets in each chain as well as the number of points in each bucket. Instead of storing the chain length, we store for each bucket a bit that says whether that bucket is the last one in the chain or not; this bit is one of the unused bits of the 4-byte integer storing the index of the first point in the corresponding bucket (i.e., if the $h_2(\cdot)$ value of the bucket is stored at position e in Y, then we use a high-order bit of the integer at position $e + 1$ in Y). For storing the length of the bucket, we use the remaining unused bits of the first point in the bucket. When the remaining bits are not enough (there are more than $2^{32-20-1} - 1 = 2^{11} - 1$ points in the bucket), we store a special value for the length (0), which means that there are more than $2^{11} - 1$ points in the bucket, and there are some additional points (that do not fit in the $2^{11} - 1$ integers allotted in Y after the $h_2(\cdot)$ value of the bucket). These additional points are also stored in Y but at a different position; their start index and number are stored in the unused bits of the remaining $2^{11} - 2$ points that follow the $h_2(\cdot)$ value of the bucket and the first point of the bucket (i.e., unused bits of the integers at positions $e + 2, \ldots e + 2^{11} - 1$).

3.5   Experimental Results

In this section we present some preliminary experimental results on the performance of E²LSH.

For the comparison, we used the MNIST data set [9]. It contains 60,000 points, each having dimension $28 \times 28 = 784$. The points were normalized so that each point has its l_2 norm equal to 1.

We compared the performance of E²LSH and ANN [2]. The latter provides an efficient implementation of a variant of the kd-tree data structure. It supports both exact and approximate nearest neighbor search (we used the former).

To compare the running times of ANN and E²LSH, we need to have E²LSH find the *nearest neighbor*, as opposed to the *near neighbor*. We achieve this by solving the near-neighbor problem for one value of R. We chose this value to ensure that all but, say, 3% of the data points have their nearest neighbor within distance R. To find such R, it suffices to find, say, the 97th percentile of the distances from points to their nearest neighbor (this can be approximated fast by sampling). In our case, we chose $R = 0.65$. Then, to find the nearest neighbor, we find the R-near neighbors and report the closest point.

We note that, in general, the value of R obtained using the above method might not lead to an efficient algorithm. This is because, for some data sets, the number of R-near neighbors of an average query point could be very large, and sifting through all of them during the query time would be inefficient. For such data sets one needs to build data structures for *several* values of R. During the query time, the data structures are queried in the

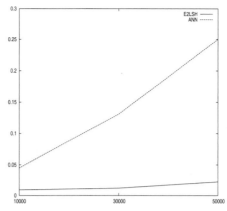

Figure 3.4 Experiments: LSH vs ANN.

increasing order of R. The process is stopped when a data structure reports an answer.

Another parameter that is required by E^2LSH is the probability of error δ. We set it to 10%. A lower probability of error would increase the running times, although not very substantially. For example, using two separate data structures in parallel (or, alternatively, doubling the number of hash functions L), would reduce the error from 10% to at most $(10\%)^2 = 1\%$.

To perform the running time comparisons, we ran the algorithms on random subsets of the original data sets of size 10,000, 30,000 and 50,000. The actual times per query are reported in fig. 3.4.

As can be observed, the running times of E^2LSH are much lower than the times of ANN. Additional experiments (not reported here) indicate that the times do not decrease substantially if ANN is allowed to report c-approximate nearest neighbor for small values of c (say, $c < 1.5$). On the other hand, setting c to a large value (say, $c = 10$) reduces running times of ANN drastically, since the search procedure is stopped at a very early stage; the resulting running times become comparable to E^2LSH. At the same time, the *actual* error of ANN is remarkably low: it reports the exact nearest neighbor for about two thirds of the query points. The fact that the kd-trees search procedure (using priority queues) reports "good" nearest neighbors, even if the search is interrupted very early, has been observed earlier in the literature (e.g., see [3]). Note, however, that any guarantees for this method are only empirical, while, for the R-near-neighbor search problem, E^2LSH provides rigorous guarantees on the probability of missing a near neighbor.

References

1. E2lsh package. `http://web.mit.edu/andoni/www/LSH/` .

2. S. Arya and D. Mount. Ann: Library for approximate nearest neighbor searching. `http://www.cs.umd.edu/~mount/ANN/`.

3. J. S. Beis and D. G. Lowe. Shape indexing using approximate nearest-neighbour search in high-dimensional space. pages 1000–1006, San Juan, PR, June 1997.

4. J. M. Chambers, C. L. Mallows, and B. W. Stuck. A method for simulating stable random variables. *Journal of the American Statistical Association*, 71:340–344, 1976.

5. M. Datar, N. Immorlica, P. Indyk, and V. Mirrokni. Locality-sensitive hashing scheme based on p-stable distributions. *DIMACS Workshop on Streaming Data Analysis and Mining*, 2003.

6. P. Indyk. Stable distributions, pseudorandom generators, embeddings and data stream computation. *Proceedings of the Symposium on Foundations of Computer Science*, 2000.

7. P. Indyk and R. Motwani. Approximate nearest neighbor: Towards removing the curse of dimensionality. *Proceedings of the Symposium on Theory of Computing*, 1998.

8. J. P. Nolan. An introduction to stable distributions. `http://www.cas.american.edu/~jpnolan/chap1.ps`.

9. H. Wang and S. Bengio. The mnist database of handwritten upper-case letters. Technical Report 04, IDIAP, 2002.

10. V.M. Zolotarev. *One-Dimensional Stable Distributions*. Volulme 65 of *Translations of Mathematical Monographs*, American Mathematical Society, Providence, R.I., 1986.

II APPLICATIONS: LEARNING

4   New Algorithms for Efficient High-Dimensional Nonparametric Classification

Ting Liu, Andrew W. Moore, and Alexander Gray

This chapter is about nonapproximate acceleration of high-dimensional nonparametric operations such as k nearest-neighbor (k-NN) classifiers. We attempt to exploit the fact that even if we want exact answers to nonparametric queries, we usually do not need to explicitly find the data points close to the query, but merely need to answer questions about the properties of that set of data points. This offers a small amount of computational leeway, and we investigate how much that leeway can be exploited. This is applicable to many algorithms in nonparametric statistics, memory-based learning, and kernel-based learning. But for clarity, this chapter concentrates on pure k-NN classification. We introduce new balltree algorithms that on real-world data sets give accelerations from 2- to 100-fold compared to highly optimized traditional balltree-based k-NN . These results include data sets with up to 10^6 dimensions and 10^5 records, and demonstrate nontrivial speedups while giving exact answers.

4.1   Introduction

This chapter is a copy of an article that is going to be published in JMLR. Nonparametric models have become increasingly popular in the statistics and probabilistic artificial intelligence communities. These models are extremely useful when the underlying distribution of the problem is unknown except that which can be inferred from samples. One simple well-known nonparametric classification method is called the k-nearest-neighbors or k-NN rule. Given a data set $V \subset R^D$ containing n points, it finds the k closest points to a query point $\mathsf{q} \in R^D$, typically under the Euclidean distance, and chooses the label corresponding to the majority. Despite the simplicity of this idea, it was famously shown by Cover and Hart [9] that asymptotically its error is within a factor of two of the optimal. Its simplicity allows it to be easily and flexibly applied to a variety of complex problems. It has applications in a wide range of real-world settings, in particular pattern recognition [15, 14]; text categorization [55]; database and data mining [26, 29]; information retrieval [10, 17, 51]; image and multimedia search [16, 47, 20, 53]; machine learning [8]; statistics and data analysis [12, 32] and also combination with other methods [57]. However, these methods all remain hampered by their computational complexity.

Several effective solutions exist for this problem when the dimension D is small, including Voronoi diagrams [48], which work well for two-dimensional (2D) data. Other methods are designed to work for problems with moderate dimension (i.e. tens of dimensions), such as k-D tree [21, 48], R-tree [26], and ball-tree [22, 43, 56, 6]. Among these tree structures, balltree, or metric-tree [43], represents the practical state of the art for achieving efficiency in the largest dimension possible [40, 7] without resorting to approximate answers. They have been used in many different ways, in a variety of tree search algorithms and with a variety of "cached sufficient statistics" decorating the internal leaves, for example in [42, 11, 59, 46, 25]. However, many real-world problems are posed with very large dimensions that are beyond the capability of such search structures to achieve sub linear efficiency, e.g., in computer vision, in which each pixel of an image represents a dimension. Thus, the high-dimensional case is the long-standing frontier of the nearest-neighbor problem.

With one exception, the proposals involving tree-based or other data structures have considered the generic nearest-neighbor problem, not that of nearest-neighbor *classification* specifically. Many proposals designed specifically for nearest-neighbor classification have been proposed, virtually all of them pursuing the idea of reducing the number of training points. In most of these approaches, such as [28], although the runningtime is reduced, so is the classification accuracy. Several similar training set reduction schemes yielding only approximate classifications have been proposed [19, 23, 5, 50, 52, 44]. Our method achieves the exact classification that would be achieved by exhaustive search for the nearest neighbors. A few training set reduction methods have the capability of yielding exact classifications. Djouadi and Bouktache [13] described both approximate and exact methods, but a speedup of only about a factor of two over exhaustive search was reported for the exact case, for simulated, low-dimensional data. The paper by Lee and Chae [35] also achieves exact classifications, but only obtained a speedup over exhaustive search of about 1.7. It is in fact common among the results reported for training set reduction methods that only 40% to 60% of the training points can be discarded, i.e., no important speedups are possible with this approach when the Bayes risk is not insignificant. Zhang and Srihari [58] pursued a combination of training set reduction and a tree data structure, but that is an approximate method.

In this chapter, we propose two new balltree based algorithms, which we will call KNS2 and KNS3. They are both designed for binary k-NN classification. We only focus the on binary case, since there are many binary classification problems, such as anomaly detection [34], drug activity detection [33], and video segmentation [49]. Liu et al. [37] applied similar ideas to many-class classification and proposed a variation of the k-NN algorithm. KNS2 and KNS3 share the same insight that the task of k-nearest-neighbor classification of a query q *need not require us to explicitly find those k nearest-neighbors.* To be more specific, there are three similar but in fact different questions: (a) *What are the k-NN of* q*?*, (b) *How many of the k-NN of* q *are from the positive class?,* and (c) *Are at least t of the k-NN from the positive class?* Many researches have focused (a), but uses of proximity queries in statistics far more frequently require (b) and (c) types of computations. In fact, for the k-NN classification problem, when the threshold t is set, it is sufficient to just answer the much simpler question (c). The triangle inequality underlying a balltree has the advantage of bounding the distances between data points, and can thus help us estimate the nearest neighbors without explicitly finding them. In this chapter, we test our algorithms on seventeen synthetic and real-world data sets, with dimensions ranging from 2 to 1.1×10^6 and the number of data points ranging from 10^4 to 4.9×10^5. We observe up to 100-fold speedup compared to highly optimized traditional balltree-based k-NN , in which the neighbors are found explicitly.

Omachi and Aso [41] proposed a fast k-NN classifier based on a branch and bound method, and the algorithm shares some ideas of KNS2, but it did not fully explore the idea of doing k-NN classification without explicitly finding the k-NN set, and the speedup of the algorithm achieved is limited. In section 4, we address Omachi and Aso's method in more detail.

We will first describe balltrees and this traditional way of using them (which we call KNS1), which computes problem a. Then we will describe a new method (KNS2) for problem b, designed for the common setting of skewed-class data. We will then describe a new method (KNS3) for problem c, which removes the skewed-class assumption, applying to arbitrary classification problems. At the end of Section 4.5 we will say a bit about the relative value of KNS2 vs. KNS3.

4.2 Balltree

A *balltree* [22, 43, 56, 6, 40] is a binary tree where each node represents a set of points, called Pts($\mathcal{N}$). Given a data set, the *root node* of a balltree represents the full set of points in the data set. A node can be either a *leaf node* or a *nonleaf node*. A leaf node explicitly contains a list of the points represented by the node. A nonleaf node has two children nodes: $\mathcal{N}.child1$ and $\mathcal{N}.child2$, where

$$Pts(\mathcal{N}.child1) \cap Pts(\mathcal{N}.child2) = \phi,$$
$$Pts(\mathcal{N}.child1) \cup Pts(\mathcal{N}.child2) = Pts(\mathcal{N}).$$

Points are organized spatially. Each node has a distinguished point called a *Pivot*. Depending on the implementation, the *Pivot* may be one of the data points, or it may be the centroid of *Pts(N)*. Each node records the maximum distance of the points it owns to its pivot. Call this the radius of the node:

$$\mathcal{N}.Radius = \max_{\mathbf{x} \in Pts(\mathcal{N})} | \mathcal{N}.Pivot - \mathbf{x} | .$$

Nodes lower down the tree have a smaller radius. This is achieved by insisting, at tree construction time, that

$$\mathbf{x} \in Pts(\mathcal{N}.child1) \;\Rightarrow\; | \mathbf{x} - \mathcal{N}.child1.Pivot | \le | \mathbf{x} - \mathcal{N}.child2.Pivot | .$$
$$\mathbf{x} \in Pts(\mathcal{N}.child2) \;\Rightarrow\; | \mathbf{x} - \mathcal{N}.child2.Pivot | \le | \mathbf{x} - \mathcal{N}.child1.Pivot | .$$

Provided that our distance function satisfies the triangle inequality, we can bound the distance from a query point $\mathbf{q}$ to any point in any balltree node. If $\mathbf{x} \in Pts(\mathcal{N})$ then we know that

$$|\mathbf{x} - \mathbf{q}| \;\ge\; |\mathbf{q} - \mathcal{N}.Pivot| - \mathcal{N}.Radius. \qquad (4.1)$$
$$|\mathbf{x} - \mathbf{q}| \;\le\; |\mathbf{q} - \mathcal{N}.Pivot| + \mathcal{N}.Radius. \qquad (4.2)$$

Here is an easy proof of the inequality. According to triangle inequality, we have $|\mathbf{x} - \mathbf{q}| \ge |\mathbf{q} - \mathcal{N}.Pivot| - |x - \mathcal{N}.Pivot|$. Given $\mathbf{x} \in Pts(\mathcal{N})$ and $\mathcal{N}.Radius$ is the maximum distance of the points it owns to its pivot, $|\mathbf{x} - \mathcal{N}.Pivot| \le \mathcal{N}.Radius$, so $|\mathbf{x} - \mathbf{q}| \ge |\mathbf{q} - \mathcal{N}.Pivot| - \mathcal{N}.Radius$. Similarly, we can prove (4.2). ∎

Balltrees are constructed topdown. There are several ways to construct them, and practical algorithms trade off the cost of construction (e.g., it can be inefficient to be $O(R^2)$ given a data set with R points) against the tightness of the radius of the balls. Moore [40] describes a fast way to construct a balltree appropriate for computational statistics. If a balltree is balanced, then the construction time is $O(CR \log R)$, where C is the cost of a point-point distance computation (which is $O(m)$ if there are m dense attributes, and $O(fm)$ if the records are sparse with only fraction f of attributes taking non-zero value). Figure 1 shows a 2D data set and the first few levels of a balltree.

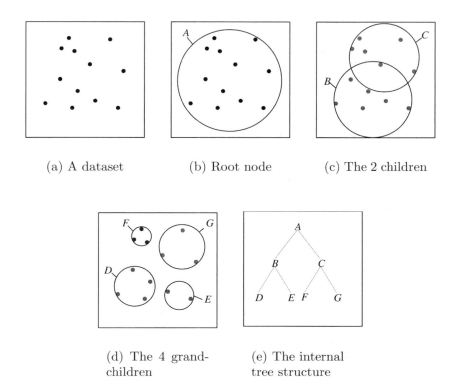

(a) A dataset   (b) Root node   (c) The 2 children

(d) The 4 grand-children   (e) The internal tree structure

Figure 4.1   An example of a balltree structure.

4.3   KNS1: Conventional k-NN Search with Balltree

In this chapter, we call the conventional balltree-based search [56] *KNS1*. Let PS be a set of data points, and $PS \subseteq V$, where V is the training set. We begin with the following definition:

Say that *PS consists of the k-NN of* q *in V* if and only if

$$| V | \geq k \quad and \quad PS \text{ are the } k\text{-NN of } \mathbf{q} \text{ in V}$$
$$or \qquad\qquad\qquad\qquad\qquad\quad (4.3)$$
$$| V | < k \quad and \quad PS == V.$$

We now define a recursive procedure called *BallKNN* with the following inputs and output.

$$PS^{out} = BallKNN(PS^{in}, \mathcal{N}).$$

Let V be the set of points searched so far, on entry. Assume that PS^{in} consists of the k-NN of q in V. This function efficiently ensures that on exit, PS^{out} consists of the k-NN of q in $V \cup Pts(\mathcal{N})$. We define

$$D_{\text{sofar}} = \begin{cases} \infty & if \ | PS^{in} | < k \\ \max_{\mathbf{x} \in PS^{in}} | \mathbf{x} - \mathbf{q} | & if \ | PS^{in} | == k. \end{cases} \qquad (4.4)$$

D_{sofar} is the minimum distance within which points become interesting to us. Let

$$D^{\mathcal{N}}_{\text{minp}} = \begin{cases} \max(|\mathbf{q} - \mathcal{N}.Pivot| - \mathcal{N}.Radius, D^{\mathcal{N}.parent}_{minp}) & if\ \mathcal{N} \neq Root \\ \max(|\mathbf{q} - \mathcal{N}.Pivot| - \mathcal{N}.Radius, 0) & if\ \mathcal{N} == Root. \end{cases}$$

$$(4.5)$$

$D^{\mathcal{N}}_{\text{minp}}$ is the minimum possible distance from any point in $\mathcal{N}$ to $\mathbf{q}$. This is computed using the bound given by (4.1) and the fact that all points covered by a node must be covered by its parent. This property implies that $D^{\mathcal{N}}_{minp}$ will never be less than the minimum distance of its ancestors. Step 2 of section 4.4 explains this optimization further. See algorithm 4.1 for details.

Procedure BallKNN $(PS^{in}, \mathcal{N})$

if $(D^{\mathcal{N}}_{\text{minp}} \geq D_{\text{sofar}})$, **then**
    /* If this condition is satisfied, then impossible
    for a point in $\mathcal{N}$ to be closer than the
    previously discovered *kth* nearest neighbor.*/
    Return PS^{in} unchanged.
else if $(\mathcal{N}$ is a leaf$)$
    $PS^{out} = PS^{in}$
    $\forall \mathbf{x} \in Pts(\mathcal{N})$
    if $(| \mathbf{x} - \mathbf{q} | < D_{\text{sofar}})$, **then**   /* If a leaf, do a naive linear scan */
      add $\mathbf{x}$ to PS^{out}
      if $(| PS^{out} | == k + 1)$, **then**
        remove furthest neighbor from PS^{out}
        update D_{sofar}
else
    /*If a nonleaf, explore the nearer of the two
    child nodes, then the further. It is likely that
    further search will immediately prune itself.*/
    $node_1$ = child of $\mathcal{N}$ closest to $\mathbf{q}$
    $node_2$ = child of $\mathcal{N}$ furthest from $\mathbf{q}$
    $PS^{temp} = BallKNN(PS^{in}, node_1)$
    $PS^{out} = BallKNN(PS^{temp}, node_2)$

Algorithm 4.1   A call of BallKNN({},Root) returns the k-NN of $\mathbf{q}$ in the balltree.

Experimental results show that KNS1 (conventional k-NN search with ball-tree) achieves significant speedup over Naive k-NN when the dimension d of the data set is moderate (less than 30). In the best case, the complexity of KNS1 can be as good as $O(d \log R)$, given a data set with R points. However, with d increasing, the benefit achieved by KNS1 degrades, and when d is really large, in the worst case, the complexity of KNS1 can be as bad as $O(dR)$. Sometimes it is even slower than Naive k-NN search, due to the curse of dimensionality.

In the following sections, we describe our new algorithms KNS2 and KNS3; these two algorithms are both based on balltree structure, but by using different search strategies, we explore how much speedup can be achieved beyond KNS1.

4.4   KNS2: Faster k-NN Classification for Skewed-Class Data

In many binary classification domains, one class is much more frequent than the other. For example, in High Throughput Screening data sets, (described in section 7.2), it is far more common for the result of an experiment to be negative than positive. In detection of fraud telephone calls [18] or credit card transactions [54], the number of legitimate transactions are far more common than fraudulent ones. In insurance risk modeling [45], a very small percentage of the policyholders file one or more claims in a given time period. There are many other examples of domains with similar intrinsic imbalance, and therefore classification with a skewed distribution is important. Various researches have been focused on designing clever methods to solve this type of problem [4, 39]. The new algorithm introduced in this section, KNS2, is designed to accelerate k-NN based classification in such skewed data scenarios.

KNS2 answers the type b question described in the introduction, namely, How many of the k-NN are in the positive class? The key idea of KNS2 is we can answer question b without explicitly finding the k-NN set.

KNS2 attacks the problem by building two balltrees: A *Postree* for the points from the positive (small) class, and a *Negtree* for the points from the negative (large) class. Since the number of points from the positive class(small) is so small, it is quite cheap to find the exact k nearest positive points of q by using KNS1. And the idea of KNS2 is to first search *Postree* using KNS1 to find the k-nearest positive neighbors set $Posset_k$, and then search *Negtree* while using $Posset_k$ as bounds to prune nodes far away, and at the same time estimate the number of negative points to be inserted to the true nearest-neighbor set. The search can be stopped as soon as we get the answer to question b. Empirically, much more pruning can be achieved by KNS2 than conventional balltree search. A concrete description of the algorithm is as follows:

Let $Root_{pos}$ be the root of *Postree*, and $Root_{neg}$ be the root of *Negtree*. Then, we classify a new query point q in the following fashion

– Step 1 " **Find positive**": Find the k nearest positive class neighbors of q (and their distances to q) using conventional balltree search.

– Step 2 — **"Insert negative"**: Do sufficient search on the negative tree to prove that the number of positive data points among k-NN is n for some value of n.

Step 2 is achieved using a new recursive search called *NegCount*. In order to describe *NegCount* we need the following four definitions.

– **The dists array.** *Dists* is an array of elements $Dists_1 \ldots Dists_k$ consisting of the distances to the k nearest positive neighbors found so far of q, sorted in increasing order of distance. For notational convenience we will also write $Dists_0 = 0$ and $Dists_{k+1} = \infty$.

– **Pointset V.** Define pointset V as the set of points in the negative balls visited so far in the search.

– **The counts array (n,C)** $(n \leq k+1)$. C is an array of counts containing n+1 array elements $C_0, C_1, \ldots C_n$. Say *(n,C)* summarize interesting negative points for pointset V if and only if

1. $\forall i = 0, 1, \ldots, n$,

$$C_i = \mid V \cap \{x : \mid x - q \mid < Dists_i\} \mid \qquad (4.6)$$

Intuitively C_i is the number of points in V whose distances to q are closer than $Dists_i$. In other words, C_i is the number of negative points in V closer than the *ith* positive neighbor to q.

2. $C_i + i \leq k (i < n)$, $C_n + n > k$.
This simply declares that the length n of the C array is as short as possible while accounting for the k members of V that are nearest to q. Such an n exists since $C_0 = 0$ and $C_{k+1} =$ total number of negative points. To make the problem interesting, we assume that the number of negative points and the number of positive points are both greater than k.

– $D^{\mathcal{N}}_{\mathbf{minp}}$ and $D^{\mathcal{N}}_{\mathbf{maxp}}$
Here we continue to use $D^{\mathcal{N}}_{\mathrm{minp}}$ which is defined in (4.4). Symmetrically, we also define $D^{\mathcal{N}}_{\mathrm{maxp}}$ as follows: Let

$$D^{\mathcal{N}}_{maxp} = \begin{cases} \min(\mid q - \mathcal{N}.Pivot \mid + \mathcal{N}.Radius, \ D^{\mathcal{N}.parent}_{maxp}) & if \ \mathcal{N} \neq Root \\ \mid q - \mathcal{N}.Pivot \mid + \mathcal{N}.Radius & if \ \mathcal{N} == Root. \end{cases}$$
$$(4.7)$$

$D^{\mathcal{N}}_{\mathrm{maxp}}$ is the maximum possible distance from any point in $\mathcal{N}$ to q. This is computed using the bound in (4.1) and the property of a balltree that all the points covered by a node must be covered by its parent. This property implies that $D^{\mathcal{N}}_{\mathrm{maxp}}$ will never be greater than the maximum possible distance of its ancestors.

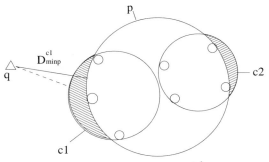

Figure 4.2   An example to illustrate how to compute $D^{\mathcal{N}}_{minp}$

Figure 4.2 gives a good example. There are three nodes: p, $c1$, and $c2$. $c1$ and $c2$ are p's children. q is the query point. In order to compute D^{c1}_{minp}, first we compute $|\mathsf{q} - c1.pivot| - c1.radius$, which is the dashed line in the figure, but D^{c1}_{minp} can be further bounded by D^{p}_{minp}, since it is impossible for any point to be in the shaded area. Similarly, we get the equation for D^{c1}_{maxp}. $D^{\mathcal{N}}_{\mathrm{minp}}$ and $D^{\mathcal{N}}_{\mathrm{maxp}}$ are used to estimate the counts array (n, C). Again we take advantage of the triangle inequality of balltree. For any $\mathcal{N}$, if there exists an i ($i \in [1, n]$) such that $Dists_{i-1} \leq D^{\mathcal{N}}_{\mathrm{maxp}} < Dists_i$, then for $\forall x \in Pts(\mathcal{N})$, $Dists_{i-1} \leq | x - \mathsf{q} | < Dists_i$. According to the definition of C, we can add $| Pts(\mathcal{N}) |$ to $C_i, C_{i+1}, ...C_n$. The function of $D^{\mathcal{N}}_{\mathrm{minp}}$ similar to KNS1, is used to help prune uninteresting nodes.

Step 2 of KNS2 is implemented by the recursive function below:

$$(n^{out}, C^{out}) = NegCount(n^{in}, C^{in}, \mathcal{N}, j_{parent}, Dists)$$

See algorithm 4.2 for the detailed implementation of NegCount.
Assume that on entry (n^{in}, C^{in}) summarize interesting negative points for pointset V, where V is the set of points visited so far during the search. This algorithm efficiently ensures that, on exit, (n^{out}, C^{out}) summarize interesting negative points for $V \cup Pts(\mathcal{N})$. In addition, j_{parent} is a temporary variable used to prevent multiple counts for the same point. This variable relates to the implementation of KNS2, and we do not want to go into the details here.

We can stop the procedure when n^{out} becomes 1 (which means all the k-NN of q are in the negative class) or when we run out of nodes. n^{out} represents the number of positive points in the k-NN of q. The top-level call is

$$NegCount(k, C^0, NegTree.Root, k + 1, Dists)$$

where C^0 is an array of zeroes and $Dists$ are defined in step 2 and obtained by applying KNS1 to the *Postree*.

Procedure NegCount $(n^{in}, C^{in}, \mathcal{N}, j_{parent}, Dists)$

$n^{out} := n^{in}$ /* Variables to be returned by the search.
$C^{out} := C^{in}$ Initialize them here. */

Compute $D^{\mathcal{N}}_{\mathrm{minp}}$ and $D^{\mathcal{N}}_{\mathrm{maxp}}$
Search for $i, j \in [1, n^{out}]$, such that
   $Dists_{i-1} \leq D^{\mathcal{N}}_{\mathrm{minp}} < Dists_i$
   $Dists_{j-1} \leq D^{\mathcal{N}}_{\mathrm{maxp}} < Dists_j$

For all indices $\in [j, j_{parent})$
   /* Re-estimate C^{out} */
   Update $C^{out}_{index} := C^{out}_{index} + |\, Pts(\mathcal{N})\, |$
/* Only update the count less than j_{parent}
to avoid counting twice. */
Update n^{out}, such that
   $C^{out}_{n^{out}-1} + (n^{out} - 1) \leq k, \; C^{out}_{n^{out}} + n^{out} > k$

Set $Dists_{n^{out}} := \infty$

(1) **if** $(n^{out} == 1)$
    /* At least k negative points closer to q
    than the closest positive one: done! */
    Return$(1, C^{out})$

(2) **if** $(i == j)$
    /* $\mathcal{N}$ is located between two adjacent
    positive points, no need to split. */
    Return(n^{out}, C^{out})

(3) **if** $(\mathcal{N}$ is a leaf)
    Forall $x \in Pts(\mathcal{N})$
       Compute $|\, x - q\, |$
    Update and return (n^{out}, C^{out})

(4) **else**
    $node_1 :=$ child of $\mathcal{N}$ closest to q
    $node_2 :=$ child of $\mathcal{N}$ furthest from q
    $(n^{temp}, C^{temp}) :=$ NegCount$(n^{in}, C^{in}, node_1, j, Dists)$
    if $(n^{temp} == 1)$
       Return $(1, C^{out})$
    else $(n^{out}, C^{out}) :=$ NegCount$(n^{temp}, C^{temp}, node_2, j, Dists)$

Algorithm 4.2   Procedure NegCount.

There are at least two situations where this algorithm can run faster than simply finding k-NN . First of all, when $n = 1$, we can stop and exit, since this means we have found at least k negative points closer than the nearest positive neighbor to q. Notice that the k negative points we have found are not necessarily the exact k-NN to q, but this will not change the answer to our question. This situation happens frequently for skewed data sets.

The second situation is as follows: An $\mathcal{N}$ can also be pruned if it is located exactly between two adjacent positive points, or it is farther away than the nth positive point. This is because that, in these situations, there is no need to figure out which negative point is closer within the $\mathcal{N}$. Especially as n gets smaller, we have more chance to prune a node, because $Dists_{n^{in}}$ decreases as n^{in} decreases.

[41] Omachin and Aso proposed a k-NN method based on branch and bound. For simplicity, we call their algorithm KNSV. KNSV is similar to KNS2, in that for the binary class case, it also builds two trees, one for each class. For consistency, let us still call them *Postree* and *Negtree*. KNSV first searches the tree whose center of gravity is closer to q. Without loses of generality, we assume *Negtree* is closer, so KNSV will search *Negtree* first. Instead of fully exploring the tree, it does a greedy depth-first search only to find k-candidate points. Then KNSV moves on to search *Postree*. The search is the same as the conventional balltree search (KNS1), except that it uses the kth candidate negative point to bound the distance. After the search of *Postree* is done, KNSV counts how many of the k-NN so far are from the negative class. If the number is more than $k/2$, the algorithm stops. Otherwise, KNSV will go back to search *Negtree* for the second time, this time to fully search the tree. KNSV has advantages and disadvantages. The first advantage is that it is simple, and thus it is easy to extend to the many-class case. Also, if the first guess of KNSV is correct and the k candidate points are good enough to prune away many nodes, it will be faster than conventional balltree search. But there are some obvious drawbacks to the algorithm. First, the guess of the winner class is only based on which class's center of gravity is the closest to q. Notice that this is a pure heuristic, and the probability of making a mistake is high. Second, using a greedy search to find the k candidate nearest neighbors has a high risk, since these candidates might not even be close to the true nearest neighbors. In that case, the chance for pruning away nodes from the other class becomes much smaller. We can imagine that in many situations, KNSV will end up searching the first tree for yet another time. Finally, we want to point out that KNSV claims it can perform well for many-class nearest neighbors, but this is based on the assumption that the winner class contains at least $k/2$ points within the nearest neighbors, which is often not true for the many-class case. Compared to KNSV, KNS2's advantages are (i) it uses the skewedness property of a data set, which can be robustly detected before the search, and (ii) more careful design gives KNS2 more chance to speedup the search.

4.5   KNS3: Are at Least t of the K-NN Positive?

In this chapter's second new algorithm, we remove KNS2's constraint of an assumed skewedness in the class distribution. Instead, we answer a weaker question: are at least t of the k-NN positive?, where the questioner must supply t and k. In the usual k-NN rule, t represents a majority with respect to k, but here we consider the slightly more general form which might be used, e.g., during classification with known false positive and false negative costs.

In KNS3, we define two important quantities:

$$D_t^{pos} = \text{ } distance \text{ } of \text{ } the \text{ } t^{th} \text{ } nearest \text{ } positive \text{ } neighbor \text{ } of \text{ } \mathsf{q}, \quad (4.8)$$
$$D_m^{neg} = \text{ } distance \text{ } of \text{ } the \text{ } m^{th} \text{ } nearest \text{ } negative \text{ } neighbor \text{ } of \text{ } \mathsf{q}. \quad (4.9)$$

where $m + t = k + 1$.

Before introducing the algorithm, we state and prove an important proposition, which relates the two quantities D_t^{pos} and D_m^{neg} with the answer to KNS3.

Proposition 4.1 *$D_t^{pos} \leq D_m^{neg}$ if and only if at least t of the k nearest neighbors of q from the positive class.*

Proof
If $D_t^{pos} \leq D_m^{neg}$, then there are at least t positive points closer than the mth negative point to q. This also implies that if we draw a ball centered at q, and with its radius equal to D_m^{neg}, then there are exactly m negative points and at least t positive points within the ball. Since $t + m = k + 1$, if we use D_k to denote the distance of the kth nearest neighbor, we get $D_k \leq D_m^{neg}$, which means that there are at most $m - 1$ of the k-NN of q from the negative class. It is equivalent to say that there are at least t of the k nearest neighbors of q are from the positive class. On the other hand, if there are at least t of the k-NN from the positive class, then $D_t^{pos} \leq D_k$, the number of negative points, is at most $k - t < m$, so $D_k \leq D_m^{neg}$. This implies that $D_t^{pos} \leq D_m^{neg}$ is true. ∎

Figure 4.3 provides an illustration. In this example, $k = 5, t = 3$. We use black circles to represent positive points, and white circles to represent negative points. The reason to redefine the problem of KNS3 is to transform a k nearest neighbor searching problem to a much simpler counting problem. In fact, in order to answer the question, we do not even have to compute the exact value of D_t^{pos} and D_m^{neg}, instead, we can estimate them. We define

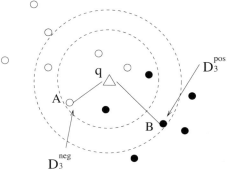

Figure 4.3   An example of D_t^{pos} and D_m^{neg}.

$Lo(D_t^{pos})$ and $Up(D_t^{pos})$ as the lower and upper bounds of D_t^{pos}, and similarly we define $Lo(D_m^{neg})$ and $Up(D_m^{neg})$ as the lower and upper bounds of D_m^{neg}. If at any point, $Up(D_t^{pos}) \leq Lo(D_m^{neg})$, we know $D_t^{pos} \leq D_m^{neg}$, on the other hand, if $Up(D_m^{neg}) \leq Lo(D_t^{pos})$, we know $D_m^{neg} \leq D_t^{pos}$.

Now our computational task is to efficiently estimate $Lo(D_t^{pos})$, $Up(D_t^{pos})$, $Lo(D_m^{neg})$ and $Up(D_m^{neg})$. And it is very convenient for a balltree structure to do so. Below is the detailed description:

At each stage of KNS3 we have two sets of balls in use called P and N, where P is a set of balls from *Postree* built from positive data points, and N consists of balls from *Negtree* built from negative data points.

Both sets have the property that if a ball is in the set, then neither its balltree ancestors nor its descendants are in the set, so that each point in the training set is a member of one or zero balls in $P \cup N$. Initially, $P = \{PosTree.root\}$ and $N = \{NegTree.root\}$. Each stage of KNS3 analyzes P to estimate $Lo(D_t^{pos})$, $Up(D_t^{pos})$, and analyzes N to estimate $Lo(D_m^{neg})$, $Up(D_m^{neg})$. If possible, KNS3 terminates with the answer, else it chooses an appropriate ball from P or N, and replaces that ball with its two children, and repeats the iteration. Figure 4.4 shows one stage of KNS3. The balls involved are labeled a through g and we have

$$P = \{a, b, c, d\}$$
$$N = \{e, f, g\}.$$

Notice that although c and d are inside b, they are not descendants of b. This is possible because when a ball is splitted, we only require that the pointset of its children be disjoint, but the balls covering the children node may be overlapped.

In order to compute $Lo(D_t^{pos})$, we need to sort the balls $u \in P$, such that

$$\forall u_i, u_j \in P, i < j \Rightarrow D_{minp}^i \leq D_{minp}^j$$

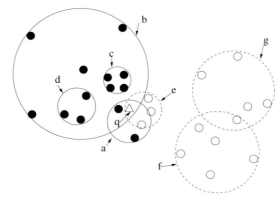

Figure 4.4   A configuration at the start of a stage.

Then

$$Lo(D_t^{pos}) = D_{minp}^{u_j}, \text{ where } \sum_{i=1}^{j-1} \mid Pts(u_i) \mid < t \text{ and } \sum_{i=1}^{j} \mid Pts(u_i) \mid \geq t$$

Symmetrically, in order to compute $Up(D_t^{pos})$, we sort $u \in P$, such that

$$\forall u_i, u_j \in P, i < j \Rightarrow D_{maxp}^i \leq D_{maxp}^j.$$

Then

$$Up(D_t^{pos}) = D_{maxp}^{u_j}, \text{ where } \sum_{i=1}^{j-1} \mid Pts(u_i) \mid < t \text{ and } \sum_{i=1}^{j} \mid Pts(u_i) \mid \geq t$$

Similarly, we can compute $Lo(D_m^{neg})$ and $Up(D_m^{neg})$.

To illustrate this, it is useful to depict a ball as an interval, where the two ends of the interval denote the minimum and maximum possible distances of a point owned by the ball to the query. Figure 4.5(a) shows an example. Notice, we also mark "+5" above the interval to denote the number of points owned by the ball B. After we have this representation, both P and N can be represented as a set of intervals, each interval corresponds to a ball. This is shown in 4.5(b). For example, the second horizontal line denotes the fact that ball B contains four positive points, and that the distance from any location in B to q lies in the range $[0, 5]$. The value of $Lo(D_t^{pos})$ can be understood as the answer to the following question: what if we tried to slide all the positive points within their bounds as far to the left as possible, where would the tth closest positive point lie? Similarly, we can estimate $Up(D_t^{pos})$ by sliding all the positive points to the right ends within their bounds.

For example, in figure 4.4, let $k = 12$ and $t = 7$. Then $m = 12 - 7 + 1 = 6$. We can estimate $(Lo(D_7^{pos}), Up(D_7^{pos}))$ and $(Lo(D_6^{neg}), Up(D_6^{neg}))$, and the

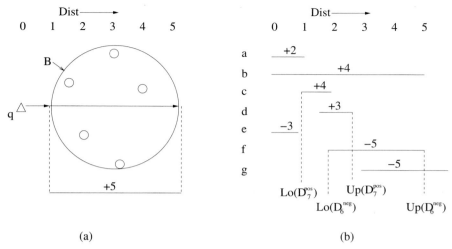

Figure 4.5 (*a*) The interval representation of a ball B. (*b*) The interval representation of the configuration in figure 4.4

results are shown in figure 4.5. Since the two intervals $(Lo(D_7^{pos}), Up(D_7^{pos}))$ and $(Lo(D_6^{neg}), Up(D_6^{neg}))$ have overlap now, no conclusion can be made at this stage. Further splitting needs to be done to refine the estimation.

Below is the pseudocode of the KNS3 algorithm: We define a loop procedure called *PREDICT* with the following input and output.

$$Answer = PREDICT(P, N, t, m)$$

The *Answer*, a boolean value, is true, if there are at least t of the k-NN from the positive class; and false otherwise. Initially, P = {*PosTree.root*} and N = {*NegTree.root*}. The threshold t is given, and $m = k - t + 1$.

Before we describe the algorithm, we first introduce two definitions.
Define
$$(Lo(D_i^S), Up(D_i^S)) = Estimate\_bound(S, i). \tag{4.10}$$

Here S is either set P or N, and we are interested in the ith nearest neighbor of q from set S. The output is the lower and upper bounds. The concrete procedure for estimating the bounds was just described.

Notice that the estimation of the upper and lower bounds could be very loose in the beginning, and will not give us enough information to answer the question. In this case, we will need to split a balltree node and re-estimate the bounds. With more and more nodes being splitted, our estimation becomes more and more precise, and the procedure can be stopped as soon as $Up(D_t^{pos}) \le Lo(D_m^{neg})$ or $Up(D_m^{neg}) \le Lo(D_t^{pos})$. The function of $Pick(P, N)$ below is to choose one node either from P or N to split. There are different strategies for picking a node, for simplicity, our implementation only randomly picks a node to split.

Define

$$split\_node = Pick(P, N). \qquad (4.11)$$

Here *split_node* is the node chosen to be split (see Algorithm 4.3).

Procedure PREDICT (P, N, t, m)

Repeat
$(Lo(D_t^{pos}), Up(D_t^{pos})) = \text{Estimate\_bound(P, t)}$ /* See definition 4.10. */
$(Lo(D_m^{neg}), Up(D_m^{neg})) = \text{Estimate\_bound(N, m)}$
if $(Up(D_t^{pos}) \leq Lo(D_m^{neg}))$ **then**
   Return TRUE
if $(Up_(m^{neg}) \leq Lo(D_m^{neg}))$ **then**
   Return FALSE

split_node = Pick(P, N)
remove split_node from P or N
insert split_node.child1 and split_node.child2 to P or N

Algorithm 4.3   Procedure PREDICT.

Our explanation of KNS3 was simplified for clarity. In order to avoid frequent searches over the full lengths of sets N and P, they are represented as priority queues. Each set in fact uses two queues: one prioritized by D_{maxp}^u and the other by D_{minp}^u. This ensures that the costs of all argmins, deletions, and splits are logarithmic in the queue size.

Some people may ask the question: It seems that KNS3 has more advantages than KNS2; it removes the assumption of skewedness of the data set. In general, it has more chances to prune away nodes, etc. Why do we still need KNS2? The answer is KNS2 does have its own advantages. It answers a more difficult question than KNS3. To know exact how many of the nearest neighbors are from the positive class can be especially useful when the threshold for deciding a class is not known. In that case, KNS3 does not work at all since we cannot provide a static t for answering the question c in section 4.1. But KNS2 can still work very well. On the other hand, the implementation of KNS2 is much simpler than KNS3. For instance, it does not need the priority queues we just described. So there do exist some cases where KNS2 is faster than KNS3.

4.6 Experimental Results

To evaluate our algorithms, we used both real data sets (from UCI and KDD repositories) and also synthetic data sets designed to exercise the algorithms in various ways.

4.6.1 Synthetic data sets

We have six synthetic data sets. The first synthetic data set we have is called `Ideal`, as illustrated in figure 4.6(a). All the data in the left upper area are assigned to the positive class, and all the data in the right lower area are assigned to the negative class. The second data set we have is called `Diag2d`, as illustrated in figure 4.6(b). The data are uniformly distributed in a 10×10 square. The data above the diagonal are assigned to the positive class; the data below the diagonal are assigned to the negative class. We made several variants of Diag2d to test the robustness of KNS3. `Diag2d(10%)` has 10% data of `Diag2d`. `Diag3d` is a cube with uniformly distributed data and classified by a diagonal plane. `Diag10d` is a 10D hypercube with uniformly distributed data and classified by a hyperdiagonal plane. `Noise-diag2d` has the same data as `Diag2d(10%)`, but 1% of the data was assigned to the wrong class.

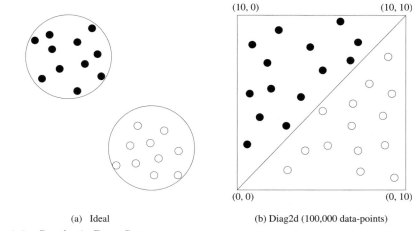

(a) Ideal   (b) Diag2d (100,000 data-points)

Figure 4.6   Synthetic Data Sets

Table 4.1 is a summary of the data sets in the empirical analysis.

Table 4.1   Synthetic Data Sets

Data Set	No. of records	No. of Dimensions	No. of positive	No.positive/No.negative
Ideal	10,000	2	5000	1
Diag2d(10%)	10,000	2	5000	1
Diag2d	100,000	2	50,000	1
Diag3d	100,000	3	50,000	1
Diag10d	100,000	10	50,000	1
Noise2d	10,000	2	5000	1

4.6.2   Real-world Data Sets

We used UCI and KDD data (listed in table 4.2), but we also experimented with data sets of particular current interest within our laboratory.

Life Sciences.
These were proprietary data sets (*ds1* and *ds2*) similar to the publicly available Open Compound Database provided by the National Cancer Institute (NCI Open Compound Database, 2000). The two data sets are sparse. We also present results on data sets derived from *ds1*, denoted *ds1.10pca*, *ds1.100pca*, and *ds2.100anchor* by linear projection using principal component analysis (PCA).

Link Detection.
The first, Citeseer, is derived from the Citeseer website (Citeseer,2002) and lists the names of collaborators on published materials. The goal is to predict whether J_Lee (the most common name) was a collaborator for each work based on who else is listed for that work. We use *J_Lee.100pca* to represent the linear projection of the data to 100 dimensions using PCA. The second link detection data set is derived from the Internet Movie Database (IMDB, 2002) and is denoted *imdb* using a similar approach, but to predict the participation of Mel Blanc (again the most common participant).

UCI/KDD data.
We use four large data sets from the KDD/UCI repository [3]. The data sets can be identified from their names. They were converted to binary classification problems. Each categorical input attribute was converted into n binary attributes by a 1-of-n encoding (where n is the number of possible values of the attribute).

1. *Letter* originally had twenty-six classes: A-Z. We performed binary classification using the letter A as the positive class and "Not A" as negative.
2. *Ipums* (from ipums.la.97). We predict *farm status*, which is binary.

3. *Movie* is a data set from [31]. The TREC-2001 Video Track organized by NIST shot boundary Task. four hours of video or 13 MPEG-1 video files at slightly over 2 GB of data.

4. *Kdd99(10%)* has a binary prediction: Normal vs. Attack.

Table 4.2   Real Data Sets

Data Set	No. of records	No. of Dimensions	No.of positive	No.positive/No.negative
ds1	26,733	6348	804	0.03
ds1.10pca	26,733	10	804	0.03
ds1.100pca	26,733	100	804	0.03
ds2	88,358	1.1×10^6	211	0.002
ds2.100anchor	88,358	100	211	0.002
J_Lee.100pca	181,395	100	299	0.0017
Blanc__Mel	186,414	10	824	0.004
Data Set	**No. records**	**No. of Dimensions**	**No.of positive**	**No.positive/No.negative**
Letter	20,000	16	790	0.04
Ipums	70,187	60	119	0.0017
Movie	38,943	62	7620	0.24
Kdd99(10%)	494,021	176	97278	0.24

4.6.3   Methodology

The data set *ds2* is particular interesting, because its dimension is 1.1×10^6. Our first experiment is especially designed for it. We use $k=9$, and $t = \lceil k/2 \rceil$, then we print out the distribution of time taken for queries of three algorithms: KNS1, KNS2, and KNS3. This is aimed at understanding the range of behavior of the algorithms under huge dimensions (some queries will be harder, or take longer, for an algorithm than other queries). We randomly took 1% negative records (881) and 50% positive records (105) as test data (total 986 points), and train on the remaining 87,372 data points.

For our second set of experiments, we did ten-fold crossvalidation on all the data sets. For each data set, we tested $k = 9$ and $k = 101$, in order to show the effect of a small value and a large value. For KNS3, we used $t = \lceil k/2 \rceil$: a data point is classified as positive if and only if the majority of its k-NN are positive. Since we use crossvalidation, each experiment required R k-NN classification queries (where R is the umber of records in the data set) and each query involved the k-NN among $0.9R$ records. A naive implementation with no ball trees would thus require $0.9R^2$ distance computations. We want to emphasize here that these algorithms are all exact. No approximations were used in the classifications.

4.6.4   Results

Figure 4.7 shows the histograms of times and speed-ups for queries on the ds2 data set. For naive k-NN , all the queries take 87,372 distance computations. For KNS1, all the queries take more than 1.0×10^4 distance computations, (the average number of distances computed is 1.3×10^5) which is greater than 87,372 and thus traditional balltree search is worse than "naive" linear scan. For KNS2, most of the queries take less than 4.0×10^4 distance computations; a few points take longer time. The average number of distances computed is 6233. For KNS3, all the queries take fewer than 1.0×10^4 distance computations; the average number of distances computed is 3411. The lower three figures illustrate speed-up achieved for KNS1, KNS2, and KNS3 over naive linear scan. The figures show the distribution of the speedup obtained for each query. From figure4.7(d) we can see that, on average, KNS1 is even slower than the naive algorithm. KNS2 can get from 2- to 250-fold speedups. On average, it has a 14-fold speedup. KNS3 can get from 2- to 2500-fold speedups. On average, it has a 26-fold speedups.

Table 4.3 on page 96 shows the results for the second set of experiments. The second column lists the computational cost of naive k-NN , both in terms of the number of distance computations and the wall-clock time on an unloaded 2 GHz Pentium. We then examine the speedups of KNS1 (traditional use of a balltree) and our two new balltree methods (KNS2 and KNS3). Generally speaking, the speedups achieved for distance computations on all three algorithms are greater than the corresponding speedup for wall-clock time. This is expected, because the wall-clock time also includes the time for building ball trees, generating priority queues, and searching. We can see that for the synthetic data sets, KNS1 and KNS2 yield 2- to 700-fold speedup over naive. KNS3 yields a 2- to 4500-fold speedup. Notice that KNS2 cannot beat KNS1 for these data sets, because KNS2 is designed to speedup k-NN search on data sets with unbalanced output classes. Since all the synthetic data sets have an equal number of data from positive and negative classes, KNS2 has no advantage.

It is notable that for some high dimensional data sets, KNS1 does not produce an acceleration over naive. KNS2 and KNS3 do, however, and in some cases they are hundreds of times faster than KNS1.

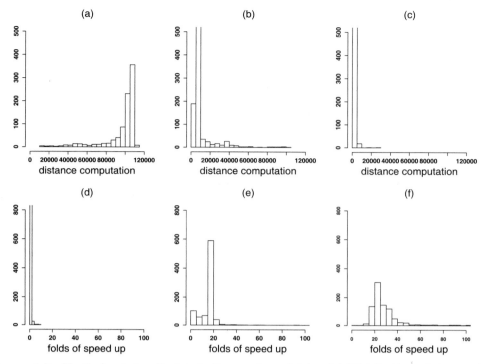

Figure 4.7 Vertical axis in all plots is the number of data. (a) Distribution of times taken for queries of KNS1. (b) Distribution of times taken for queries of KNS2. (c) Distribution of times taken for queries of KNS3. (d) Distribution of speedup for queries achieved for KNS1. (e) Distribution of speedup for queries achieved for KNS2. (f) Distribution of speedup for queries achieved for KNS3.

4.7 Comments and related work

Why k-NN ?

k-NN is an old classification method, often not achieving the highest possible accuracies when compared to more complex methods. Why study it? There are many reasons. k-NN is a useful sanity check or baseline against which to check more sophisticated algorithms *provided* k-NN is tractable. It is often the first line of attack in a new complex problem, due to its simplicity and flexibility. The user need only provide a sensible distance metric. The method is easy to interpret once this distance metric is understood. We have already mentioned its compelling theoretical properties, which explains its surprisingly good performance in practice in many cases. For these reasons and others, k-NN is still popular in some fields that need classification, e.g., computer vision and QSAR analysis of high throughput screening data, e.g., trps:nove. Finally, we believe that the same insights that accelerate k-NN will apply to more modern algorithms. From a theoretical viewpoint, many classification algorithms can be viewed simply as the nearest-neighbor method with a certain broader notion of distance func-

Table 4.3 Number of distance computations and wall-clock time for naive k-NN classification (second column). Acceleration for normal use of KNS1 (in terms of number. distances and time). Accelerations of new methods KNS2 and KNS3 in other columns. Naive times are independent of k.

	k	NAIVE		KNS1		KNS2		KNS3	
		dists	Time	Dists	Time	Dists	Time	Dists	Time
			(sec)	Speedup	Speedup	Speedup	Speedup	Speedup	Speedup
ideal	9	9.0×10^7	30	96.7	56.5	112.9	78.5	4500	**486**
	101			23.0	10.2	24.7	14.7	4500	**432**
Diag2d(10%)	9	9.0×10^7	30	91	51.1	88.2	**52.4**	282	27.1
	101			22.3	8.7	21.3	9.3	167.9	**15.9**
Diag2d	9	9.0×10^9	3440	738	366	664	**372**	2593	287
	101			202.9	104	191	107.5	2062	**287**
Diag3d	9	9.0×10^9	4060	361	**184.5**	296	**184.5**	1049	176.5
	101			111	56.4	95.6	48.9	585	**78.1**
Diag10d	9	9.0×10^9	6080	7.1	**5.3**	7.3	5.2	12.7	2.2
	101			3.3	**2.5**	3.1	1.9	6.1	0.7
Noise2d	9	9.0×10^7	40	91.8	20.1	79.6	30.1	142	**42.7**
	101			22.3	4	16.7	4.5	94.7	**43.5**
ds1	9	6.4×10^8	4830	1.6	1.0	4.7	3.1	12.8	**5.8**
	101			1.0	0.7	1.6	1.1	10	**4.2**
ds1.10pca	9	6.4×10^8	420	11.8	11.0	33.6	**21.4**	71	20
	101			4.6	3.4	6.5	4.0	40	**6.1**
ds1.100pca	9	6.4×10^8	2190	1.7	1.8	7.6	7.4	23.7	**29.6**
	101			0.97	1.0	1.6	1.6	16.4	**6.8**
ds2	9	8.5×10^9	105,500	0.64	0.24	14.0	2.8	25.6	**3.0**
	101			0.61	0.24	2.4	0.83	28.7	**3.3**
ds2.100-	9	7.0×10^9	24,210	15.8	14.3	185.3	144	580	311
	101			10.9	14.3	23.0	19.4	612	**248**
J_Lee.100-	9	3.6×10^{10}	142,000	2.6	2.4	28.4	**27.2**	15.6	12.6
	101			2.2	1.9	12.6	11.6	37.4	**27.2**
Blanc_Mel	9	3.8×10^{10}	44,300	3.0	3.0	47.5	**60.8**	51.9	60.7
	101			2.9	3.1	7.1	33	203	**134.0**
Letter	9	3.6×10^8	290	8.5	7.1	42.9	**26.4**	94.2	25.5
	101			3.5	2.6	9.0	5.7	45.9	**9.4**
Ipums	9	4.4×10^9	9520	195	136	665	501	1003	**515**
	101			69.1	50.4	144.6	121	5264	**544**
Movie	9	1.4×10^9	3100	16.1	13.8	29.8	**24.8**	50.5	22.4
	101			9.1	7.7	10.5	8.1	33.3	**11.6**
Kddcup99	9	2.7×10^{11}	167,000	4.2	4.2	574	**702**	4	4.1
(10%)	101			4.2	4.2	187.7	**226.2**	3.9	3.9

tion; see, e.g., [2] for such a broad notion. RKHS kernel methods use another example of a broadened notion of distance function. More concretely, we have applied similar ideas to speed up nonparametric Bayes classifiers, in work to be submitted.

Applicability of other Proximity Query Work.

For the problem of find the k nearest data points (as opposed to our question of "perform k-NN or kernel classification") in high dimensions, the frequent failure of a traditional balltree to beat naive has led to some very ingenious and innovative alternatives, based on random projections, hashing discretized cubes, and acceptance of approximate answers. For example, [24] gives a hashing method that was demonstrated to provide speedups over a balltree-based approach in sixty-four dimensions by a factor of two to five depending on how much error in the approximate answer was permitted. Another approximate k-NN idea is in [1], one of the first k-NN approaches to use a priority queue of nodes, in this case achieving a three-fold speedup with an approximation to the true k-NN . In [36], we introduced a variant of balltree structures which allow nonbacktracking search to speed up approximate nearest neighbor, and we observed up to 700-fold accelerations over conventional balltree based k-NN . A similar idea has been proposed by [30]. However, these approaches are based on the notion that any points falling within a factor of $(1+\epsilon)$ times the true nearest-neighbor distance are acceptable substitutes for the true nearest neighbor. Noting in particular that distances in high-dimensional spaces tend to occupy a decreasing range of continuous values [27], it remains unclear whether schemes based upon the absolute values of the distances rather than their *ranks* are relevant to the classification task. Our approach, because it need not find the k-NN to answer the relevant statistical question, finds an answer without approximation. The fact that our methods are easily modified to allow $(1 + \epsilon)$ approximation in the manner of [1] suggests an obvious avenue for future research.

No free lunch

For uniform high dimensional data no amount of trickery can save us. The explanation for the promising empirical results is that all the interdependencies in the data mean we are working in a space of much lower intrinsic dimensionality [38]. Note though, that in experiments not reported here, QSAR and vision k-NN classifiers give better performance on the original data than on PCA-projected low dimensional data, indicating that some of these dependencies are non-linear.

Summary

This chapter has introduced and evaluated two new algorithms for more effectively exploiting spatial data structures during k-NN classification. We have shown significant speedups on high-dimensional data sets without resorting to approximate answers or sampling. The result is that the k-NN method now scales to many large high-dimensional data sets that previously were not tractable for it, and are still not tractable for many popular methods such as support vector machines.

Notes

[1]Note that the exact shape context distance is different from exact EMD. It first solves the optimal assignment problem, and then given those correspondences, it estimates the thin-plate spline transformation that best aligns the two shapes. The scalar measure of dissimilarity is then the sum of the matching errors between the corresponding points, plus the magnitude of the aligning transform [2].

References

1. S. Arya, D. M. Mount, N. S. Netanyahu, R. Silverman, and A. Y. Wu. An optimal algorithm for approximate nearest neighbor searching fixed dimensions. *Journal of the ACM*, 45(6):891–923, 1998.

2. J. Baxter and P. Bartlett. The Canonical Distortion Measure in Feature Space and 1-NN Classification. In *Advances in Neural Information Processing Systems 10*. Morgan Kaufmann, 1998.

3. S. D. Bay. UCI KDD Archive [http://kdd.ics.uci.edu]. Irvine, CA: University of California, Dept of Information and Computer Science, 1999.

4. C. Cardie and N. Howe. Improving minority class prediction using case-specific feature weights. In *Proceedings of 14th International Conference on Machine Learning*, pages 57–65. Morgan Kaufmann, 1997.

5. C. L. Chang. Finding prototypes for nearest neighbor classifiers. *IEEE Trans. Computers*, C-23(11):1179–1184, November 1974.

6. P. Ciaccia, M. Patella, and P. Zezula. M-tree: An efficient access method for similarity search in metric spaces. In *Proceedings of the 23rd VLDB International Conference*, September 1997.

7. K. Clarkson. Nearest Neighbor Searching in Metric Spaces: Experimental Results for sb(S).   , 2002.

8. S. Cost and S. Salzberg. A Weighted Nearest Neighbour Algorithm for Learning with Symbolic Features. *Machine Learning*, 10:57–67, 1993.

9. T. M. Cover and P. E. Hart. Nearest neighbor pattern classification. *IEEE Trans. Information Theory*, IT-13,no.1:21–27, 1967.

10. Scott C. Deerwester, Susan T. Dumais, Thomas K. Landauer, George W. Furnas, and Richard A. Harshman. Indexing by latent semantic analysis. *Journal of the American Society of Information Science*, 41(6):391–407, 1990.

11. K. Deng and A. W. Moore. Multiresolution Instance-based Learning. In *Proceedings of the Twelfth International Joint Conference on Artificial Intelligence*, pages 1233–1239, San Francisco, 1995. Morgan Kaufmann.

12. L. Devroye and T. J. Wagner. *Nearest neighbor methods in discrimination*, volume 2. P.R. Krishnaiah and L. N. Kanal, eds., North-Holland, 1982.

13. A. Djouadi and E. Bouktache. A fast algorithm for the nearest-neighbor classifier. *IEEE Trans. Pattern Analysis and Machine Intelligence*, 19(3):277–282, March 1997.

14. N. R. Draper and H. Smith. *Applied Regression Analysis, 2nd ed.* John Wiley, New York, 1981.

15. R. O. Duda and P. E. Hart. *Pattern Classification and Scene Analysis*. John Wiley & Sons, 1973.

16. Christos Faloutsos, Ron Barber, Myron Flickner, Jim Hafner, Wayne Niblack, Dragutin Petkovic, and William Equitz. Efficient and effective querying by image content. *Journal of Intelligent Information Systems*, 3(3/4):231–262, 1994.

17. Christos Faloutsos and Douglas W. Oard. A survey of information retrieval and filtering methods. Technical Report CS-TR-3514, Carnegie Mellon University Computer Science Department, 1995.

18. T. Fawcett and F. J. Provost. Adaptive fraud detection. *Data Mining and Knowledge Discovery*, 1(3):291–316, 1997.

19. F. P. Fisher and E. A. Patrick. A preprocessing algorithm for nearest neighbor decision rules. In *Proc. Nat'l Electronic Conf.*, volume 26, pages 481–485, December 1970.

20. M. Flickner, H. Sawhney, W. Niblack, J. Ashley, Q. Huang, B. Dom, M. Gorkani, J. Hafner, D. Lee, D. Petkovic, D. Steele, and P. Yanker. Query by image and video content: the qbic system. *IEEE Computer*, 28:23–32, 1995.

21. J. H. Friedman, J. L. Bentley, and R. A. Finkel. An algorithm for finding best matches in logarithmic expected time. *ACM Transactions on Mathematical Software*, 3(3):209–226, September 1977.

22. K. Fukunaga and P.M. Narendra. A Branch and Bound Algorithm for Computing K-Nearest Neighbors. *IEEE Trans. Computers*, C-24(7):750–753, 1975.

23. G. W. Gates. The reduced nearest neighbor rule. *IEEE Trans. Information Theory*, IT-18(5):431–433, May 1972.

24. A. Gionis, P. Indyk, and R. Motwani. Similarity Search in High Dimensions via Hashing. In *Proceedings of the 25th VLDB Conference*, 1999.

25. A. Gray and A. W. Moore. N-Body Problems in Statistical Learning. In Todd K. Leen, Thomas G. Dietterich, and Volker Tresp, editors, *Advances in Neural Information Processing Systems 13*. MIT Press, 2001.

26. A. Guttman. R-trees: A dynamic index structure for spatial searching. In *Proceedings of the Third ACM SIGACT-SIGMOD Symposium on Principles of Database Systems*. Assn for Computing Machinery, April 1984.

27. J. M. Hammersley. The Distribution of Distances in a Hypersphere. *Annals of Mathematical Statistics*, 21:447–452, 1950.

28. P. E. Hart. The condensed nearest neighbor rule. *IEEE Trans. Information Theory*, IT-14(5):515–516, May 1968.

29. T. Hastie and R. Tibshirani. Discriminant adaptive nearest neighbor classification. *IEEE Trans. Pattern Analysis and Machine Intelligence*, 18(6):607–615, June 1996.

30. P. Indyk. On approximate nearest neighbors under l_∞ norm. 63(4), 2001.

31. CMU informedia digital video library project. The trec-2001 video trackorganized by nist shot boundary task, 2001.

32. V. Koivune and S. Kassam. Nearest neighbor filters for multivariate data. In *IEEE Workshop on Nonlinear Signal and Image Processing*, 1995.

33. P. Komarek and A. W. Moore. Fast robust logistic regression for large sparse datasets with binary outputs. In *Artificial Intelligence and Statistics*, 2003.

34. C. Kruegel and G. Vigna. Anomaly detection of web-based attacks. In *Proceedings of the 10th ACM conference on Computer and communications security table of contents*, pages 251–261, 2003.

35. E. Lee and S. Chae. Fast design of reduced-complexity nearest-neighbor classifiers using triangular inequality. *IEEE Trans. Pattern Analysis and Machine Intelligence*, 20(5):562–566, May 1998.

36. T. Liu, A. W. Moore, A. Gray, and K. Yang. An investigation of practical approximate nearest neighbor algorithms. In *Proceedings of Neural Information Processing Systems*, 2004.

37. T. Liu, K. Yang, and A. Moore. The ioc algorithm: Efficient many-class non-parametric classification for high-dimensional data. In *Proceedings of the conference on Knowledge Discovery in Databases (KDD)*, 2004.

38. S. Maneewongvatana and D. M. Mount. The analysis of a probabilistic approach to nearest neighbor searching. In *In Proceedings of WADS 2001*, 2001.

39. M. C. Monard and G. E. A. P. A. Batista. Learning with skewed class distribution. In J. M. Abe and J. I. da Silva Filho, editors, *Advances in Logic, Artificial Intelligence and Robotics*, pages 173–180, São Paulo, SP, 2002. IOS Press.

40. A. W. Moore. The Anchors Hierarchy: Using the Triangle Inequality to Survive High-Dimensional Data. In *Twelfth Conference on Uncertainty in Artificial Intelligence*. AAAI Press, 2000.

41. S. Omachi and H. Aso. A fast algorithm for a k-nn classifier based on branch and bound method and computational quantity estimation. In *In Systems and Computers in Japan, vol.31, no.6, pp.1-9*, 2000.

42. S. M. Omohundro. Efficient Algorithms with Neural Network Behaviour. *Journal of Complex Systems*, 1(2):273–347, 1987.

43. S. M. Omohundro. Bumptrees for Efficient Function, Constraint, and Classification Learning. In R. P. Lippmann, J. E. Moody, and D. S. Touretzky, editors, *Advances in Neural Information Processing Systems 3*. Morgan Kaufmann, 1991.

44. A. M. Palau and R. R. Snapp. The labeled cell classifier: A fast approximation to k nearest neighbors. In *Proceedings of the 14th International Conference on Pattern Recognition*, 1998.

45. E. P. D. Pednault, B. K. Rosen, and C. Apte. Handling imbalanced data sets in insurance risk modeling, 2000.

46. D. Pelleg and A. W. Moore. Accelerating Exact *k*-means Algorithms with Geometric Reasoning. In *Proceedings of the Fifth International Conference on Knowledge Discovery and Data Mining*. ACM, 1999.

47. A. Pentland, R. Picard, and S. Sclaroff. Photobook: Content-based manipulation of image databases, 1994.

48. F. P. Preparata and M. Shamos. *Computational Geometry*. Springer-Verlag, 1985.

49. Y. Qi, A. Hauptman, and T. Liu. Supervised classification for video shot segmentation. In *Proceedings of IEEE International Conference on Multimedia and Expo*, 2003.

50. G. L. Ritter, H. B. Woodruff, S. R. Lowry, and T. L. Isenhour. An algorithm for a selective nearest neighbor decision rule. *IEEE Trans. Information Theory*, IT-21(11):665–669, November 1975.

51. G. Salton and M. McGill. *Introduction to Modern Information Retrieval.* McGraw-Hill Book Company, New York, NY, 1983.

52. I. K. Sethi. A fast algorithm for recognizing nearest neighbors. *IEEE Trans. Systems, Man, and Cybernetics*, SMC-11(3):245–248, March 1981.

53. A.W.M. Smeulders, R. Jain, and editors. Image databases and multi-media search. In *Proceedings of the First International Workshop, IDB-MMS'96*, 1996.

54. S. Stolfo, W. Fan, W. Lee, A. Prodromidis, and P. Chan. Credit card fraud detection using meta-learning: Issues and initial results, 1997.

55. Y. Hamamoto S. Uchimura and S. Tomita. A bootstrap technique for nearest neighbor classifier design. *IEEE Trans. Pattern Analysis and Machine Intelligence*, 19(1):73–79, 1997.

56. J. K. Uhlmann. Satisfying general proximity/similarity queries with metric trees. *Information Processing Letters*, 40:175–179, 1991.

57. K. Woods, K. Bowyer, and W. P. Kegelmeyer Jr. Combination of multiple classifiers using local accuracy estimates. *IEEE Trans. Pattern Analysis and Machine Intelligence*, 19(4):405–410, 1997.

58. B. Zhang and S. Srihari. Fast k-nearest neighbor classification using cluster-based trees. *IEEE Trans. Pattern Analysis and Machine Intelligence*, 26(4):525–528, April 2004.

59. T. Zhang, R. Ramakrishnan, and M. Livny. BIRCH: An Efficient Data Clustering Method for Very Large Databases. In *Proceedings of the Fifteenth ACM SIGACT-SIGMOD-SIGART Symposium on Principles of Database Systems : PODS 1996*. ACM, 1996.

5 Approximate Nearest Neighbor Regression in Very High Dimensions

Sethu Vijayakumar, Aaron D'Souza, and Stefan Schaal

Fast and approximate nearest-neighbor search methods have recently become popular for scaling nonparameteric regression to more complex and high-dimensional applications. As an alternative to fast nearest neighbor search, training data can also be incorporated online into appropriate sufficient statistics and adaptive data structures, such that approximate nearest-neighbor predictions can be accelerated by orders of magnitude by means of exploiting the compact representations of these sufficient statistics. This chapter describes such an approach for locally weighted regression with locally linear models. Initially, we focus on *local* dimensionality reduction techniques in order to scale locally weighted learning to domains with very high dimensional input data. The key issue here revolves around obtaining a statistically robust and computationally inexpensive estimation of local linear models in such large spaces, despite potential irrelevant and redundant inputs. We develop a local version of partial least squares regression that fulfills all of these requirements, and embed it in an incremental nonlinear regression algorithm that can be shown to work efficiently in a number of complex applications. In the second part of the chapter, we introduce a novel Bayesian formulation of partial least squares regression that converts our nonparametric regression approach to a probabilistic formulation. Some of the heuristic components inherent in partial least squares can be eliminated with this new algorithm by means of efficient Bayesian regularization techniques. Evaluations are provided for all algorithms on various synthetic data sets and real-time learning examples with anthropomorphic robots and complex simulations.

5.1 Introduction

Despite the recent progress in statistical learning, nonlinear function approximation with high-dimensional input data remains a nontrivial problem, especially in incremental and real-time formulations. There is, however, an increasing number of problem domains where both these properties are important. Examples include the online modeling of dynamic processes observed by visual surveillance, user modeling for advanced computer interfaces and game playing, and the learning of value functions, policies, and models for learning control, particularly in the context of high-dimensional movement systems like humans or humanoid robots. An ideal algorithm for such tasks needs to avoid potential numerical problems from redundancy in the input data, eliminate irrelevant input dimensions, keep the computational complexity of learning updates low while remaining data efficient, allow for online incremental learning, and, of course, achieve accurate function approximation and adequate generalization.

When looking for a learning framework to address these goals, one can identify two broad classes of function approximation methods: (i) methods which fit nonlinear functions *globally*, typically by input space expansions with predefined or parameterized basis functions and subsequent linear combinations of the expanded inputs, and (ii) methods which fit nonlinear functions *locally*, usually by using spatially localized simple (e.g., low-order polynomial) models in the original input space and automatically adjusting the complexity (e.g., number of local models and their locality) to accurately account for the nonlinearities and distributions of the target function. Interestingly, the current trends in statistical learning have concentrated on methods that fall primarily in the first class of global nonlinear function approximators, for example, Gaussian process regression(GPR)[48], support vector machine regression(SVMR)[40] and variational Bayes for mixture models[1](VBM)[13]. In spite of the solid theoretical foundations that these approaches possess in terms of generalization and convergence, they are not necessarily the most suitable for online learning in high-dimensional spaces. First, they require an a priori determination of the right modeling biases. For instance, in the case of GPR and SVMR, these biases involve selecting the right function space in terms of the choice of basis or kernel functions[44], and in VBM the biases are concerned with the the right number of latent variables and proper initialization.[2] Second, all these recent function approximator methods were developed primarily for batch data analysis and are not easily or efficiently adjusted for incrementally arriving data. For instance, in SVMR, adding a new data point can drastically change the outcome of the global optimization problem in terms of which data points actually become support vectors, such that all (or a carefully selected subset) of data has to be kept in memory for reevaluation. Thus, adding a new data point in SVMR is computationally rather expensive, a property that is also shared by GPR. VBM suffers from similar problems due to the need for storing and reevaluating data when adding new mixture components[43]. In general, it seems that most suggested Bayesian learning algorithms are computationally too expensive for real-time learning because they tend to represent the complete joint distribution of the data, albeit as a conditionally independent factored representation. As a last point, incremental approximation of functions with global methods is prone to lead to negative interference when input distributions change[35]; such changes are, however, a typical scenario in many online learning tasks.

In contrast to the global learning methods described above, function approximation with spatially localized models, that is, nearest-neighbor(NN) techniques, are rather well suited for incremental and real-time learning[2]. Such nonparametric methods are very useful when there is limited knowledge about the model complexity such that the model resources need to be increased in a purely incremental and data-driven fashion, as demonstrated in previous work[35]. However, since these techniques allocate resources to cover the input space in a localized fashion, in general, with an increasing number of input dimensions, they encounter an exponential explosion in the number of local models required for accurate approximation, often referred to as the "curse of dimensionality"[31]. Hence, at the outset, high-dimensional function approximation seems to be computationally infeasible for local nonparametric learning.

Nonparametric learning in high-dimensional spaces with *global* methods, however, has been employed successfully by using techniques of projection regression (PR). PR copes with high-dimensional inputs by decomposing multivariate regressions into a superposition of single variate regressions along a few selected projections in input space. The major difficulty of PR lies in the selection of efficient projections, that is, how to achieve the best fitting result with as few univariate regressions as possible. Among the best known PR algorithms are projection pursuit regression [11], and its generalization in the form of generalized additive models[16]. Sigmoidal neural networks can equally be conceived of as a method of projection regression, in particular when new projections are added sequentially, e.g., as in cascade correlation[9].

In this chapter we suggest a method of extending the beneficial properties of *local nonparametric learning* to high-dimensional function approximation problems. The prerequisite of our approach is that the high-dimensional learning problems we address have locally low dimensional distributions, an assumption that holds for a large class of real-world data (see below). If distributions are locally low-dimensional, the allocation of local models can be restricted to these thin distributions, and only a tiny part of the entire high dimensional space needs to be filled with local models. Thus, the curse of dimensionality of spatially localized model fitting can be avoided. Under these circumstances, an alternative method of projection regression can be derived, focusing on finding efficient *local* projections. Local projections can be used to accomplish local function approximation in the neighborhood of a given query point with traditional local nonparametric approaches, thus inheriting most of the statistical properties from the well established methods of locally weighted learning and nearest-neighbor regression[15, 2]. As this chapter will demonstrate, the resulting learning algorithm combines the fast, efficient, and incremental capabilities of the nonparametric techniques while alleviating the problems faced due to high-dimensional input domains through local projections.

In the following sections, we first motivate why many high dimensional learning problems have locally low-dimensional data distributions such that the prerequisites of our local learning system are justified. Second, we address the question of how to find good local projections by looking into various schemes for performing dimensionality reduction for regression. Third, we embed the most efficient and robust of these projection algorithms in an incremental nonlinear function approximator[45] capable of automatically adjusting the model complexity in a purely data-driven fashion. Finally, a new Bayesian approach is suggested to reformulate our algorithms in a probabilistic framework, thus removing several levels of open parameters in the techniques. In several evaluations, in both on synthetic and real world data, in the resulting incremental learning system demonstrates high accuracy for function fitting in very high-dimensional spaces, robustness toward irrelevant and redundant inputs, as well as low computational complexity. Comparisons will prove the competitiveness with other state-of-the-art learning systems.

5.2   Evidence for Low-Dimensional Distributions

The development of our learning system in the next sections relies on the assumption that high-dimensional data sets have locally low dimensional distributions, an assumption that requires some clarification. Across domains like vision, speech, motor control, climate patterns, human gene distributions, and a range of other physical and biological sciences, various researchers have reported evidence that corroborate the fact that the true intrinsic dimensionality of high-dimensional data is often very low[42, 27, 47]. We interpret these findings as evidence that the physical world has a significant amount of coherent structure that expresses itself in terms of a strong correlations between different variables that describe the state of the world at a particular moment in time. For instance, in computer vision it is quite obvious that neighboring pixels of an image of a natural scene have redundant information. Moreover, the probability distribution of natural scenes in general has been found to be highly structured such that it lends itself to a sparse encoding in terms of set of basis functions[24, 3]. Another example comes from our own research on human motor control. In spite of the fact that humans can accomplish movement tasks in almost arbitrary ways, thus possibly generating arbitrary distributions of the variables that describe their movements, behavioral research has discovered a tremendous amount of regularity within and across individuals[20, 32]. These regular-

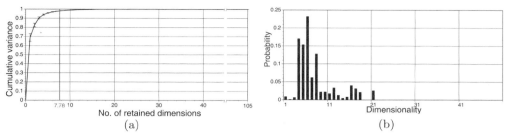

Figure 5.1 Dimensionality Analysis. (*a*) The cumulative variance accounted vs. the local dimensionality (averaged across all mixture models). (*b*) The distribution of the effective dimensionality across all mixture models.

ities lead to a locally low-dimensional data distribution, as illustrated in the example in figure5.1. In this analysis[6], we assessed the intrinsic dimensionality of data collected from full body movement of several human subjects, collected with a special full-body exoskeleton that recorded simultaneously 35 degrees of freedom(DOF) of the joint angular movement of the subjects at 100Hz sampling frequency. Subjects performed a variety of daily-life tasks (e.g., walking, object manipulation, reaching, etc.) until about a gigabyte of data was accumulated. Our analysis examined the local dimensionality of the joint distribution of positions, velocities, and accelerations of the collected data, that is, a 105-dimensional data set, as would be needed as inputs to learn an inverse dynamics model for motor control[20]. As an analysis tool, we employed a variational Bayesian mixture of factor analyzers that automatically estimated the required number of mixture components[13]. As demonstrated in figure 5.1(a), the local dimensionality was around five to eight dimensions, computed based on the average number of significant latent variables per mixture component. Figure 5.1(b) shows the distribution of the effective dimensionality across all mixture models.

In summary, the results from our analysis and other sources in the literature show that there is a large class of high-dimensional problems that can be treated locally in much lower dimensions if one can determine appropriate regions of locality and the local projections that model the corresponding low-dimensional distributions. As a caveat, however, it may happen that such low dimensional distributions are embedded in additional dimensions that are irrelevant to the problem at hand but have considerable variance. In the context of regression, it will thus be important to only model those local dimensions that carry information that is important for the regression and eliminate all other dimensions, that is, to perform local dimensionality reduction with regression in mind and not just based on input or joint input-output distributions, as discussed in the next section.

5.3   Local Dimensionality Reduction

Assuming that data are characterized by locally low dimensional distributions, efficient algorithms are needed to exploit this property. For this purpose, we will focus on locally weighted learning (LWL) methods[2] because they allow us to adapt a variety of linear dimensionality reduction techniques for the purpose of nonlinear function approximation (see section 5.4) and because they are easily modified for incremental learning. LWL-related methods have also found widespread application in mixture models [19, 50, 13] such that the results of this section can contribute to this field, too.

In pursuit of the question of what is the "right" method to perform local dimensionality reduction for regression, Schaal et al.[36] examined several candidate techniques theoretically and empirically. In particular, the authors focused on locally weighted versions of principal component regression (LWPCR), joint data principal component analysis (LWPCA), factor analysis (LWFA), and partial least squares (LWPLS). We will briefly revisit some main insights of this work before moving on to the development of our key learning algorithm.

5.3.1   The Locally Weighted Regression Model

The learning problems considered here assume the standard regression model:

$$y = f(\mathbf{x}) + \epsilon,$$

where $\mathbf{x}$ denotes the d-dimensional input vector, y the (for simplicity) scalar output, and ϵ a mean-zero random noise term. When only a local subset of data in the vicinity of a point $\mathbf{x}_c$ is considered and the locality is chosen appropriately, a low-order polynomial can be employed to model this local subset. Due to a favorable compromise between computational complexity and quality of function approximation[15], we choose linear models

$$y = \boldsymbol{\beta}^T \mathbf{x} + \epsilon.$$

A measure of locality for each data point, the weight w_i, is computed from a Gaussian kernel:

$$w_i = \exp(-0.5(\mathbf{x}_i - \mathbf{x}_c)^T \mathbf{D}(\mathbf{x}_i - \mathbf{x}_c)), \quad \mathbf{W} \equiv diag\{w_1, \ldots, w_M\}, \quad (5.1)$$

where $\mathbf{D}$ is a positive semidefinite distance metric which determines the size and shape of the neighborhood contributing to the local model[2]. The weights w_i will enter all following algorithms to assure spatial localization in input space. In particular, zero mean prerequisites of several algorithms are ensured by subtracting the weighted mean $\overline{\mathbf{x}}$ or $\overline{y}$ from the data, where

$$\overline{\mathbf{x}} = \sum_{i=1}^{M} w_i \mathbf{x}_i / \sum_{i=1}^{M} w_i, \text{ and } \overline{y} = \sum_{i=1}^{M} w_i y_i / \sum_{i=1}^{M} w_i, \qquad (5.2)$$

and M denotes the number of data points. For simplicity, and without loss of generality, we will thus assume in the derivations in the next sections that all input and output data have a weighted mean of zero with respect to a particular weighting kernel. The input data are summarized in the rows of the matrix $\mathbf{X} = [\mathbf{x}_1\ \mathbf{x}_2\ ...\mathbf{x}_M]^T$, the corresponding outputs are the coefficients of the vector $\mathbf{y}$, and the corresponding weights, determined from (5.1), are in the diagonal matrix $\mathbf{W}$. In some cases, we need the joint input and output data, denoted as $\mathbf{Z} = [\mathbf{z}_1\ \mathbf{z}_2...\mathbf{z}_M]^T = [\mathbf{X}\ \mathbf{y}]$.

5.3.2 Locally Weighted Factor Analysis

Factor analysis[8] is a density estimation technique that assumes that the observed data $\mathbf{z}$ were actually generated from a lower-dimensional process, characterized by *k-latent* or *hidden* variables $\mathbf{v}$ that are all independently distributed with mean zero and unit variance. The observed variables are generated from the latent variables through the transformation matrix $\mathbf{U}$ and additive mean zero independent noise $\boldsymbol{\epsilon}$ with diagonal covariance matrix $\boldsymbol{\Omega}$:

$$\mathbf{z} = \mathbf{U}\mathbf{v} + \boldsymbol{\epsilon}, \qquad (5.3)$$

where

$$\mathbf{z} = \begin{bmatrix} \mathbf{x} \\ y \end{bmatrix}, \boldsymbol{\epsilon} = \begin{bmatrix} \boldsymbol{\epsilon}_x \\ \epsilon_y \end{bmatrix}, E\{\boldsymbol{\epsilon}\boldsymbol{\epsilon}^T\} = \boldsymbol{\Omega}, \qquad (5.4)$$

and $E\{.\}$ denotes the expectation operator. If both $\mathbf{v}$ and $\boldsymbol{\epsilon}$ are normally distributed, the parameters $\boldsymbol{\Omega}$ and $\mathbf{U}$ can be obtained iteratively by the expectation-maximization (EM) algorithm[28].

Factor analysis can be adapted for linear regression problems by assuming that $\mathbf{z}$ was generated with

$$\mathbf{U} = [\mathbf{I}^d\ \boldsymbol{\beta}]^T, \qquad (5.5)$$
$$\mathbf{v} = \mathbf{x}, \qquad (5.6)$$

where $\boldsymbol{\beta}$ denotes the vector of regression coefficients of the linear model $y = \boldsymbol{\beta}^T \mathbf{x}$ and $\mathbf{I}^d$ the *d*-dimensional identity matrix. For the standard regression model, $\boldsymbol{\epsilon}_x$ would be zero, that is, we consider noise contamination in the output only; for numerical reasons, however, some remaining variance needs to be permitted and we prefer to leave it to the EM algorithm to find the optimal values of the covariance $\boldsymbol{\Omega}$. After calculating $\boldsymbol{\Omega}$ and $\mathbf{U}$ with EM in joint data space as formulated in (5.3), an estimate of $\boldsymbol{\beta}$ can be derived from the conditional probability $p(y|\mathbf{x})$. Let us denote $\mathbf{Z}=[\mathbf{z}_1 \ \mathbf{z}_2...\mathbf{z}_M]^T$ and $\mathbf{V}=[\mathbf{v}_1 \ \mathbf{v}_2...\mathbf{v}_M]^T$. The locally weighted version (LWFA) of $\boldsymbol{\beta}$ can be obtained together with an estimate of the factors $\mathbf{v}$ from the joint weighted covariance matrix $\boldsymbol{\Psi}$ of $\mathbf{z}$ and $\mathbf{v}$ as

$$E\left\{\begin{bmatrix} y \\ \mathbf{v} \end{bmatrix} |\mathbf{x}\right\} = \begin{bmatrix} \boldsymbol{\beta}^T \\ \mathbf{B} \end{bmatrix} \mathbf{x} = \Psi_{21}\Psi_{11}^{-1}\mathbf{x}, \tag{5.7}$$

where

$$\boldsymbol{\Psi} = [\mathbf{Z}^T \ \mathbf{V}^T]\mathbf{W} \begin{bmatrix} \mathbf{Z} \\ \mathbf{V} \end{bmatrix} / \sum_{i=1}^{M} w_i = \begin{bmatrix} \Omega + \mathbf{U}\mathbf{U}^T & \mathbf{U} \\ \mathbf{U}^T & \mathbf{I}^d \end{bmatrix} = \begin{bmatrix} \Psi_{11} & \Psi_{12} \\ \Psi_{21} & \Psi_{22} \end{bmatrix},$$

and $\mathbf{B}$ is a matrix of coefficients involved in estimating the factors $\mathbf{v}$. Note that unless the noise $\boldsymbol{\epsilon}_x$ is zero, the estimated $\boldsymbol{\beta}$ is different from the true $\boldsymbol{\beta}$ as it tries to optimally average out the noise in the data. Thus, factor analysis can also be conceived of as a tool for linear regression with noise-contaminated inputs.

5.3.3 Partial Least Squares

Partial least squares (PLS)[49, 10], a technique used extensively in chemometrics, recursively computes orthogonal projections of the input data and performs single variable regressions along these projections on the residuals of the previous iteration step. It is outlined in algorithm 5.1. The key ingredient in PLS is to use the direction of maximal correlation between the residual error and the input data as the projection direction at every regression step. Additionally, PLS regresses the inputs of the previous step against the projected inputs $\mathbf{s}$ in order to ensure the orthogonality of all the projections $\mathbf{u}$ (step 2c). Actually, this additional regression could be avoided by replacing $\mathbf{p}$ with $\mathbf{u}$ in step 2c, similar to techniques used in PCA[30]. However, using this regression step leads to better performance of the algorithm as PLS chooses the most effective projections if the input data have a spherical distribution: in the spherical case, with only one projection, PLS will find the direction of the gradient and achieve optimal regression results. The regression step in 2(c) in algorithm 5.1 chooses the reduced input data $\mathbf{X}_{res}$ such that the resulting data vectors have minimal norms and, hence, push the distribution of $\mathbf{X}_{res}$ to become more spherical. An additional consequence of 2(c) is that all the projections $\mathbf{s}_i$ become uncorrelated, that is, $\mathbf{s}_j^T\mathbf{s}_i = 0 \ \forall i \neq j$, a property which will be important in the derivations below.

5.3.4 Other Techniques

There are several other approaches to local dimensionality reduction, including principal component regression[22, 45], and principal component in

---

1. Initialize: $\mathbf{X}_{res} = \mathbf{X}$, $\mathbf{y}_{res} = \mathbf{y}$
2. **for** $i = 1$ **to** k **do**
   - (a) $\mathbf{u}_i = \mathbf{X}_{res}^T \mathbf{y}_{res}$.
   - (b) $\beta_i = \mathbf{s}_i^T \mathbf{y}_{res}/(\mathbf{s}_i^T \mathbf{s}_i)$ where $\mathbf{s}_i = \mathbf{X}_{res}\mathbf{u}_i$.
   - (c) $\mathbf{y}_{res} = \mathbf{y}_{res} - \mathbf{s}_i\beta_i$, $\mathbf{X}_{res} = \mathbf{X}_{res} - \mathbf{s}_i\mathbf{p}_i^T$
     where $\mathbf{p}_i = \mathbf{X}_{res}^T \mathbf{s}_i/(\mathbf{s}_i^T \mathbf{s}_i)$.

Algorithm 5.1 Outline of PLS regression algorithm

joint space(LWPCA_J). Both of these methods can be regarded as locally weighted factor analysis models with specific constraints on the structure of the data generating model, and restrictive assumptions about the generative probabilistic model. As shown in [36], the methods are always inferior to the full formulation of factor analysis from the previous section.

5.3.5 Which Approach to Choose?

Schaal et al.[36] demonstrated that both LWPLS and LWFA perform approximately the same under a large variety of evaluation sets. This result was originally slightly surprising, as LWPLS has more of a heuristic component than the theoretically principled factor analysis, a fact that leads to naturally favoring factor analysis models. However, there are two components that lift LWPLS above LWFA for our approximate nearest-neighbor approach. First, we wish to learn incrementally and remain computationally inexpensive in high dimensions. For this purpose, one would like to have a constructive approach to factor analysis, that is, an approach that adds latent variables as needed, a pruning approach, starting from the maximal latent variable dimensionality, would be unacceptably expensive. Empirically, [36] found that LWFA performs a lot worse if the latent variable space is underestimated, meaning that a constructive approach to LWFA would have transients of very bad performance until enough data were encountered to correctly estimate the latent space. For applications in robot control, for instance, such behavior would be inappropriate.

Second, besides redundant variables, we also expect a large number of irrelevant variables in our input data. This scenario, however, is disadvantageous for LWFA, as in the spirit of a density estimation technique, it needs to model the full dimensionality of the latent space, and not just those dimensions that matter for regression. In empirically evaluations (not shown here) similar to [36], we confirmed that LWFA's performance degrades strongly if it does not have enough latent variables to represent the irrelevant inputs. LWPLS, in contrast, uses the projection step based on input-output correlation to exclude irrelevant inputs, which exhibits very reliable and good performance even if there are many irrelevant and redundant inputs.

Table 5.1   Legend of indexes and symbols used for LWPR

Notation	Affectation
M	No. of training data points
N	Input dimensionality (i.e., dim. of $\mathbf{x}$)
$k = (1:K)$	No. of local models
$r = (1:R)$	No. of local projections used by PLS
$\{\mathbf{x}_i, y_i\}_{i=1}^{M}$	Training data
$\{\mathbf{z}_i\}_{i=1}^{M}$	Lower-dimensional projection of input data $\mathbf{x}_i$
$\{z_{i,r}\}_{r=1}^{R}$	Elements of projected input
$\mathbf{X}, \mathbf{Z}$	Batch representations of input and projected data
w	Weight or activation of data $(\mathbf{x}, y)$ with respect to local model or receptive field(RF) center $\mathbf{c}$
$\mathbf{W}$	Weight matrix: $\mathbf{W} \equiv diag\{w_1, \dots, w_N\}$
W^n	Cumulative weights seen by local model
$a_{var,r}^{n}$	Trace variable for incremental computation of rth dimension of variable var after seeing n data points

These considerations make LWPLS a superior choice for approximate nearest-neighbors in high dimensions. In the next section, we embed LW-PLS in an incremental nonlinear function approximator to demonstrate its abilities for nontrivial function-fitting problems.

5.4   Locally Weighted Projection Regression

For nonlinear function approximation, the core concept of our learning system - locally weighted projection regression (LWPR)- is to find approximations by means of piecewise linear models[2]. Learning involves automatically determining the appropriate *number* of local models K, the parameters $\boldsymbol{\beta}_k$ of the *hyperplane* in each model, and also the *region of validity*, called receptive field (RF), parameterized as a distance metric $\mathbf{D}_k$ in a Gaussian kernel:

$$w_k = exp(-\frac{1}{2}(\mathbf{x} - \mathbf{c}_k)^T \mathbf{D}_k (\mathbf{x} - \mathbf{c}_k)). \qquad (5.8)$$

Given a query point $\mathbf{x}$, every linear model calculates a prediction $\hat{y}_k(\mathbf{x})$. The total output of the learning system is the normalized weighted mean of all K linear models:

$$\hat{y} = \sum_{k=1}^{K} w_k \hat{y}_k / \sum_{k=1}^{K} w_k, \qquad (5.9)$$

also illustrated in Figure 5.2. The centers $\mathbf{c}_k$ of the RFs remain fixed in order to minimize negative interference during incremental learning that could occur due to changing input distributions[35]. Local models are created on an "as-needed" basis as described in sub-section 5.4.2. Table 5.1 provides a

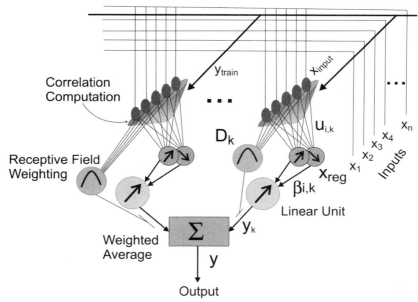

Figure 5.2 Information processing unit of LWPR.

reference list of indices and symbols that are used consistently across the description of the LWPR algorithm.

5.4.1 Learning with Locally Weighted Projection Regression

Despite its appealing simplicity, the "piecewise linear modeling" approach becomes numerically brittle and computationally too expensive in high-dimensional input spaces when using ordinary linear regression to determine the local model parameters[35]. Given the empirical observation (cf. section 5.2) that high-dimensional data often lie on locally low-dimensional distributions, and given the algorithmic results in section 5.3, we will thus use local projection regression, that is, LWPLS, within each local model to fit the hyperplane. As a significant computational advantage, we expect that far fewer projections than the actual number of input dimensions are needed for accurate learning. The next sections will describe the necessary modifications of LWPLS for this implementation, embed the local regression into the LWL framework, explain a method of automatic distance metric adaptation, and finish with a complete nonlinear learning scheme, called locally weighted projection regression (LWPR).

Incremental Computation of Projections and Local Regression

For incremental learning, that is, a scheme that does not explicitly store any training data, the sufficient statistics of the learning algorithm need to be accumulated in appropriate variables. Algorithm 5.2[46] provides suitable incremental update rules. The variables $a_{zz,r}$, $a_{zres,r}$, and $\mathbf{a}_{xz,r}$ are sufficient

1. Initialization: (# data points seen $n = 0$)
$\mathbf{x}_0^0 = \mathbf{0}$, $\beta_0^0 = 0$, $W^0 = 0$, $\mathbf{u}_r^0 = \mathbf{0}$; $r = 1 : R$

2. Incorporating new data: Given training point $(\mathbf{x}, y)$

2a. Compute activation and update the means

      1. $w = exp(-\frac{1}{2}(\mathbf{x} - \mathbf{c})^T \mathbf{D}(\mathbf{x} - \mathbf{c}))$; $W^{n+1} = \lambda W^n + w$

      2. $\mathbf{x}_0^{n+1} = (\lambda W^n \mathbf{x}_0^n + w\mathbf{x})/W^{n+1}$; $\beta_0^{n+1} = (\lambda W^n \beta_0^n + wy)/W^{n+1}$

2b. Compute the current prediction error

    $\mathbf{x}_{res,1} = \mathbf{x} - \mathbf{x}_0^{n+1}$, $\hat{y} = \beta_0^{n+1}$

    Repeat for $r = 1 : R$ (# projections)

      1. $z_r = \mathbf{x}_{res,r}^T \mathbf{u}_r^n / \sqrt{\mathbf{u}_r^{n\,T} \mathbf{u}_r^n}$

      2. $\hat{y} \leftarrow \hat{y} + \beta_r^n z_r$

      3. $\mathbf{x}_{res,r+1} = \mathbf{x}_{res,r} - z_r \mathbf{p}_r^n$

      4. $MSE_r^{n+1} = \lambda MSE_r^n + w\,(y - \hat{y})^2$

    $e_{cv} = y - \hat{y}$

2c. Update the local model

$res_1 = y - \beta_0^{n+1}$

For $r = 1 : R$ (# projections)

    2c.1 *Update the local regression and compute residuals*

      1. $a_{zz,r}^{n+1} = \lambda\, a_{zz,r}^n + w\, z_r^2$; $a_{zres,r}^{n+1} = \lambda\, a_{zres,r}^n + w\, z_r\, res_r$

      2. $\beta_r^{n+1} = a_{zres,r}^{n+1}/a_{zz,r}^{n+1}$

      3. $res_{r+1} = res_r - z_r \beta_r^{n+1}$

      4. $\mathbf{a}_{xz,r}^{n+1} = \lambda\, \mathbf{a}_{xz,r}^n + w\mathbf{x}_{res,r} z_r$

    2c.2 *Update the projection directions*

      1. $\mathbf{u}_r^{n+1} = \lambda\, \mathbf{u}_r^n + w\mathbf{x}_{res,r}\, res_r$

      2. $\mathbf{p}_r^{n+1} = \mathbf{a}_{xz,r}^{n+1}/a_{zz,r}^{n+1}$

$e = res_{r+1}$

3. Predicting with novel data ($\mathbf{x}_q$):

Initialize: $y_q = \beta_0$, $\mathbf{x}_q = \mathbf{x}_q - \mathbf{x}_0$

Repeat for $r = 1 : R$

    1. $y_q \leftarrow y_q + \beta_r s_r$ where $s_r = \mathbf{u}_r^T \mathbf{x}_q$

    2. $\mathbf{x}_q \leftarrow \mathbf{x}_q - s_r \mathbf{p}_r^n$

Note: The subscript k referring to the kth local model is omitted throughout this table since we are referring to updates in one local model or RF.

Algorithm 5.2   Incremental locally weighted PLS for one RF centered at $\mathbf{c}$

statistics that enable us to perform the univariate regressions in step 2c.1.2 and step 2c.2.2, similar to recursive least squares, that is, a fast Newton-like incremental learning technique. $\lambda \in [0, 1]$ denotes a forgetting factor that allows exponential forgetting of older data in the sufficient statistics. Forgetting is necessary in incremental learning since a change of some learning parameters will affect a change in the sufficient statistics; such forgetting factors are a standard technique in recursive system identification [21]. It can be shown that the prediction error of step 2b corresponds to the leave-one-out cross-validation error of the current point *after* the regression parameters were updated with the data point; hence, it is denoted by e_{cv}.

In algorithm 5.2, for $R = N$, that is, the same number of projections as the input dimensionality, the entire input space would be spanned by the projections $\mathbf{u}_r$ and the regression results would be identical to that of ordinary linear regression[49]. However, once again, we would like to emphasize the important properties of the local projection scheme. First, if all the input variables are statistically independent and have equal variance,[3] PLS will find the optimal projection direction $\mathbf{u}_r$ in roughly a single sweep through the training data; the optimal projection direction corresponds to the gradient of the local linearization parameters of the function to be approximated. Second, choosing the projection direction from correlating the input and the output data in step 2b.1 automatically excludes irrelevant input dimensions. And third, there is no danger of numerical problems due to redundant input dimensions as the univariate regressions can easily be prevented from becoming singular.

Given that we will adjust the distance metric to optimize the local model approximation (see below), it is also possible to perform LWPR with only *one* projection direction (denoted as LWPR-1). In this case, this distance metric will have to be adjusted to find the optimal receptive field size for a local linearization as well as to make the locally weighted input distribution spherical. An appropriate learning rule of the distance metric can accomplish this adjustment, as explained below. It should be noted that LWPR-1 is obtained from algorithm5.2 by setting $R = 1$.

Adjusting the Shape and Size of the Receptive Field

The distance metric $\mathbf{D}$ and hence the locality of the receptive fields can be learned for each local model individually by stochastic gradient descent in a penalized leave-one-out cross-validation cost function[35]:

$$J = \frac{1}{\sum_{i=1}^{M} w_i} \sum_{i=1}^{M} w_i (y_i - \hat{y}_{i,-i})^2 + \frac{\gamma}{N} \sum_{i,j=1}^{N} D_{ij}^2, \qquad (5.10)$$

where M denotes the number of data points in the training set. The first term of the cost function is the mean leave-one-out cross-validation error of the local model (indicated by the subscript $i, -i$) which ensures proper

Table 5.2   Derivatives for distance metric update

For the current data point $\mathbf{x}$, its PLS projection $\mathbf{z}$ and activation w:
(Refer to table 5.2 for some of the variables)

$$\frac{\partial J}{\partial \mathbf{M}} \approx \left(\sum_{i=1}^{M} \frac{\partial J_1}{\partial w}\right)\frac{\partial w}{\partial \mathbf{M}} + \frac{w}{W^{n+1}}\frac{\partial J_2}{\partial \mathbf{M}} \quad \text{[stochastic update of (5.12)]}$$

$$\frac{\partial w}{\partial M_{kl}} = -\frac{1}{2}w(\mathbf{x}-\mathbf{c})^T\frac{\partial \mathbf{D}}{\partial M_{kl}}(\mathbf{x}-\mathbf{c}); \quad \frac{\partial J_2}{\partial M_{kl}} = 2\frac{\gamma}{N}\sum_{i,j=1}^{N}D_{ij}\frac{\partial D_{ij}}{\partial M_{kl}}$$

$$\frac{\partial D_{ij}}{\partial M_{kl}} = M_{kj}\delta_{il} + M_{ki}\delta_{jl}; \quad \text{where } \delta_{ij}=1 \text{ if } i=j, \text{ else } \delta_{ij}=0.$$

$$\sum_{i=1}^{M}\frac{\partial J_1}{\partial w} = \frac{e_{cv}^2}{W^{n+1}} - \frac{2\,e}{W^{n+1}}\mathbf{q}^T\mathbf{a}_H^n - \frac{2}{W^{n+1}}\mathbf{q}^{2T}\mathbf{a}_G^n - \frac{a_E^{n+1}}{(W^{n+1})^2}$$

$$\text{where } \mathbf{z}=\begin{bmatrix} z_1 \\ \vdots \\ z_R \end{bmatrix} \quad \mathbf{z}^2=\begin{bmatrix} z_1^2 \\ \vdots \\ z_R^2 \end{bmatrix} \quad \mathbf{q}=\begin{bmatrix} z_1/a_{zz,1}^{n+1} \\ \vdots \\ z_R/a_{zz,R}^{n+1} \end{bmatrix}$$

$$\mathbf{a}_H^{n+1} = \lambda\mathbf{a}_H^n + \frac{w\,e_{cv}\mathbf{z}}{(1-h)}; \quad \mathbf{a}_G^{n+1} = \lambda\mathbf{a}_G^n + \frac{w^2e_{cv}^2\mathbf{z}^2}{(1-h)}$$

$$\text{where } h = w\mathbf{z}^T\mathbf{q}$$

$$a_E^{n+1} = \lambda a_E^n + we_{cv}^2$$

---

generalization[35]. The second term, the penalty term, makes sure that receptive fields cannot shrink indefinitely in case of large amounts of training data; such shrinkage would be statistically correct for asymptotically unbiased function approximation, but it would require maintaining an ever increasing number of local models in the learning system, which is computationally too expensive. The tradeoff parameter γ can be determined either empirically or from assessments of the maximal local curvature of the function to be approximated[34]; in general, results are not very sensitive to this parameter[35] as it primarily affects resource efficiency.

It should be noted that due to the *local* cost function in (5.10), learning becomes entirely localized, too, that is, no parameters from other local models are needed for updates as, for instance, in competitive learning with mixture models. Moreover, minimizing (5.10) can be accomplished in an incremental way *without* keeping data in memory[35]. This property is due to a reformulation of the leave-one-out cross-validation error as the PRESS residual error[4]. As detailed in[35] the bias-variance tradeoff is thus resolved for every local model *individually* such that an increasing number of local models will not lead to overfitting; indeed, it leads to better approximation results due to model averaging [e.g. (5.9)]in the sense of committee machines[25].

In ordinary weighted linear regression, expanding (5.10) with the PRESS residual error results in

$$J = \frac{1}{\sum_{i=1}^{M} w_i} \sum_{i=1}^{M} \frac{w_i(y_i - \hat{y}_i)^2}{(1 - w_i \mathbf{x}_i^T \mathbf{P} \mathbf{x}_i)^2} + \frac{\gamma}{N} \sum_{i,j=1}^{N} D_{ij}^2, \tag{5.11}$$

where $\mathbf{P}$ corresponds to the inverted weighted covariance matrix of the input data. Interestingly, the PRESS residuals of (5.11) can be *exactly* formulated in terms of the PLS projected inputs $\mathbf{z}_i \equiv [z_{i,1} \ldots z_{i,R}]^T$ (algorithm 5.2) as

$$
\begin{aligned}
J &= \frac{1}{\sum_{i=1}^{M} w_i} \sum_{i=1}^{M} \frac{w_i(y_i - \hat{y}_i)^2}{(1 - w_i \mathbf{z}_i^T \mathbf{P}_z \mathbf{z}_i)^2} + \frac{\gamma}{N} \sum_{i,j=1}^{N} D_{ij}^2 \\
&\equiv \frac{1}{\sum_{i=1}^{M} w_i} \sum_{i=1}^{M} J_1 + \frac{\gamma}{N} J_2,
\end{aligned}
\tag{5.12}
$$

where $\mathbf{P}_z$ corresponds to the covariance matrix computed from the projected inputs $\mathbf{z}_i$ for $R = N$, that is, the $\mathbf{z}_i$'s span the same full-rank input space[4] as the $\mathbf{x}_i$'s in (5.11). It can also been deduced that $\mathbf{P}_z$ is diagonal, which greatly contributes to the computational efficiency of our update rules. Based on this cost function, the distance metric in LWPR is learned by gradient descent:

$$\mathbf{M}^{n+1} = \mathbf{M}^n - \alpha \frac{\partial J}{\partial \mathbf{M}} \text{ where } \mathbf{D} = \mathbf{M}^T \mathbf{M} \text{ (for positive definiteness)},$$

where $\mathbf{M}$ is an upper triangular matrix resulting from a Cholesky decomposition of $\mathbf{D}$. Following[35], a stochastic approximation of the gradient $\frac{\partial J}{\partial \mathbf{M}}$ of (5.12) can be derived by keeping track of several sufficient statistics as shown in table 5.2. It should be noted that in these update laws, we treated the PLS projection direction and hence $\mathbf{z}$ as if it were independent of the distance metric, such that chain rules need not be taken throughout the entire PLS recursions. Empirically, this simplification did not seem to have any negative impact and reduced the update rules significantly.

5.4.2   The Complete LWPR Algorithm

All update rules can be combined in an incremental learning scheme that automatically allocates new locally linear models as needed. The concept of the final learning network is illustrated in figure 5.2 and an outline of the final LWPR algorithm is shown in algorithm 5.3.

In this pseudocode, w_{gen} is a threshold that determines when to create a new receptive field, as discussed in [35], w_{gen} is a computational efficiency parameter and not a complexity parameter as in mixture models. The closer w_{gen} is set to 1, the more overlap local models will have, which is beneficial in the spirit of committee machines (cf. [35, 25]) but more costly to compute; in

---

```
1:   Initialize the LWPR with no receptive field (RF)
2:   for every new training sample (x,y) do
3:       for k=1 to K(# of receptive fields) do
4:           calculate the activation from (5.8)
5:           update projections and regression (algorithm 5.2) and distance metric (table 5.2),
6:           check if number of projections needs to be increased (cf. subsection 5.4.2).
7:       end for
8:       if no RF was activated by more than w_{gen} then
9:           create a new RF with R = 2, c = x, D = D_{def}.
10:      end if
11:  end for
```

Algorithm 5.3   Pseudocode of the complete LWPR algorithm

general, the more overlap is permitted, the better the function fitting results, without any danger that the increase in overlap can lead to overfitting. $\mathbf{D}_{def}$ is the initial (usually diagonal) distance metric in (5.8). The initial number of projections is set to $R = 2$. The algorithm has a simple mechanism of determining whether R should be increased by recursively keeping track of the mean-squared error (MSE) as a function of the number of projections included in a local model, that is, step 2b.4 in algorithm 5.2. If the MSE at the next projection does not decrease more than a certain percentage of the previous MSE, that is, $\frac{MSE_{r+1}}{MSE_r} > \phi$, where $\phi \in [0, 1]$, the algorithm will stop adding new projections locally. As MSE_r can be interpreted as an approximation of the leave-one-out cross-validation error of each projection, this threshold criterion avoids problems due to overfitting. Due to the need to compare the MSE of two successive projections, LWPR needs to be initialized with at least two projection dimensions.

Speedup for Learning from Trajectories

If in incremental learning, training data are generated from trajectories, that is, data are temporally correlated, it is possible to accelerate lookup and training times by taking advantage of the the fact that two consecutively arriving training points are close neighbors in input space. For such cases, we added a special data structure to LWPR that allows restricting updates and lookups only to a small fraction of local models instead of exhaustively sweeping through all of them. For this purpose, each local model maintains a list of all other local models that overlap sufficiently with it. Sufficient overlap between two models i and j can be determined from the centers and distance metrics. The point $\mathbf{x}$ in input space that is the closest to both centers in the sense of a Mahalanobis distance is $\mathbf{x} = (\mathbf{D}_i + \mathbf{D}_j)^{-1}(\mathbf{D}_i \mathbf{c}_i + \mathbf{D}_j \mathbf{c}_j)$. Inserting this point into (5.8) of one of the local models gives the activation w due to this point. The two local models are listed as sufficiently overlapping if $w \geq w_{gen}$ (cf. algorithm 5.3). For diagonal distance metrics, the overlap computation is linear in the number of inputs. Whenever a new data point is added to LWPR, one neighborhood relation is checked for the maximally activated RF. An appropriate counter for each local model ensures that overlap with all other local models is checked exhaustively. Given this "nearest-neighbor" data structure, lookup and learning can be confined to only a few RFs. For every lookup (update), the identification number of the maximally activated RF is returned. The next lookup (update) will only consider the neighbors of this RF. It can be shown that this method performs as well as an exhaustive lookup (update) strategy that excludes RFs that are activated below a certain threshold w_{cutoff}.

Pruning of Local Models

As in the RFWR algorithm[35], it is possible to prune local models depending upon the level of overlap between two local models and the accumulated locally weighted mean-squared error; the pruning strategy is virtually identical as in [[35], section 3.14]. However, due to the numerical robustness of PLS, we have noticed that the need for pruning or merging is almost nonexistent in the LWPR implementation, such that we do not expand on this possible feature of the algorithm.

Computational Complexity

For a diagonal distance metric $\mathbf{D}$ and under the assumption that the number of projections R remains small and bounded, the computational complexity of one incremental update of all parameters of LWPR is linear in the number of input dimensions N. To the best of our knowledge, this property makes LWPR one of the computationally most efficient algorithms that have been suggested for high-dimensional function approximation. This low computational complexity sets LWPR apart from our earlier work on the RFWR algorithm[35], which was cubic in the number of input dimensions. We thus accomplished one of our main goals, that is, maintaining the appealing function approximation properties of RFWR while eliminating its problems in high-dimensional learning problems.

Confidence Intervals

Under the classical probabilistic interpretation of weighted least squares[12], that is, that each local model's conditional distribution is normal with heteroscedastic variances $p(y|\mathbf{x}; w_k) \sim N(\mathbf{z}_k{}^T \beta_k, s_k{}^2/w_k)$, it is possible to derive the predictive variances $\sigma^2_{pred,k}$ for a new query point $\mathbf{x}_q$ for each local model in LWPR.[5] The derivation of this measure is in analogy with ordinary linear regression[33, 23] and is also consistent with the Bayesian formulation of predictive variances [12]. For each individual local model,

$\sigma^2_{pred,k}$ can be estimated as (see table 5.2 and algorithm 5.2 for variable definitions):

$$\sigma^2_{pred,k} = s_k^2(1 + w_k \mathbf{z}_{q,k}^T \mathbf{q}_k), \tag{5.13}$$

where $\mathbf{z}_{q,k}$ is the projected query point $\mathbf{x}_q$ under the kth local model, and

$$s_k^2 \approx MSE_{k,R}^{n=M}/(M_k' - p_k'); \quad M_k' \equiv \sum_{i=1}^{M} w_{k,i} \approx W_k^{n=M},$$

$$p_k' \equiv \sum_{i=1}^{M} w_{k,i}^2 \mathbf{z}_{k,i}^T \mathbf{q}_{k,i} \approx a_{p_k'}^{n=M},$$

$$\text{with incremental update of } a_{p_k'}^{n+1} = \lambda a_{p_k'}^n + w_k^2 \mathbf{z}_k^T \mathbf{q}_k.$$

The definition of M' in terms of the sum of weights reflects the effective number of data points entering the computation of the local variance s_k^2[33] after an update of M training points has been performed. The definition of p', also referred to the as the *local* degrees of freedom, is analogous to the global degrees of freedom of linear smoothers [16, 33].

In order to obtain a predictive variance measure for the averaging formula (5.9), one could just compute the weighed average of the predictive variance in (5.13). While this approach is viable, it nevertheless ignores important information that can be obtained from variance of the individual predictions $\hat{y}_{q,k}$ and is thus potentially too optimistic. To remedy this issue, we postulate that from the view of combining individual $\hat{y}_{q,k}$, each contributing $y_{q,k}$ was generated from the process

$$y_{q,k} = y_q + \epsilon_1 + \epsilon_{2,k},$$

where we assume two separate noise processes: (i) one whose variance σ^2 is independent of the local model, that is, $\epsilon_1 \sim N(0, \sigma^2/w_k)$ (and accounts for the differences between the predictions of the local models), and (ii) another, which is the noise process $\epsilon_{2,k} \sim N(0, \sigma^2_{pred,k}/w_k)$ of the individual local models. It can be shown that (5.9) is a consistent way of combining prediction from multiple models under the noise model we just described and that the combined predictive variance over all models can be approximated as

$$\sigma^2_{pred} = \frac{\sum_k w_k \, \sigma^2}{(\sum_k w_k)^2} + \frac{\sum_k w_k \, \sigma^2_{pred,k}}{(\sum_k w_k)^2}. \tag{5.14}$$

The estimate of $\sigma_{pred,k}$ is given in (5.13). The global variance across models can be approximated as $\sigma^2 = \sum_k w_k(\hat{y}_q - \hat{y}_{k,q})^2/\sum_k w_k$. Inserting these values in (5.14), we obtain

$$\sigma^2_{pred} = \frac{1}{(\sum_k w_k)^2} \sum_{k=1}^{K} w_k[(\hat{y}_q - \hat{y}_{k,q})^2 + s_k^2(1 + w_k \mathbf{z}_k^T \mathbf{q}_k)]. \tag{5.15}$$

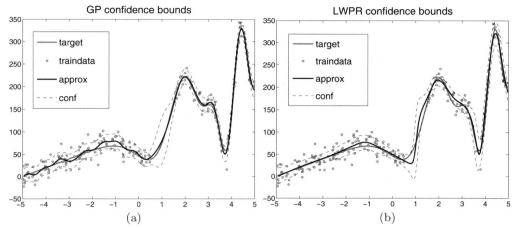

Figure 5.3 Function approximation with 200 noisy data points along with plots of confidence intervals for *(a)* Gaussian Process Regression and *(b)* LWPR algorithms. Note the absence of data in the range [0.5 1.5]

A one-standard-deviation-based confidence interval would thus be

$$I_c = \hat{y}_q \pm \sigma_{pred}. \tag{5.16}$$

The variance estimate in (5.14) is consistent with the intuitive requirement that when only one local model contributes to the prediction, the variance is entirely attributed to the predictive variance of that single model. Moreover, a query point that does not receive a high weight from any local model will have a large confidence interval due to the small squared sum-of-weight value in the denominator. Figure 5.3 illustrates comparisons of confidence interval plots on a toy problem with 200 noisy data points. Data from the range [0.5 1.5] was excluded from the training set. Both GPR and LWPR show qualitatively similar confidence interval bounds and fitting results.

5.5 Empirical Evaluation

The following sections provide an evaluation of our proposed LWPR learning algorithm over a range of artificial and real-world data sets. Whenever useful and feasible, comparisons to state-of-the-art alternative learning algorithms are provided, in particular SVMR and GPR. SVMR and GPR were chosen due to their generally acknowledged excellent performance in nonlinear regression on finite data sets. However, it should be noted, that both SVMR and GPR are batch learning systems, while LWPR was implemented as a fully incremental algorithm, as described in the previous sections.

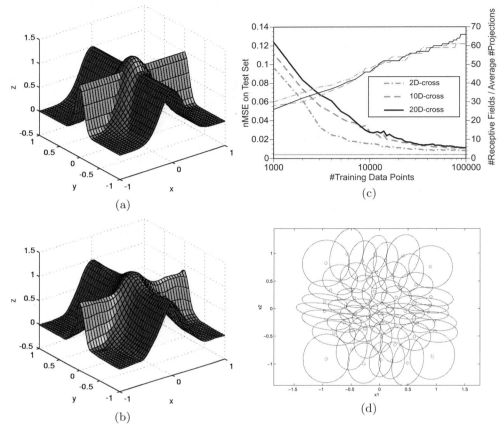

Figure 5.4 *(a)* Target and *(b)* learned nonlinear cross-function. *(c)* Learning curves for 2D, 10D and 20D data. *(d)* The automatically tuned distance metric.

5.5.1   Function Approximation with Redundant and Irrelevant Data

We implemented the LWPR algorithm as outlined in section 5.4. In each local model, the projection regressions are performed by (locally weighted) PLS, and the distance metric $\mathbf{D}$ is learned by stochastic incremental cross-validation; all learning methods employed second-order learning techniques, that is, incremental PLS uses recursive least squares, and gradient descent in the distance metric was accelerated as described in [35]. In all our evaluations, an initial (diagonal) distance metric of $\mathbf{D}_{def} = 30\mathbf{I}$ was chosen; the activation threshold for adding local models was $w_{gen} = 0.2$, and the threshold for adding new projections was $\phi = 0.9$ (cf. subsection 5.4.2). As a first test, we ran LWPR on 500 noisy training data drawn from the two-dimensional function (cross 2D) generated from

$$y = \max\{\exp(-10x_1^2), \exp(-50x_2^2, 1.25\exp(-5(x_1^2 + x_2^2)))\} + \mathrm{N}(0, 0.01),$$

as shown in figure 5.4(a). This function has a mixture of areas of rather high and rather low curvature and is an interesting test of the learning and generalization capabilities of a learning algorithm: learning models with low complexity find it hard to capture the nonlinearities accurately, while more complex models easily overfit, especially in linear regions. A second test added eight constant (i.e., redundant) dimensions to the inputs and rotated this new input space by a random 10D rotation matrix to create a 10D input space with high rank deficiency (cross 10D). A third test added another ten (irrelevant) input dimensions to the inputs of the second test, each having $N(0, 0.05^2)$ Gaussian noise, thus obtaining a data set with 20D input space (cross 20D). Typical learning curves with these data sets are illustrated in figure 5.4(c). In all three cases, LWPR reduced the normalized mean squared error (thick lines) on a noiseless test set (1681 points on a 41x41 grid in the unit-square in input space) rapidly in ten to twenty epochs of training to less than $nMSE = 0.05$, and it converged to the excellent function approximation result of $nMSE = 0.015$ after 100,000 data presentations or 200 epochs.[6] Figure 5.4(b) illustrates the reconstruction of the original function from the 20D test data, visualized in 3D - a highly accurate approximation. The rising lines in figure 5.4(c) show the number of local models that LWPR allocated during learning. The lines at the bottom of the graph indicate the average number of projections that the local models allocated: the average settled at a value of around two local projections, as is appropriate for this originally 2D data set. This set of tests demonstrate that LWPR is able to recover a low-dimensional nonlinear function embedded in high-dimensional space despite irrelevant and redundant dimensions, and that the data efficiency of the algorithm does not degrade in higher-dimensional input spaces. The computational complexity of the algorithm only increased linearly with the number of input dimensions, as explained in section 5.4.

The results of these evaluations can be directly compared with our earlier work on the RFWR algorithm[35], in particular figures 4 and 5 of this earlier paper. The learning speed and the number of allocated local models for LWPR is essentially the same as for RFWR in the 2D test set. Applying RFWR to the 10D and 20D data set of this paper, however, is problematic, as it requires a careful selection of initial ridge regression parameters to stabilize the highly rank-deficient full covariance matrix of the input data, and it is easy to create too much bias or too little numerical stabilization initially, which can trap the local distance metric adaptation in local minim. While the LWPR algorithm just computes about a factor ten times longer for the 20D experiment in comparison to the 2D experiment, REFER requires a 1000-fold increase of computation time, thus rendering this algorithm unsuitable for high-dimensional regression.

In order to compare LWPR's results to other popular regression methods, we evaluated the 2D, 10D, and 20D cross data sets with GPR and SVMR in addition to our LWPR method. It should be noted that neither SVMR nor GPR methods is an incremental method, although they can be considered

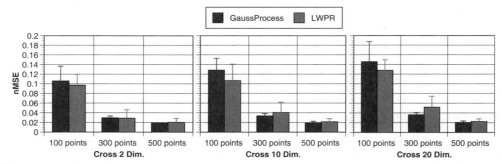

Figure 5.5 Normalized mean squared error comparisons between LWPR and Gaussian Processes for 2D, 10D and 20D Cross data sets

the state-of-the-art for batch regression under relatively small number of training data and reasonable input dimensionality. The computational complexity of these methods are prohibitively high for realtime applications. The GPR algorithm[14] used a generic covariance function and optimized over the hyperparameters. The SVMR was performed using a standard available package[29] and optimized for kernel choices.

Figure 5.5 compares the performance of LWPR and GPR for the above mentioned data sets using 100, 300, and 500 training data points.[7] As in figure 5.4, the test data set consisted of 1681 data points corresponding to the vertices of a $41x41$ grid over the unit square; the corresponding output values were the exact function values. The approximation error was measured as a normalized weighted mean squared error, $nMSE$, i.e, the weighted MSE on the test set normalized by the variance of the outputs of the test set; the weights were chosen as $1/\sigma^2_{pred,i}$ for each test point $\mathbf{x}_i$. Using such a weighted $nMSE$ was useful to allow the algorithms to incorporate their confidence in the prediction of a query point, which is especially useful for training data sets with few data points where query points often lie far away from any training data and require strong extrapolation to form a prediction. Multiple runs on ten randomly chosen training data sets were performed to accumulate the statistics.

As can be seen from figure 5.5, the performance differences between LWPR and GPR were largely statistically insignificant across training data sizes and input dimensionality. LWPR had a tendency to perform slightly better on the 100-point data sets, most likely due to its quickly decreasing confidence when significant extrapolation is required for a test point. For the 300-point data sets, GPR had a minor advantage and less variance in its predictions, while for 500-point data sets both algorithms achieved equivalent results. While GPRs used all the input dimensions for predicting the output (deduced from the final converged coefficients of the covariance matrix), LWPR stopped at an average of two local projections, reflecting that it exploited the low dimensional distribution of the data. Thus, this comparison illustrates that LWPR is a highly

Table 5.3 Comparison of $nMSE$ on Boston and Abalone data sets

	Gaussian Process	**Support Vectors**	**LWPR**
Boston	0.0806 ± 0.0195	0.1115 ± 0.09	0.0846 ± 0.0225
Abalone	0.4440 ± 0.0209	0.4830 ± 0.03	0.4056 ± 0.0131

competitive learning algorithm in terms of its generalization capabilities and accuracy of results, despite it being a truly incremental, computationally efficient and real-time implementable algorithm.

5.5.2 Comparisons on Benchmark Regression Data Sets

While LWPR is specifically geared toward real-time incremental learning in high dimensions, it can nevertheless also be employed for traditional batch data analysis. Here we compare its performance on two natural real-world benchmark datasets, using again GPR and SVMR as competitors.

The data sets we used were the Boston housing data and the Abalone data set, both available from the UCI Machine Learning Repository[18]. The Boston housing data, which had fourteen attributes, was split randomly (10 random splits) into disjoint sets of 404 training and 102 testing data. The Abalone data set, which had nine attributes, was downsampled to yield ten disjoint sets of 500 training data points and 1177 testing points.[8]

The GPR used hyperparameter estimation for the open parameters of the covariance matrix while for SVMR, the results were obtained by employing a Gaussian kernel of width 3.9 and 10 for the Boston and Abalone data sets, respectively, based on the optimized values suggested in [38]. Table 5.3 shows the comparisons of the $nMSE$ achieved by GPR, SVMR and LWPR on both these data sets. Once again, LWPR was highly competitive on these real-world data sets, consistently outperforming SVMR and achieving very similar $nMSE$ results as GPR.

5.5.3 Sensorimotor Learning in High Dimensional Space

In this section, we look at the application of LWPR to realtime learning in high-dimensional spaces in a data-rich environment - an example of which is learning for robot control. In such domains, LWPR is -to the best of our knowledge - one of the only viable and practical options for principled statistical learning. The goal of learning in this evaluation is to estimate the inverse dynamics model (also referred to as an *internal model*) of the robotic system such that it can be used as a component of a feedforward controller for executing fast accurate movements.

Before demonstrating the applicability of LWPR in realtime, a comparison with alternative learning methods will serve to demonstrate the complexity of the learning task. We collected 50,000 data points from various movement

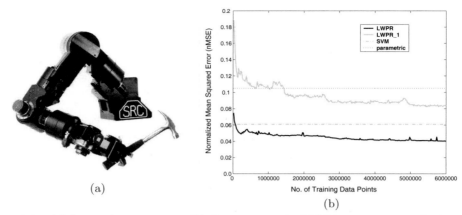

(a)

(b)

Figure 5.6 *(a)* Sarcos dextrous arm. *(b)* Comparison of $nMSE$ learning curves for learning the robot's inverse dynamics model for the shoulder DOF.

patterns from a 7DOF anthropomorphic robot arm [figure 5.6(a)], sampled at 50 Hz. The learning task was to fit the the inverse dynamics model of the robot, a mapping from seven joint positions, seven joint velocities, and seven joint accelerations to the corresponding seven joint torques (i.e, a 21D to 7D function). Ten percent of these data were excluded from training as a test set. The training data were approximated by four different methods: (i) parameter estimation based on an analytical rigid-body dynamics model[1], (ii) SVMR[29] (using a ten-fold downsampled training set for computational feasibility), (iii) LWPR-1, that is, LWPR that used only one single projection (cf. 5.4.1), and (iv) full LWPR. It should be noted that neither (i) nor (ii) is an incremental method. Using a parametric rigid-body dynamics model as suggested in (i) and just approximating its open parameters from data results in a global model of the inverse dynamics that is theoretically the most powerful method. However, given that our robot is actuated hydraulically and is rather lightweight and compliant, we know that the rigid body dynamics assumption is not fully justified. In all our evaluations, the inverse dynamics model of each DOF was learned separately, that is, all models had a univariate output and twenty-one inputs. LWPR employed a diagonal distance metric.

Figure 5.6 illustrates the function approximation results for the shoulder motor command graphed over the number of training iterations (one iteration corresponds to the update from one data point). Surprisingly, rigid-body parameter estimation achieved the worst results. LWPR-1 outperformed parameter estimation, but fell behind SVMR. Full LWPR performed the best. The results for all other DOFs were analogous and are not shown here. For the final result, LWPR employed 260 local models, using an average of 3.2 local projections. LWPR-1 did not perform better because we used a diagonal distance metric. The abilities of a diagonal distance metric to "carve out" a locally spherical distribution are too limited to accomplish

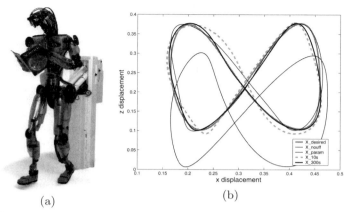

(a)   (b)

Figure 5.7   *(a)* The 30-DOF Sarcos humanoid robot. *(b)* Results of online learning of the inverse dynamics with LWPR on the humanoid robot.

better results; a full distance metric can remedy this problem, but would make the learning updates quadratic in the number of inputs. As in the previous sections, these results demonstrate that LWPR is a competitive function approximation technique that can be applied successfully in real world applications.

Online Learning for Humanoid Robots

We implemented LWPR on the realtime operating system (vxWorks) for two of our robotic setups, the 7DOF Sarcos dextrous arm mentioned above in figure 5.6(a), and the Sarcos humanoid robot in figure 5.7(a), a 30DOF system. Out of the four parallel processors of the system, one 366 MHz PowerPC processor was completely devoted to lookup and learning with LWPR.

For the dexterous arm, each DOF had its own LWPR learning system, resulting in seven parallel learning modules. In order to accelerate lookup and training times, the nearest-neighbor data lookup described on page 118 was utilized. The LWPR models were trained online while the robot performed a randomly drifting figure-eight pattern in front of its body. Lookup proceeded at 480 Hz, while updating the learning model was achieved at about 70 Hz. At 10-second intervals, learning was stopped and the robot attempted to draw a planar figure eight in the x-z plane of the robot end effector at 2 Hz frequency for the entire pattern. The quality of these drawing patterns is illustrated in figure 5.8. In figure 5.8(a), X_{des} denotes the desired figure eight pattern, X_{sim} illustrates the figure eight performed by our robot simulator that uses a perfect inverse dynamics model (but not necessarily a perfect tracking and numerical integration algorithm), X_{param} is the performance of the estimated rigid-body dynamics model, and X_{lwpr} shows the results of LWPR. While the rigid-body model has the worst

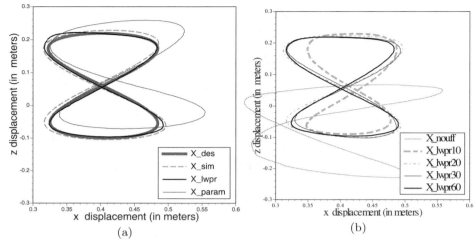

Figure 5.8 *(a)* Trajectories of robot end effector: X_{des} is the desired trajectory, X_{sim} is a trajectory obtained from a robot simulator that had a perfect controller but numerical inaccuracy due to the integration of the equations of motion, X_{lwpr} is the result of a computed torque controller using LWPR's approximated inverse model, and X_{param} is the trajectory using an inverse model due to rigid body parameter estimation. *(b)* Results of online learning with LWPR starting from scratch, that is, initially with no functional inverse model; the improvement of control due to LWPR learning is shown at intervals of 10 seconds over the first minute of learning.

performance, LWPR obtained the best results, even slightly better than the simulator. Figure 5.8(b) illustrates the speed of LWPR learning. The X_{nouff} trace demonstrates the figure eight patterns performed without any inverse dynamics model, just using a low-gain PD controller. The other traces show how rapidly LWPR learned the figure eight pattern during training: they denote performance after 10, 20, 30, and 60 *seconds* of training. After 60 seconds, the figure eight is hardly distinguishable from the desired trace.

In order to demonstrate the complexity of functions that can be learned in realtime with LWPR, we repeated the same training and evaluation procedure with the Sarcos humanoid robot, which used its right hand to draw a lying figure eight pattern. In this case, learning of the inverse dynamics model required learning in a 90D input space, and the outputs were the thirty torque commands for each of the DOFs. As the learning of thirty parallel LWPR models would have exceeded the computational power of our 366 MHz real-time processors, we chose to learn one single LWPR model with a 30D output vector, that is, each projection of PLS in LWPR regressed all outputs vs. the projected input data. The projection direction was chosen as the mean projection across all outputs at each projection stage of PLS. This approach is suboptimal, as it is quite unlikely that all output dimensions agree on one good projection direction; essentially, one assumes that the gradients of all outputs point roughly in the same direction. On the other hand, section 5.2 demonstrated that movement data of actual physical systems lie on locally low-dimensional distributions, such that one can hope that LWPR with multiple outputs can still work successfully by simply spanning this locally low-dimensional input space with all projections. Figure 5.7(b) demonstrates the result of learning in a similar way as figure 5.8(b); the notation for the different trajectories in this figure follow as explained above for the 7DOF robot. Again, LWPR very rapidly improves over a control system with no inverse dynamics controller, that is, within 10 seconds of movement, the most significant inertial perturbation have been compensated. Convergence to low error tracking of the figure eight takes slightly longer, that is, about 300 seconds [X_{300} in figure 5.7(b)], but is reliably achieved. About fifty local models were created for this task. The learned inverse dynamics outperformed a model estimated by rigid-body dynamics methods significantly [cf. X_{param} in figure 5.7(b)].

Online Learning for Autonomous Airplane Control

The online learning abilities of LWPR are ideally suited to be incorporated in algorithms of provably stable adaptive control. The control theoretic development of such an approach was presented in Nakanishi et al.[26]. In essence, the problem formulation begins with a specific class of equations of motion of the form

$$\dot{\mathbf{x}} = f(\mathbf{x}) + g(\mathbf{x})\mathbf{u}, \tag{5.17}$$

where $\mathbf{x}$ denotes the state of the control system, the control inputs, and $f(\mathbf{x})$ and $g(\mathbf{x})$ are nonlinear function to approximated. A suitable control law for such a system is

$$\mathbf{u} = \hat{g}(\mathbf{x})^{-1}\left(-\hat{f}(\mathbf{x}) + \dot{\mathbf{x}}_c + \mathbf{K}(\mathbf{x}_c - \mathbf{x})\right), \tag{5.18}$$

where $\mathbf{x}_c, \dot{\mathbf{x}}_c$ are a desired reference trajectory to be tracked, and the "hat" notation indicates that these are the approximated version of the unknown function.

We applied LWPR in this control framework to learn the unknown function f and g for the problem of autonomous airplane control on a high-fidelity simulator. For simplicity, we only considered a planar version of the airplane, governed by the differential equation[41]:

$$\begin{aligned}
\dot{V} &= \tfrac{1}{m}(T\cos\alpha - D) - g\sin\gamma, \\
\dot{\alpha} &= -\tfrac{1}{mV}(L + T\sin\alpha) + \tfrac{g\cos\gamma}{V} + Q, \\
\dot{Q} &= cM.
\end{aligned} \tag{5.19}$$

In these equations, V denotes the forward speed of the airplane, m the mass, T the thrust, α the angle of attack, g the gravity constant, γ the flight path angle with respect to the horizontal world coordinate system axis, Q the pitch rate, and c an inertial constant. The complexity of these equations is hidden in $D, L,$ and M, which are the unknown highly nonlinear aerodynamic lift force, drag force, and pitch moment terms, which are specific to every airplane.

While we will not go into the details of provably stable adaptive control with LWPR in this chapter and how the control law (5.18) is applied to for airplane control, from the viewpoint of learning the main components to learn are the lift and drag forces and the pitch moment. These can be obtained by rearranging (5.19) to

$$
\begin{aligned}
D &= T\cos\alpha - \left(\dot{V} + g\sin\gamma\right)m = \\
&\quad f_D\left(\alpha, Q, V, M, \gamma, \delta_{OFL}, \delta_{OFR}, \delta_{MFL}, \delta_{MFR}, \delta_{SPL}, \delta_{SPR}\right) \\
L &= \left(\tfrac{g\cos\gamma}{V} + Q - \dot{\alpha}\right)mV - T\sin\alpha = \\
&\quad f_L\left(\alpha, Q, V, M, \gamma, \delta_{OFL}, \delta_{OFR}, \delta_{MFL}, \delta_{MFR}, \delta_{SPL}, \delta_{SPR}\right) \\
M &= \tfrac{Q}{c} = f_M\left(\alpha, Q, V, M, \gamma, \delta_{OFL}, \delta_{OFR}, \delta_{MFL}, \delta_{MFR}, \delta_{SPL}, \delta_{SPR}\right).
\end{aligned}
\tag{5.20}
$$

The δ terms denote the control surface angles of the airplane, with indices midboard-flap-left/right (MFL,MFR), outboard-flap-left/right(OFL,OFR), and left and right spoilers (SPL,SPR). All terms on the right hand side of (5.20) are known, such that we have to cope with three simultaneous function approximation problems in an 11D input space, an ideal application for LWPR.

We implemented LWPR for the three functions above in a high-fidelity simulink simulation of an autonomous airplane using the adaptive control approach of[26]. The airplane started with no initial knowledge, just the proportional controller term in (5.18) (i.e., the term multiplied by **K**). The task of the controller was to fly doublets, that is, up-and-down trajectories, which are essentially sinusoid like variations of the flight path angle γ

Figure 5.9 demonstrates the results of this experiment. Figure 5.9(a) shows the desired trajectory in γ and its realization by the controller. Figure 5.9(b-d) illustrate the online function approximation of D, L, and M. As can be seen, the control of γ achieves almost perfect tracking after just a very few seconds. The function approximation of D and L is very accurate after a very short time. The approximation M requires a longer time for convergence, but progresses fast. About ten local models were needed for learning f_D and f_L, while about twenty local models were allocated for f_M.

An interesting element of figure 5.9 happens after 400 seconds of flight, where we simulated a failure of the airplane mechanics by locking the MFR to 17-degree deflection. As can be seen, the function approximators very quickly reorganize after this change, and the flight is successfully continued, although γ tracking has some error for a while until it converges back to good tracking performance. The strong signal changes in the first seconds after the failure are due to oscillations of the control surfaces, and not a problem in function approximation. Without adaptive control, the airplane would have crashed.

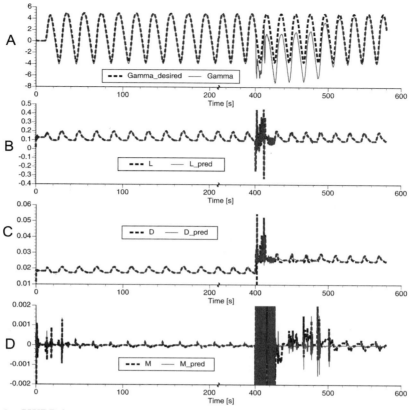

Figure 5.9 LWPR learning results for adaptive learning control on a simulated autonomous airplane *(a)* Tracking of flight angle γ. *(b)* Approximation of lift force. *(c)* Approximation of drag force, *(d)* Approximation of pitch moment. At 400 seconds into the flight, a failure is simulated that locks one control surface to a 17-degree angle. Note that for reasons of clearer illustration, an axis break was inserted after 200 seconds.

5.6 Bayesian Backfitting

The PLS algorithm described in subsection 5.3.3 has an attractive feature: rather than reduce the dimensionality of the input data to the most relevant subspace, it deals with the complete dimensionality, and structures its computation efficiently such that successive computationally inexpensive univariate regressions suffice rather than expensive matrix inversion techniques. However, PLS also has two heuristic components, that is, the way the projection directions are selected by an input-output correlation analysis, and the decision on when to stop adding new projection directions. In this section we suggest a Bayesian algorithm to replace PLS.

Another algorithm similar in vein to PLS is *backfitting* [16]. The backfitting algorithm estimates additive models of the form

$$y(\mathbf{x}) = \sum_{m=1}^{d} g_m(\mathbf{x}; \theta_m),$$

```
1:  Init: X = [x₁ ... x_N]^T, y = [y₁ ... y_N]^T, g_{m,i} = g_m(x_i; θ_m), g_m = [g_{m,1} ... g_{m,N}]^T
2:  repeat
3:      for m = 1 to d do
4:          r_m ← y − Σ_{k≠m} g_k    {compute partial residual (fake target)}
5:          θ_m ← arg min_{θ_m} (g_m − r_m)²    {optimize to fit partial residual}
6:      end for
7:  until convergence of θ_m
```

Algorithm 5.4   Algorithm for backfitting.

where the functions g_m are adjustable basis functions (e.g., splines), parameterized by θ_m. As shown in algorithm 5.4, backfitting decomposes the statistical estimation problem into d individual estimation problems by using partial residuals as "fake supervised targets" for each function g_m. At the cost of an iterative procedure, this strategy effectively reduces the computational complexity of multiple input settings, and allows easier numerical robustness control since no matrix inversion is involved.

For all its computational attractiveness, backfitting presents two serious drawbacks. There is no guarantee that the iterative procedure outlined in algorithm 5.4 will converge as this is heavily dependent on the nature of the functions g_m. The updates have no probabilistic interpretation, making backfitting difficult to insert into the current framework of statistical learning which emphasizes confidence measures, model selection, and predictive distributions. It should be mentioned that a Bayesian version of backfitting has been proposed in [17]. This algorithm however, relies on Gibbs sampling, which is more applicable when dealing with the nonparametric spline models discussed there, and is quite useful when one wishes to generate samples from the posterior additive model.

5.6.1   A Probabilistic Derivation of Backfitting

Consider the graphical model shown in figure 5.10(a), which represents the statistical model for *generalized* linear regression (GLR)[16]:

$$y|\mathbf{x} \sim \text{Normal}\left(y; \sum_{m=1}^{d} b_m f_m(\mathbf{x}; \boldsymbol{\theta}_m), \psi_y\right)$$

Given a data set $\mathbf{x}_{\mathcal{D}} = \{(\mathbf{x}_i, y_i)\}_{i=1}^{N}$, we wish to determine the most likely regression vector $\mathbf{v} = \begin{bmatrix} b_1 & b_2 & \cdots & b_d \end{bmatrix}^T$ which linearly combines the basis functions f_m to generate the output y. Since computing the ordinary least squares (OLS) solution $(\mathbf{v} = (\mathbf{F}^T\mathbf{F})^{-1}\mathbf{F}^T\mathbf{y})$ is an $O(d^3)$ task that grows computationally expensive and numerically brittle as the dimensionality of the input increases, we introduce a simple modification of the graphical model of figure 5.10(a), which enables us to create the desired algorithmic decoupling of the predictor functions, and gives backfitting a probabilistic interpretation. Consider the introduction of random variables z_{im} as shown

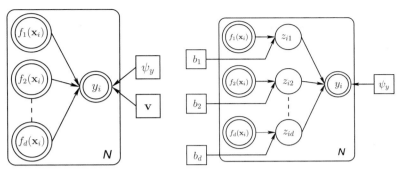

(a) Graphical model for generalized linear regression.

(b) Graphical model for probabilistic backfitting.

Figure 5.10 We modify the original graphical model for generalized linear regression by inserting hidden variables z_{im} in each branch of the fan-in. This modified model can be solved using the EM framework to derive a probabilistic version of backfitting.

in figure 5.10(b). These variables are analogous to the output of the g_m function of algorithm 5.4, and can also be interpreted as an unknown *fake target* for each branch of the regression fan-in. For the derivation of our algorithm, we assume the following conditional distributions for each variable in the model:

$$
\begin{aligned}
y_i | \mathbf{z}_i &\sim \text{Normal} \left(y_i; \mathbf{1}^T \mathbf{z}_i, \psi_y \right) \\
z_{im} | \mathbf{x}_i &\sim \text{Normal} \left(z_{im}; b_m f_m(\mathbf{x}_i), \psi_{zm} \right)
\end{aligned}
\tag{5.21}
$$

where $\mathbf{1} = [1, 1, \ldots, 1]^T$. With this modification in place, we are essentially in a situation where we wish to optimize the parameters

$$
\phi = \left\{ \{b_m, \psi_{zm}\}_{m=1}^d, \psi_y \right\},
$$

given that we have observed variables $\mathbf{x}_{\mathcal{D}} = \{(\mathbf{x}_i, y_i)\}_{i=1}^N$ and that we have unobserved variables $\mathbf{x}_{\mathcal{H}} = \{\mathbf{z}_i\}_{i=1}^N$ in our graphical model. This situation fits very naturally into the framework of maximum-likelihood estimation via the EM algorithm, by maximizing the expected *complete* log likelihood $\langle \ln p(\mathbf{x}_{\mathcal{D}}, \mathbf{x}_{\mathcal{H}}; \phi) \rangle$ which, from figure 5.10(b), can be expressed as

$$\ln p(\mathbf{x}_{\mathcal{D}}, \mathbf{x}_{\mathcal{H}}; \boldsymbol{\phi}) = -\frac{N}{2}\ln \psi_y - \frac{1}{2\psi_y}\sum_{i=1}^{N}\left(y_i - \mathbf{1}^T\mathbf{z}_i\right)^2$$

$$-\sum_{m=1}^{d}\left[\frac{N}{2}\ln \psi_{zm} + \frac{1}{2\psi_{zm}}\sum_{i=1}^{N}\left(z_{im} - b_m f_m(\mathbf{x}_i; \boldsymbol{\theta}_m)\right)^2\right]$$

$$+ \, const. \tag{5.22}$$

The resulting EM update equations are summarized below:

M-Step :

$$b_m = \frac{\sum_{i=1}^{N}\langle z_{im}\rangle f_m(\mathbf{x}_i)}{\sum_{i=1}^{N} f_m(\mathbf{x}_i)^2}$$

$$\psi_y = \frac{1}{N}\sum_{i=1}^{N}\left(y_i - \mathbf{1}^T\langle \mathbf{z}_i\rangle\right)^2 + \mathbf{1}^T\boldsymbol{\Sigma}_{\mathbf{z}}\mathbf{1}$$

$$\psi_{zm} = \frac{1}{N}\sum_{i=1}^{N}\left(\langle z_{im}\rangle - b_m f_m(\mathbf{x}_i)\right)^2 + \sigma_{zm}^2$$

E-Step :

$$\mathbf{1}^T\boldsymbol{\Sigma}_{\mathbf{z}}\mathbf{1} = \left(\sum_{m=1}^{d}\psi_{zm}\right)\left[1 - \frac{1}{s}\left(\sum_{m=1}^{d}\psi_{zm}\right)\right]$$

$$\sigma_{zm}^2 = \psi_{zm}\left(1 - \frac{1}{s}\psi_{zm}\right)$$

$$\langle z_{im}\rangle = b_m f_m(\mathbf{x}_i) + \frac{1}{s}\psi_{zm}\left(y_i - \mathbf{v}^T\mathbf{f}(\mathbf{x}_i)\right)$$

where we define $s \equiv \psi_y + \sum_{m=1}^{d}\psi_{zm}$. In addition, the parameters $\boldsymbol{\theta}_m$ of each function f_m can be updated by setting:

$$\sum_{i=1}^{N}\left(\langle z_{im}\rangle - b_m f_m\left(\mathbf{x}_i; \boldsymbol{\theta}_m\right)\right)\frac{\partial f_m\left(\mathbf{x}_i; \boldsymbol{\theta}_m\right)}{\partial \boldsymbol{\theta}_m} = 0 \tag{5.23}$$

and solving for $\boldsymbol{\theta}_m$. As this step depends on the particular choice of f_m, e.g., splines, kernel smoothers, parametric models, etc., we will not pursue it any further and just note that *any* statistical approximation mechanism could be used. Importantly, all equations in both the expectation and maximization steps are algorithmically $O(d)$ where d is the number of predictor functions f_m, and no matrix inversion is required.

To understand our EM solution as probabilistic backfitting, we note that backfitting can be viewed as a formal Gauss-Seidel algorithm; an equivalence that becomes exact in the special case of linear models[16]. For the linear system $\mathbf{F}^T\mathbf{F}\mathbf{v} = \mathbf{F}^T\mathbf{y}$, the Gauss-Seidel updates for the individual b_m are

$$b_m = \frac{\sum_{i=1}^{N} \left(y_i - \sum_{k \neq m}^{d} b_k f_k(\mathbf{x}_i) \right) f_m(\mathbf{x}_i)}{\sum_{i=1}^{N} f_m(\mathbf{x}_i)^2}. \tag{5.24}$$

Note that (5.24) - if used naively - only guarantees convergence for very specially structured matrices. An extension to the Gauss-Seidel algorithm adds a fraction $(1 - \omega)$ of b_m to the update and gives us the well-known *relaxation* algorithms:

$$b_m^{(n+1)} = (1 - \omega)b_m^{(n)} + \omega \frac{\sum_{i=1}^{N} \left(y_i - \sum_{k \neq m}^{d} b_k f_k(\mathbf{x}_i) \right) f_m(\mathbf{x}_i)}{\sum_{i=1}^{N} f_m(\mathbf{x}_i)^2}, \tag{5.25}$$

which has improved convergence rates for *overrelaxation* $(1 < \omega < 2)$, or improved stability for *underrelaxation* $(0 < \omega < 1)$. For $\omega = 1$, the standard Gauss-Seidel/backfitting of equation (5.24) is recovered. The appropriate value of ω, which allows the iterations to converge while still maintaining a reasonable convergence rate can only be determined by treating (5.24) as a discrete dynamical system, and analyzing the eigenvalues of its system matrix - an $O(d^3)$ task. If, however, we substitute the expression for $\langle z_{im} \rangle$ in the maximization equation for b_m, and set $\omega = \omega_m = \psi_{zm}/s$ in (5.25), it can be shown that (after some algebraic rearrangement,) the two equations are identical, that is, we indeed derive a probabilistic version of backfitting.

This allows us to now place backfitting within the wider context of Bayesian machine learning algorithms. In particular, we can place individual priors over the regression coefficients:

$$b_m \sim \text{Normal}\left(b_m; 0, 1/\alpha_m\right),$$
$$\alpha_m \sim \text{Gamma}\left(\alpha_m; a_\alpha, b_\alpha\right),$$

where a_α and b_α are small enough to select an uninformative Gamma prior over the precisions α_m. Figure 5.11(a) shows the graphical model with the added priors, while figure 5.11(b) shows the resulting marginal prior over $\mathbf{v}$. This prior structure favors solutions which have as few nonzero regression coefficients as possible, and thus performs an automatic relevance determination (ARD) sparsification of the input dimensions.

We compared the use of PLS and ARD Bayesian backfitting to analyze the following real-world data set collected from neuroscience. The data set consists of simultaneous recordings (2400 data points) of firing-rate coded activity in seventy-one motor cortical neurons and the electromyograms(EMGs) of eleven muscles. The goal is to determine which neurons are responsible for the activity of each muscle. The relationship between neural and muscle activity is assumed to be linear, such that the basis functions in backfitting are simply a copy of the respective input dimensions, that is $f_m(\mathbf{x}) = x_m$.

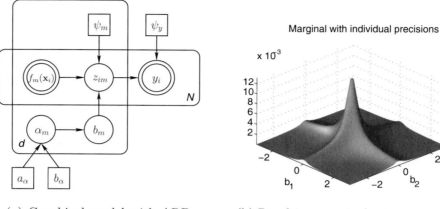

(a) Graphical model with ARD prior

(b) Resulting marginal prior over **v**

Figure 5.11 By associating an individual gamma distributed precision with each regression coefficient, we create a marginal prior over **v** that favors sparse solutions which lie along the (hyper)-spines of the distribution.

Table 5.4 Results on the neuron-muscle data set

	Bayesian backfitting	**PLS**	**Baseline**
neuron match	93.6%	18%	—
$nMSE$	0.8446	1.77	0.84

A brute-force study (conducted by our research collaborators) painstakingly considered every possible combination of neurons (up to groups of twenty for computational reasons; i.e., even this reduced analysis required several weeks of computation on a thirty-node cluster computer), to determine the optimal neuron-muscle correlation as measured on various validation sets. This study provided us with a baseline neuron-muscle correlation matrix that we hoped to duplicate with PLS and Bayesian backfitting, although with much reduced computational effort.

The results shown in table 5.4 demonstrate two points:

– The relevant neurons found by Bayesian backfitting contained over 93% of the neurons found by the baseline study, while PLS fails to find comparable correlations. The neuron match in backfitting is easily inferred from the resulting magnitude of the precision parameters α, while for PLS, the neuron match was inferred based on the subspace spanned by the projections that PLS employed.

– The regression accuracy of Bayesian backfitting (as determined by eight-fold crossvalidation), is comparable to that of the baseline study, while PLS's failure to find the correct correlations causes it to have significantly higher generalization errors. The analysis for both backfitting and PLS was carried out using the same validation sets as those used for the baseline analysis.

The performance of Bayesian backfitting on this particularly difficult data set shows that it is a viable alternative to traditional generalized linear regression tools. Even with the additional Bayesian inference for ARD, it maintains its algorithmic efficiency since no matrix inversion is required.

As an aside it is useful to note that Bayesian backfitting and PLS required of the order of 8 hours of computation on a standard PC (compared with several weeks on a cluster for the brute-force study), and evaluated the contributions of all seventy-one neurons.

An alternative form of prior in which a *single* precision parameter is shared among the regression coefficients results in a shrinkage of the norm of the regression vector solution, similar to ridge regression. In this case, however, no additional crossvalidation is required to determine the ridge parameters, as these are automatically inferred. The Bayesian backfitting algorithm is also applicable within the framework of sparse Bayesian learning [7], and provides a competitive and robust nonlinear supervised learning tool.

Bayesian Backfitting can thus completely replace PLS in LWPR, thus reducing the number of open parameters in LWPR and facilitating its probabilistic interpretation.

5.7   Discussion

Nearest-neighbor regression with spatially localized models remains one of the most data efficient and computationally efficient methods for incremental learning with automatic determination of the model complexity. In order to overcome the curse of dimensionality of local learning systems, we investigated methods of linear projection regression and how to employ them in spatially localized nonlinear function approximation for high-dimensional input data that have redundant and irrelevant components. We compared various local dimensionality reduction techniques - an analysis that resulted in choosing a localized version of Partial Least Squares regression at the core of a novel nonparametric function approximator, Locally Weighted Projection Regression (LWPR). The proposed technique was evaluated on a range of artificial and real-world data sets in up to 90D input spaces. Besides showing fast and robust learning performance due to second-order learning methods based on stochastic leave-one-out cross-validation, LWPR excelled by its low computational complexity: updating each local model with a new data point remained *linear* in its computational cost in the number of inputs since the algorithm accomplishes good approximation results with only three to four projections irrespective of the number of input dimensions. To our knowledge, this is the first spatially localized incremental learning system that can efficiently work in high-dimensional spaces and that is thus suited for online and realtime applications. In addition, LWPR compared favorably in its generalization performance with state-of-the-art batch regression methods like Gaussian process regression, and can provide qualitatively similar estimates of confidence bounds and predictive variances. Finally, a new algorithm, Bayesian backfitting, was suggested to replace partial least squares in the future. Bayesian backfitting is a Bayesian treatment of linear regression with automatic relevance detection of inputs and a robust EM-like incremental updating technique. Future work will investigate this algorithm in the nonlinear setting of LWPR on the way to a full Bayesian approach to approximate nearest-neighbor regression.

Notes

[1]Mixture models are actually somehow in between global and local function approximators since they use local model fitting but employ a global optimization criterion.

[2]It must be noted that there has been some recent work[39] that has started to look at model selection for SVMs and GPRs and automatic determination of the number of latent models for VBM[13]

[3]It should be noted that we could insert one more preprocessing step in algorithm 5.2 that independently scales all inputs to unit variance; empirically, however, we did not notice a significant improvement of the algorithm, so that we omit this step for the sake of simplicity.

[4]For rank-deficient input spaces, the equivalence of (5.11) and (5.12) holds in the space spanned by X

[5]Note that w_k is used here as an abbreviated version of $w_{\{q,k\}}$ -the weight contribution due to query point $\mathbf{q}$ in model k- for the sake of simplicity.

[6]Since LWPR is an incremental algorithm, data presentations in this case refer to repeated, random-order presentations of training data from our noisy data set of size 500

[7]We have not plotted the results for SVMR since it was found to consistently perform worse that GPR for the given number of training data.

[8]The GPR algorithm had problems of convergence and numerical stability for training data sizes above 500 points.

References

1. C.H. An, C. Atkeson, and J. Hollerbach. *Model Based Control of a Robot Manipulator.* Cambridge, MA, MIT Press, 1988.

2. C. Atkeson, A. Moore, and S.Schaal. Locally weighted learning. *Artificial Intelligence Review*, 11(4):76–113, 1997.

3. A. Bell and T. Sejnowski. The "independent components" of natural scenes are edge filters. *Vision Research*, 37(23):3327–3338, 1997.

4. D.A. Belsley, E. Kuh and D. Welsch. *Regression Diagnostics.* New York, John Wiley & Sons, 1980.

5. C. Bishop *Neural Networks for Pattern Recognition.* Oxford, Oxford University Press, 1995.

6. A. D'Souza, S. Vijayakumar and S. Schaal. Are internal models of the entire body learnable? *Society for Neuroscience Abstracts.* Volume 27, Program No. 406.2, 2001.

7. A. D'Souza, S. Vijayakumar and S. Schaal. The Bayesian backfitting relevance vector machine. In *Proceedings of the Twenty-first International Conference on Machine Learning.* New York, ACM Press, 2004.

8. B.S. Everitt. *An Introduction to Latent Variable Models.* London, Chapman & Hall, 1984.

9. S.E. Fahlman and C. Lebiere. The cascade correlation learning architecture. *Advances in NIPS 2*, 1990.

10. I.E. Frank and J.H. Friedman. A statistical view of some chemometric regression tools. *Technometrics*, 35(2):109–135, 1993.

11. J.H. Friedman and W. Stutzle. Projection pursuit regression. *Journal of the American Statistical Association*, 76:817-823, 1981.

12. A.B. Gelman, J.S. Carlin, H.S. Stern and D.B. Rubin. *Bayesian Data Analysis.* London, Chapman & Hall, 1995.

13. Z. Ghahramani and M.J. Beal. Variational inference for Bayesian mixtures of factor analysers. In editors, S. A. Solla, T. K. Leen and K. Muller, *Advances in Neural Information Processing Systems 12*, pages 449-455, Cambridge, MA, MIT Press, 2000.

14. M. Gibbs and D.J.C., MacKay. Efficient implementation of Gaussian processes. Technical Report, Cavendish Laboratory, Cambridge, UK, 1997.

15. T.J. Hastie and C. Loader. Local regression: Automatic kernel carpentry. *Statistical Science*, 8(2):120–143, 1993.

16. T.J. Hastie and R.J. Tibshirani. *Generalized Additive Models.* No. 43 in *Monographs on Statistics and Applied Probability.* London, Chapman & Hall, 1990.

17. T.J. Hastie and R.J. Tibshirani. Bayesian backfitting. *Statistical Science*, 15(3):196–213, August 2000.

18. S. Hettich and S. D. Bay. The UCI KDD archive. Irvine, CA, University of California, Dept. of Information and Computer Science, [http://kdd.ics.uci.edu], 1999.

19. M.I. Jordan and R. Jacobs. Hierarchical mixture of experts and the EM algorithm. *Neural Computation*, 6(2):181–214, 1994.

20. M. Kawato. Internal models for motor control and trajectory planning. *Current Opinion in Neurobiology*, 9:718–727, 1999.

21. L. Ljung and T. Soderstrom. *Theory and Practice of Recursive Identification.* Cambridge, MA, MIT Press, 1986.

22. W.F. Massy. Principal component regression in exploratory statistical research. *Journal of the American Statistical Association*, 60:234–246, 1965.

23. R.H. Myers. *Classical and Modern Regression with Applications* Boston: Duxbury Press, 1990.

24. B.A. Olshausen and D.J. Field. Emergence of simple cell receptive field properties by learning a sparse code for natural images. *Nature*, 381:607-609, 1996.

25. M.P. Perrone and L.N. Cooper. When networks disagree: Ensemble methods for hybrid neural networks. In editor, R. J. Mammone, *Neural Networks for Speech and Image Processing*. London, Chapman & Hall, 1993.

26. J. Nakanishi, J.A. Farrell and S. Schaal, Learning composite adaptive control for a class of nonlinear systems. In *IEEE International Conference on Robotics and Automation*, pages 2647-2652, New Orleans, 2004.

27. S. Roweis and L. Saul. Nonlinear dimensionality reduction by locally linear embedding. *Science*, 290:2323-2326, 2000.

28. D.B. Rubin and D.T. Thayer. EM algorithms for ML factor analysis. *Psychometrika*, 47(1):69–76, 1982.

29. C. Saunders, M.O. Stitson, J. Weston, L. Bottou, B. Schoelkopf and A. Smola. *Support Vector Machine - Reference Manual*. TR CSD-TR-98-03, Dept. of Computer Science, Royal Holloway, University of London, 1998.

30. T.D. Sanger. Optimal unsupervised learning in a single layer feedforward neural network. *Neural Networks*, 2:459–473, 1989.

31. D.W. Scott. *Multivariate Density Estimation*, Hoboken, NJ, John Wiley & Sons, 1992.

32. S. Schaal and D. Sternad. Origins and violations of the 2/3 power law in rhythmic 3D movements. *Experimental Brain Research*. 136:60-72, 2001.

33. S. Schaal, S. Vijayakumar and C.G. Atkeson. Assessing the quality of learned local models. *Advances in Neural Information Processing Systems 6*, pages 160-167. San Mateo, CA, Morgan Kaufmann, 1994.

34. S.Schaal & C.G.Atkeson Receptive field weighted regression, *Technical Report TR-H-209, ATR Human Information Processing Labs.*, Kyoto, Japan.

35. S. Schaal and C.G. Atkeson. Constructive incremental learning from only local information. *Neural Computation*, 10(8):2047–2084, 1998.

36. S. Schaal, S. Vijayakumar and C.G. Atkeson. Local dimensionality reduction. *Advances in NIPS, 10*, 1998.

37. S. Schaal, C.G. Atkeson and S. Vijayakumar. Realtime robot learning with locally weighted statistical learning. In *Proceedings of International Conference on Robotics and Automation ICRA2000*, San Francisco, CA, pages 288–293, 2000.

38. B. Scholkopf, A. Smola, R. Williamson, R and P. Bartlett. New Support Vector Algorithms. *Neural Computation*, (12)5:1207-1245, 2000.

39. B. Scholkopf, C. Burges and A. Smola. *Advances in Kernel Methods: Support Vector Learning*. Cambridge, MA, MIT Press, 1999.

40. A. Smola and B. Scholkopf. A tutorial on support vector regression. NeuroCOLT Technical Report NC-TR-98-030, Royal Holloway College, University of London, 1998.

41. B.L. Stevens and F.L. Lewis. *Aircraft Control and Simulation.* Hoboken, NJ, John Wiley & Sons, 2003.

42. J. Tenenbaum, V. de Silva and J. Langford. A global geometric framework for nonlinear dimensionality reduction *Science,* 290:2319-2323, 2000.

43. N. Ueda, R. Nakano, Z. Ghahramani and G. Hinton, SMEM Algorithm for Mixture Models *Neural Computation,* 12, pp. 2109-2128, 2000.

44. S. Vijayakumar and H. Ogawa. RKHS based Functional Analysis for Exact Incremental Learning *Neurocomputing : Special Issue on Theoretical Analysis of Real Valued Function Classes,* 29(1-3):85-113, 1999.

45. S. Vijayakumar and S. Schaal. Local adaptive subspace regression. *Neural Processing Letters,* 7(3):139–149, 1998.

46. S. Vijayakumar and S. Schaal. Locally Weighted Projection Regression : An $O(n)$ algorithm for incremental real time learning in high dimensional space. In *Proceedings of International Conference in Machine Learning (ICML),* pages 1079-1086, 2000.

47. N. Vlassis, Y. Motomura and B. Krose. Supervised dimension reduction of intrinsically low-dimensional data. *Neural Computation,* Cambridge, MA, MIT Press, 2002.

48. C.K.I. Williams and C. Rasmussen. Gaussian processes for regression. In D.S. Touretsky, M. Mozer and M.E. Hasselmo, editors, *Advances in Neural Information Processing Systems 8,* Cambridge, MA, MIT Press, 1996.

49. H. Wold. Soft modeling by latent variables: The nonlinear iterative partial least squares approach. In J. Gani (Ed.), *Perspectives in probability and statistics, papers in honour of M. S. Bartlett,* pages 520–540. London, Academic Press, 1975.

50. L. Xu, M.I. Jordan and G.E. Hinton. An alternative model for mixtures of experts. In G. Tesauro, D. Touretzky, and T. Leen, editors, *Advances in Neural Information Processing Systems 7,* pages 633–640. Cambridge, MA, MIT Press, 1995.

6   Learning Embeddings for Fast Approximate Nearest Neighbor Retrieval

Vassilis Athitsos, Jonathan Alon, Stan Sclaroff,
and George Kollios

We present an embedding method that can signficantly reduce nearest neighbor retrieval time when the underlying distance measure is computationally expensive. Database and query objects are embedded into a Euclidean space, in which similarities can be rapidly measured using a weighted Manhattan distance. Embedding construction is formulated as a machine learning task, where AdaBoost is used to combine many simple, 1D embeddings into a multidimensional embedding that preserves a significant amount of the proximity structure in the original space. Performance is evaluated in a hand pose estimation system, and a dynamic gesture recognition system, where the proposed method is used to retrieve approximate nearest neighbors under expensive similarity measures. In both systems, BoostMap significantly increases efficiency, with minimal losses in accuracy. Moreover, the experiments indicate that BoostMap compares favorably with existing embedding methods that have been employed in computer vision and database applications, such as FastMap and Lipschitz embeddings.

6.1   Introduction

Many important applications require efficient nearest-neighbor retrieval in non-Euclidean, and often nonmetric spaces. Finding nearest neighbors efficiently in such spaces can be challenging, because the underlying distance measures can take time superlinear to the length of the data, and also because most indexing methods are not applicable in such spaces. For example, most tree-based and hash-based indexing methods typically assume that objects live in a Euclidean space, or at least a so-called "coordinate-space", where each object is represented as a feature vector of fixed dimensions. There is a wide range of non-Euclidean spaces that violate those assumptions. Some examples of such spaces are proteins and DNA in biology, time series data in various fields, and edge images in computer vision.

Euclidean embeddings (like Bourgain embeddings [17] and FastMap [8]) provide an alternative for indexing non-Euclidean spaces. Using embeddings, we associate each object with a Euclidean vector, so that distances between objects are related to distances between the vectors associated with those objects. Database objects are embedded offline. Given a query object q, its embedding $F(q)$ is computed efficiently online, by measuring distances between q and a small number of database objects. To retrieve the nearest neighbors of q, we first find a small set of candidate matches using distances in the Euclidean space, and then we refine those results by measuring distances in the original space. Euclidean embeddings can significantly improve retrieval time in domains where evaluating the distance measure in the original space is computationally expensive.

This chapter presents BoostMap, a machine learning method for constructing Euclidean embeddings. The algorithm is domain-independent and can be applied to *arbitrary* distance measures, metric or nonmetric. With respect to existing embedding methods for efficient approximate nearest-neighbor methods, BoostMap has the following advantages:

– Embedding construction explicitly optimizes a quantitative measure of how well the embedding preserves similarity rankings. Existing methods (like Bourgain embeddings [11] and FastMap [8]) typically use random choices and heuristics, and do not attempt to optimize some measure of embedding quality.

– Our optimization method does not make any assumptions about the original distance measure. For example, no Euclidean or metric properties are required.

Embeddings are seen as classifiers, which estimate for any three objects a, b, c if a is closer to b or to c. Starting with a large family of simple, one-dimensional (1D) embeddings, we use AdaBoost [20] to combine those embeddings into a single, high-dimensional embedding that can give highly accurate similarity rankings.

6.2   Related Work

Various methods have been employed for similarity indexing in multidimensional data sets, including hashing and tree structures [29]. However, the performance of such methods degrades in high dimensions. This phenomenon is one of the many aspects of the "curse of dimensionality." Another problem with tree-based methods is that they typically rely on Euclidean or metric properties, and cannot be applied to arbitrary spaces.

Approximate nearest-neighbor methods have been proposed in [12] and scale better with the number of dimensions. However, those methods are available only for specific sets of metrics, and they are not applicable to arbitrary distance measures. In [9], a randomized procedure is used to create a locality-sensitive hashing (LSH) structure that can report a $(1 + \epsilon)$-approximate nearest neighbor with a constant probability. In [32] M-trees are used for approximate similarity retrieval, while [16] proposes clustering the data set and retrieving only a small number of clusters (which are stored sequentially on disk) to answer each query. In [4, 7, 13] dimensionality reduction techniques are used where lower-bounding rules are ignored when dismissing dimensions and the focus is on preserving close approximations of distances only. In [27] the authors used VA-files [28] to find nearest neighbors by omitting the refinement step of the original exact search algorithm and estimating approximate distances using only the lower and upper bounds computed by the filtering step. Finally, in [23] the authors partition the data space into clusters and then the representatives of each cluster are compressed using quantization techniques. Other similar approaches include [15, 19]. However, all these techniques can be employed mostly for distance functions defined using L_p norms.

Various techniques appeared in the literature for robust evaluation of similarity queries on time-series databases when using nonmetric distance functions [14, 25, 30]. These techniques use the filter-and-refine approach where an approximation of the original distance that can be computed efficiently is utilized in the filtering step. Query speedup is achieved by pruning a large part of the search space before the original, accurate, but more expensive distance measure needs to be applied on few remaining candidates during the refinement step. Usually, the distance approximation function is designed to be metric (even if the original distance is not) so that traditional indexing techniques can be applied to index the database in order to speed up the filtering stage as well.

In domains where the distance measure is computationally expensive, significant computational savings can be obtained by constructing a distance-approximating embedding, which maps objects into another space with a more efficient distance measure. A number of methods have been proposed for embedding arbitrary metric spaces into a Euclidean or pseudo-Euclidean space [3, 8, 11, 18, 22, 26, 31]. Some of these methods, in particular multi-dimensional scaling (MDS) [31], Bourgain embeddings [3, 10], locally linear embeddings (LLE) [18], and Isomap [22] are not targeted at speeding up online similarity retrieval, because they still need to evaluate exact distances between the query and most or all database objects. Online queries can be handled by Lipschitz embeddings [10], FastMap [8], MetricMap [26] and SparseMap [11], which can readily compute the embedding of the query, measuring only a small number of exact distances in the process. These four methods are the most related to our approach. The goal of BoostMap is to achieve better indexing performance in domains where those four methods are applicable.

6.3   Background on Embeddings

Let X be a set of objects, and $D_X(x_1, x_2)$ be a distance measure between objects $x_1, x_2 \in X$. D_X can be metric or nonmetric. A Euclidean embedding $F : X \to \mathbb{R}^d$ is a function that maps objects from X into the d-dimensional Euclidean space $\mathbb{R}^d$, where distance is measured using a measure $D_{\mathbb{R}^d}$. $D_{\mathbb{R}^d}$ is typically an L_p or weighted L_p norm. Given X and D_X, our goal is to construct an embedding F that can be used for efficient and accurate approximate k-nearest neighbor (k-NN) retrieval, for previously unseen query objects, and for different values of k.

In this section we describe some existing methods for constructing Euclidean embeddings. We briefly go over Lipschitz embeddings [10], Bourgain embeddings [3, 10], FastMap [8], and MetricMap [26]. All these methods, with the exception of Bourgain embeddings, can be used for efficient approximate nearest-neighbor retrieval. Although Bourgain embeddings require too many distance computations in the original space X in order to embed the query, there is a heuristic approximation of Bourgain embeddings called SparseMap [11] that can also be used for efficient retrieval.

6.3.1   Lipschitz Embeddings

We can extend D_X to define the distance between elements of X and subsets of X. Let $x \in X$ and $R \subset X$. Then,

$$D_X(x, R) = \min_{r \in R} D_X(x, r) \ . \tag{6.1}$$

Given a subset $R \subset X$, a simple 1D Euclidean embedding $F^R : X \to \mathbb{R}$ can be defined as follows:

$$F^R(x) = D_X(x, R) \ . \tag{6.2}$$

The set R that is used to define F^R is called a *reference set*. In many cases R can consist of a single object r, which is typically called a *reference object* or a *vantage object* [10]. In that case, we denote the embedding as F^r:

$$F^r(x) = D_X(x, r) \ . \tag{6.3}$$

If D_X obeys the triangle inequality, F^R intuitively maps nearby points in X to nearby points on the real line $\mathbb{R}$. In many cases D_X may violate the triangle inequality for some triples of objects (an example is the chamfer distance [2]), but F^R may still map nearby points in X to nearby points in $\mathbb{R}$, at least most of the time [1]. On the other hand, distant objects may also map to nearby points (fig. 6.1).

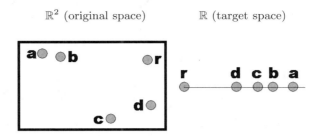

Figure 6.1 A set of five 2D points (shown on the left), and an embedding F^r of those five points into the real line (shown on the right), using r as the reference object. The target of each 2D point on the line is labeled with the same letter as the 2D point. The classifier $\tilde{F}^r$ (6.7) classifies correctly 46 out of the 60 triples we can form from these five objects (assuming no object occurs twice in a triple). Examples of misclassified triples are: $(b, a, c), (c, b, d), (d, b, r)$. For example, b is closer to a than it is to c, but $F^r(b)$ is closer to $F^r(c)$ than it is to $F^r(a)$.

In order to make it less likely for distant objects to map to nearby points, we can define a multidimensional embedding $F : X \to \mathbb{R}^k$, by choosing k different reference sets $R_1, ..., R_k$:

$$F(x) = (F^{R_1}(x), ..., F^{R_k}(x)) \ . \tag{6.4}$$

These embeddings are called *Lipschitz embeddings* [3, 10, 11]. Bourgain embeddings [3, 10] are a special type of Lipschitz embeddings. For a finite space X containing $|X|$ objects, we choose $\lfloor \log |X| \rfloor^2$ reference sets. In particular, for each $i = 1, ..., \lfloor \log |X| \rfloor$ we choose $\lfloor log |X| \rfloor$ reference sets, each with 2^i elements. The elements of each set are picked randomly. Bourgain embeddings are optimal in some sense: using a measure of embedding quality called *distortion*, if D_X is a metric, Bourgain embeddings achieve $O(\log(|X|))$ distortion, and there exist metric spaces X for which no embedding can achieve lower distortion [10, 17]. However, we should emphasize that if D_X is nonmetric, then Bourgain embeddings can have distortion higher than $O(\log(|X|))$.

A weakness of Bourgain embeddings is that, in order to compute the embedding of an object, we have to compute its distances D_X to almost all objects in X. This happens because some of the reference sets contain at least half of the objects in X. In database applications, computing all those distances is exactly what we want to avoid. SparseMap [11] is a heuristic simplification of Bourgain embeddings, in which the embedding of an object can be computed by measuring only $O(\log^2 |X|)$ distances. The penalty for this heuristic is that SparseMap no longer guarantees $O(\log(|X|))$ distortion for metric spaces.

Another way to speed up retrieval using a Bourgain embedding is to define this embedding using a relatively small random subset $X' \subset X$. That is, we

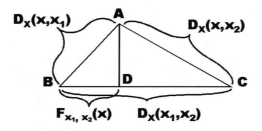

Figure 6.2 Computing $F^{x_1,x_2}(x)$, as defined in Equation 6.5: we construct a triangle ABC so that the sides AB, AC, BC have lengths $D_X(x, x_1), D_X(x, x_2)$ and $D_X(x_1, x_2)$ respectively. We draw from A a line perpendicular to BC, and D is the intersection of that line with BC. The length of the line segment BD is equal to $F^{x_1,x_2}(x)$.

choose $\lfloor \log |X'| \rfloor^2$ reference sets, which are subsets of X'. Then, to embed any object of X we only need to compute its distances to all objects of X'. We use this method to produce Bourgain embeddings of different dimensions in the experiments we describe in this chapter. We should note that, if we use this method, the optimality of the embedding only holds for objects in X', and there is no guarantee about the distortion attained for objects of the larger set X. We should also note that, in general, defining an embedding using a smaller set X' can in principle also be applied to Isomap [22], LLE [18], and even MDS [31], so that it takes less time to embed new objects.

The theoretical optimality of Bourgain embeddings with respect to distortion does not mean that Bourgain embeddings actually outperform other methods in practice. Bourgain embeddings have a worst-case bound on distortion, but that bound is very loose, and in actual applications the quality of embeddings is often much better, both for Bourgain embeddings and for embeddings produced using other methods.

A simple and attractive alternative to Bourgain embeddings is to simply use Lipschitz embeddings in which all reference sets are singleton, as in (6.3). In that case, if we have a d-dimensional embedding, in order to compute the embedding of a previously unseen object we only need to compute its distance to d reference objects.

6.3.2   FastMap and MetricMap

A family of simple, 1D embeddings is proposed in [8] and used as building blocks for FastMap. The idea is to choose two objects $x_1, x_2 \in X$, called pivot objects, and then, given an arbitrary $x \in X$, define the embedding F^{x_1,x_2} of x to be the *projection* of x onto the "line" $x_1 x_2$. As illustrated in fig. 6.2, the projection can be defined by treating the distances between x, x_1, and x_2 as specifying the sides of a triangle in R^2:

$$F^{x_1,x_2}(x) = \frac{D_X(x,x_1)^2 + D_X(x_1,x_2)^2 - D_X(x,x_2)^2}{2D_X(x_1,x_2)} . \qquad (6.5)$$

If X is Euclidean, then F^{x_1,x_2} will map nearby points in X to nearby points in $\mathbb{R}$. In practice, even if X is non-Euclidean, $F^{(x_1,x_2)}$ often still preserves some of the proximity structure of X.

FastMap [8] uses multiple pairs of pivot objects to project a finite set X into $\mathbb{R}^k$ using only $O(kn)$ evaluations of D_X. The first pair of pivot objects (x_1, x_2) is chosen using a heuristic that tends to pick points that are far from each other. Then the rest of the distances between objects in X are "updated," so that they correspond to projections into the "hyperplane" perpendicular to the "line" x_1x_2. Those projections are computed again by treating distances between objects in X as Euclidean distances in some $\mathbb{R}^m$. After distances are updated, FastMap is recursively applied again to choose a next pair of pivot objects and apply another round of distance updates. Although FastMap treats X as a Euclidean space, the resulting embeddings can be useful even when X is non-Euclidean, or even nonmetric. We have seen that in our own experiments (Section 6.6).

MetricMap [26] is an extension of FastMap that maps X into a a pseudo-Euclidean space. The experiments in [26] report that MetricMap tends to do better than FastMap when X is non-Euclidean. So far we have no conclusive experimental comparisons between MetricMap and our method, partly because some details of the MetricMap algorithm have not been fully specified (as pointed out in [10]), and therefore we could not be sure how close our MetricMap implementation was to the implementation evaluated in [26].

6.3.3   Embedding Application: Filter-and-refine Retrieval

In applications where we are interested in retrieving the k-NN for a query object q, a d-dimensional Euclidean embedding F can be used in a filter-and-refine framework [10], as follows:

– Offline preprocessing step: compute and store vector $F(x)$ for every database object x.

– Embedding step: given a query object q, compute $F(q)$. Typically this involves computing distances D_X between q and a small number of objects of X.

– Filter step: find the database objects whose vectors are the p most similar vectors to $F(q)$. This step involves measuring distances in $\mathbb{R}^d$.

– Refine step: sort those p candidates by evaluating the exact distance D_X between q and each candidate.

The assumption is that distance measure D_X is computationally expensive and evaluating distances in Euclidean space is much faster. The filter step discards most database objects by comparing Euclidean vectors. The refine step applies D_X only to the top p candidates. This is much more efficient than brute-force retrieval, in which we compute D_X between q and the entire database.

To optimize filter-and-refine retrieval, we have to choose p, and often we also need to choose d, which is the dimensionality of the embedding. As p increases, we are more likely to get the true k-NN in the top p candidates found at the filter step, but we also need to evaluate more distances D_X at the refine step. Overall, we trade accuracy for efficiency. Similarly, as d increases, computing $F(q)$ becomes more expensive (because we need to measure distances to more objects of X), and measuring distances between vectors in $\mathbb{R}^d$ also becomes more expensive. At the same time, we may get more accurate results in the filter step, and we may be able to decrease p. The best choice of p and d will depend on domain-specific parameters like k, the time it takes to compute the distance D_X, the time it takes to compare d-dimensional vectors, and the desired retrieval accuracy (i.e., how often we are willing to miss some of the true k-NN).

6.4   Associating Embeddings with Classifiers

In this section we define a quantitative measure of embedding quality, that is directly related to how well an embedding preserves the similarity structure of the original space. The BoostMap learning algorithm will then be shown to directly optimize this quantitative measure.

As previously, X is a set of objects, and $D_X(x_1, x_2)$ is a distance measure between objects $x_1, x_2 \in X$. Let (q, x_1, x_2) be a triple of objects in X. We define the *proximity order* $P_X(q, x_1, x_2)$ to be a function that outputs whether q is closer to x_1 or to x_2:

$$P_X(q, x_1, x_2) = \begin{cases} 1 & \text{if } D_X(q, x_1) < D_X(q, x_2) \\ 0 & \text{if } D_X(q, x_1) = D_X(q, x_2) \\ -1 & \text{if } D_X(q, x_1) > D_X(q, x_2) \end{cases} \quad (6.6)$$

If F maps space X into $\mathbb{R}^d$ (with associated distance measure $D_{\mathbb{R}^d}$), then F can be used to define a *proximity classifier* $\tilde{F}$ that estimates, for any triple (q, x_1, x_2), whether q is closer to x_1 or to x_2, simply by checking whether $F(q)$ is closer to $F(x_1)$ or to $F(x_2)$:

$$\tilde{F}(q, x_1, x_2) = D_{\mathbb{R}^d}(F(q), F(x_2)) - D_{\mathbb{R}^d}(F(q), F(x_1)) . \quad (6.7)$$

If we define $\text{sign}(x)$ to be 1 for $x > 0$, 0 for $x = 0$, and -1 for $x < 0$, then $\text{sign}(\tilde{F}(q, x_1, x_2))$ is an estimate of $P_X(q, x_1, x_2)$.

We define the classification error $G(\tilde{F}, q, x_1, x_2)$ of applying $\tilde{F}$ on a particular triple (q, x_1, x_2) as

$$G(\tilde{F}, q, x_1, x_2) = \frac{|P_X(q, x_1, x_2) - \text{sign}(\tilde{F}(q, x_1, x_2))|}{2} . \qquad (6.8)$$

Finally, the overall classification error $G(\tilde{F})$ is defined to be the expected value of $G(\tilde{F}, q, x_1, x_2)$, over X^3, i.e., the set of triples of objects of X. If X contains a finite number of objects, we get

$$G(\tilde{F}) = \frac{\sum_{(q, x_1, x_2) \in X^3} G(\tilde{F}, q, x_1, x_2)}{|X|^3} . \qquad (6.9)$$

Using the definitions in this section, our problem definition is very simple: we want to construct an embedding $F_{\text{out}} : X \to \mathbb{R}^d$ in a way that minimizes $G(\tilde{F}_{\text{out}})$. If an embedding F has error rate $G(\tilde{F}) = 0$, then F perfectly preserves nearest-neighbor structure, meaning that for any $x_1, x_2 \in X$, and any integer $k > 0$, x_1 is the kth NN of x_2 in X if and only if $F(x_1)$ is the kth NN of $F(x_2)$ in the set $F(X)$. Overall, the lower the error rate $G(\tilde{F})$ is, the better the embedding F is in terms of preserving the similarity structure of X.

We address the problem of minimizing $G(\tilde{F}_{\text{out}})$ as a problem of combining classifiers. As building blocks we use a family of simple, 1D embeddings. Then, we apply AdaBoost to combine many 1D embeddings into a high-dimensional embedding F_{out} with a low error rate.

6.5 Constructing Embeddings via AdaBoost

The 1D embeddings that we use as building blocks in our algorithm are of two types: embeddings of type F^r as defined in (6.3), and embeddings of type F^{x_1, x_2}, as defined in (6.5). Each 1D embedding F corresponds to a binary classifier $\tilde{F}$. These classifiers estimate, for triples (q, x_1, x_2) of objects in X, if q is closer to x_1 or x_2. If F is a 1D embedding, we expect $\tilde{F}$ to behave as a *weak classifier* [20], meaning that it will have a high error rate, but it should still do better than a random classifier. We want to combine many 1D embeddings into a multidimensional embedding that behaves as a *strong classifier*, i.e., that has relatively high accuracy. To choose which 1D embeddings to use, and how to combine them, we use the AdaBoost framework [20].

6.5.1 Overview of the Training Algorithm

The training algorithm for BoostMap is an adaptation of AdaBoost to the problem of embedding construction. The inputs to the training algorithm are the following:

– A training set $T = ((q_1, a_1, b_1), ..., (q_t, a_t, b_t))$ of t triples of objects from X.

– A set of labels $Y = (y_1, ..., y_t)$, where $y_i \in \{-1, 1\}$ is the class label of (q_i, a_i, b_i). If $D_X(q_i, a_i) < D_X(q_i, b_i)$, then $y_i = 1$, else $y_i = -1$. The training set includes no triples where q_i is equally far from a_i and b_i.

– A set $C \subset X$ of candidate objects. Elements of C can be used to define 1D embeddings.

– A matrix of distances from each $c \in C$ to each q_i, a_i, and b_i included in one of the training triples in T.

The training algorithm combines many classifiers $\tilde{F}_j$ associated with 1D embeddings F_j, into a classifier $H = \sum_{j=1}^{d} \alpha_j \tilde{F}_j$. The classifiers $\tilde{F}_j$ and weights α_j are chosen so as to minimize the classification error of H. Once we get the classifier H, its components $\tilde{F}_j$ are used to define a high-dimensional embedding $F = (F_1, ..., F_d)$, and the weights α_j are used to define a weighted L_1 distance, that we will denote as $D_{\mathbb{R}^d}$, on $\mathbb{R}^d$. We are then ready to use F and $D_{\mathbb{R}^d}$ to embed objects into $\mathbb{R}^d$ and compute approximate similarity rankings.

Training is done in a sequence of rounds. At each round, the algorithm either modifies the weight of an already chosen classifier, or selects a new classifier. Before we describe the algorithm in detail, here is an intuitive, high-level description of what takes place at each round:

1. Go through the classifiers $\tilde{F}_j$ that have already been chosen, and try to identify a weight α_j that, if modified, decreases the training error. If such an α_j is found, modify it accordingly.

2. If no weights were modified, consider a set of classifiers that have not been chosen yet. Identify, among those classifiers, the classifier $\tilde{F}$ which is the best at correcting the mistakes of the classifiers that have already been chosen.

3. Add that classifier $\tilde{F}$ to the set of chosen classifiers, and compute its weight. The weight that is chosen is the one that maximizes the corrective effect of $\tilde{F}$ on the output of the previously chosen classifiers.

Intuitively, weak classifiers are chosen and weighted so that they complement each other. Even when individual classifiers are highly inaccurate, the combined classifier can have very high accuracy, as evidenced in several applications of AdaBoost (e.g., in [24]).

Trying to modify the weight of an already chosen classifier before adding in a new classifier is a heuristic that reduces the number of classifiers that we need to achieve a given classification accuracy. Since each classifier corresponds to a dimension in the embedding, this heuristic leads to lower-dimensional embeddings, which reduce database storage requirements and retrieval time.

6.5.2 The Training Algorithm in Detail

This subsection, together with the original AdaBoost reference [20], provides enough information to allow implementation of BoostMap, and it can be skipped if the reader is more interested in a high-level description of our method.

The training algorithm performs a sequence of training rounds. At the jth round, it maintains a weight $w_{i,j}$ for each of the t triples (q_i, a_i, b_i) of the training set, so that $\sum_{i=1}^{t} w_{i,j} = 1$. For the first round, each $w_{i,1}$ is set to $\frac{1}{t}$.

At the jth round, we try to modify the weight of an already chosen classifier or add a new classifier, in a way that improves the overall training error. A key measure that is used to evaluate the effect of choosing classifier $\tilde{F}$ with weight α is the function Z_j:

$$Z_j(\tilde{F}, \alpha) = \sum_{i=1}^{t} (w_{i,j} \exp(-\alpha y_i \tilde{F}(q_i, a_i, b_i))) . \qquad (6.10)$$

The full details of the significance of Z_j can be found in [20]. Here it suffices to say that $Z_j(\tilde{F}, \alpha)$ is a measure of the benefit we obtain by adding $\tilde{F}$ with weight α to the list of chosen classifiers. The benefit increases as $Z_j(\tilde{F}, \alpha)$ decreases. If $Z_j(\tilde{F}, \alpha) > 1$, then adding $\tilde{F}$ with weight α is actually expected to increase the classification error.

A frequent operation during training is identifying the pair $(\tilde{F}, \alpha)$ that minimizes $Z_j(\tilde{F}, \alpha)$. For that operation we use the shorthand $Z_{\min}$, defined as follows:

$$Z_{\min}(B, j) = \mathrm{argmin}_{(\tilde{F}, \alpha) \in B \times \mathbb{R}} Z_j(\tilde{F}, \alpha) . \qquad (6.11)$$

In (6.11), B is a set of classifiers.

At training round j, the training algorithm goes through the following steps:

1. Let B_j be the set of classifiers chosen so far. Set $(\tilde{F}, \alpha) = Z_{\min}(B_j, j)$. If $Z_j(\tilde{F}, \alpha) < .9999$ then modify the current weight of $\tilde{F}$, by adding α to it, and proceed to the next round. We use .9999 as a threshold, instead of 1, to avoid minor modifications with insignificant numerical impact.

2. Construct a set of 1D embeddings $\mathbb{F}_{j1} = \{F^r \mid r \in C\}$ where F^r is defined in (6.3), and C is the set of candidate objects that is one of the inputs to the training algorithm (see subsection 6.5.1).

3. For a fixed number m, choose randomly a set C_j of m pairs of elements of C, and construct a set of embeddings $\mathbb{F}_{j2} = \{F^{x_1, x_2} \mid (x_1, x_2) \in C_j\}$, where F^{x_1, x_2} is as defined in (6.5).

4. Define $\mathbb{F}_j = \mathbb{F}_{j1} \cup \mathbb{F}_{j2}$. We set $\tilde{\mathbb{F}}_J = \{\tilde{F} \mid F \in \mathbb{F}_j\}$.

5. Set $(\tilde{F}, \alpha) = Z_{\min}(\tilde{\mathbb{F}}_j, j)$.

6. Add $\tilde{F}$ to the set of chosen classifiers, with weight α.

7. Set training weights $w_{i,j+1}$ as follows:

$$w_{i,j+1} = \frac{w_{i,j} \exp(-\alpha y_i \tilde{F}(q_i, a_i, b_i))}{Z_j(\tilde{F}, \alpha)} \ . \tag{6.12}$$

Intuitively, the more $\alpha \tilde{F}(q_i, a_i, b_i)$ disagrees with class label y_i, the more $w_{i,j+1}$ increases with respect to $w_{i,j}$. This way triples that get misclassified by many of the already chosen classifiers will carry a lot of weight and will influence the choice of classifiers in the next rounds.

The algorithm can terminate when we have chosen a desired number of classifiers, or when, at a given round j, no combination of $\tilde{F}$ and α makes $Z_j(\tilde{F}, \alpha) < 1$.

6.5.3   Training Output: Embedding and Distance

The output of the training stage is a classifier $H = \sum_{j=1}^{d} \alpha_j \tilde{F}_j$, where each $\tilde{F}_j$ is associated with a 1D embedding F_j. The final output of BoostMap is an embedding $F_{\text{out}} : X \to \mathbb{R}^d$ and a weighted Manhattan (L_1) distance $D_{\mathbb{R}^d} : \mathbb{R}^d \times \mathbb{R}^d \to \mathbb{R}$:

$$F_{\text{out}}(x) = (F_1(x), ..., F_d(x)) \ . \tag{6.13}$$

$$D_{\mathbb{R}^d}((u_1, ..., u_d), (v_1, ..., v_d)) = \sum_{j=1}^{d} (\alpha_j |u_j - v_j|) \ . \tag{6.14}$$

It is important to note (and easy to check) that the way we define F_{out} and $D_{\mathbb{R}^d}$, if we apply (6.7) to obtain a classifier $\tilde{F}_{\text{out}}$ from F_{out}, then $\tilde{F}_{\text{out}} = H$, i.e., $\tilde{F}_{\text{out}}$ is equal to the output of AdaBoost. This means that the output of AdaBoost, which is a classifier, is mathematically equivalent to the embedding F_{out}: given a triple (q, a, b), both the embedding and the classifier give the exact same answer as to whether q is closer to a or to b. If AdaBoost has been successful in learning a good classifier, the embedding F_{out} inherits the properties of that classifier, with respect to preserving the proximity order of triples.

Also, we should note that this equivalence between classifier and embedding relies on the way we define $D_{\mathbb{R}^d}$. For example, if $D_{\mathbb{R}^d}$ were defined without using weights α_j, or if $D_{\mathbb{R}^d}$ were defined as an L_2 metric, the equivalence would not hold.

6.5.4   Complexity

If C is the set of candidate objects, and n is the number of database objects, we need to compute $|C|n$ distances D_X to learn the embedding and compute the embeddings of all database objects. At each training round, we evaluate classifiers defined using $|C|$ reference objects and m pivot pairs. Therefore,

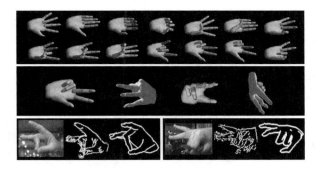

Figure 6.3 Top: 14 of the 26 hand shapes used to generate the hand database. Middle: four of the 4128 3D orientations of a hand shape. Bottom: for two test images we see, from left to right: the original hand image, the extracted edge image that was used as a query, and a correct match (noise-free computer-generated edge image) retrieved from the database.

the computational time per training round is $O((|C| + m)t)$, where t is the number of training triples. In our experiments we always set $m = |C|$.

Computing the d-dimensional embedding of a query object takes $O(d)$ time and requires $O(d)$ evaluations of D_X. Overall, query processing time is not worse than that of FastMap [8], SparseMap [11], and MetricMap [26].

6.6 Experiments

We used two data sets to compare BoostMap to FastMap [8] and Bourgain embeddings [3, 11]: a database of hand images, and an ASL (American Sign Language) database, containing video sequences of ASL signs. In both data sets the test queries were not part of the database, and not used in the training.

The hand database contains 107,328 hand images, generated using computer graphics. Twenty-six hand shapes were used to generate those images. Each shape was rendered under 4128 different 3D orientations (fig. 6.3). As queries we used 703 real images of hands. Given a query, we consider a database image to be correct if it shows the same hand shape as the query, in a 3D orientation within 30 degrees of the 3D orientation of the query [1]. The queries were manually annotated with their shape and 3D orientation. For each query there are about 25 to 35 correct matches among the 107,328 database images. Similarity between hand images is evaluated using the symmetric chamfer distance [2], applied to edge images. Evaluating the exact chamfer distance between a query and the entire database takes about 260 seconds.

The ASL database contains 880 gray-scale video sequences. Each video sequence depicts a sign, as signed by one of three native ASL signers (fig. 6.4). As queries we used 180 video sequences of ASL signs, signed by a single

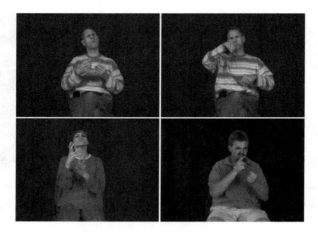

Figure 6.4   Four sample frames from the video sequences in the ASL database.

signer who was not included in the database. Given a query, we consider a database sequence to be a correct match if it is labeled with the same sign as the query. For each query, there are exactly 20 correct matches in the database. Similarity between video sequences is measured as follows: first, we use the similarity measure proposed in [6], which is based on optical flow, as a measure of similarity between single frames. Then, we use dynamic time warping [5] to compute the optimal time alignment and the overall matching cost between the two sequences. Evaluating the exact distance between the query and the entire database takes about 6 minutes.

In all experiments, the training set for BoostMap was 200,000 triples. For the hand database, the size of C (subsection 6.5.2) was 1000 elements, and the elements of C were chosen randomly at each step from among 3282 objects, i.e., C was different at each training round (a slight deviation from the description in section 6.5), to speed up training time. For the ASL database, the size of C was 587 elements. The objects used to define FastMap and Bourgain embeddings were also chosen from the same 3282 and 587 objects respectively. Also, in all experiments, we set $m = |C|$, where m is the number of embeddings based on pivot pairs that we consider at each training round. Learning a 256D BoostMap embedding of the hand database took about 2 days, using a 1.2 GHz Athlon processor.

To evaluate the accuracy of the approximate similarity ranking for a query, we used two measures: exact nearest-neighbor rank (ENN rank) and highest ranking correct match rank (HRCM rank). The ENN rank is computed as follows: let b be the database object that is the nearest neighbor to the query q under the exact distance D_X. Then, the ENN rank for that query in a given embedding is the rank of b in the similarity ranking that we get using the embedding. The HRCM rank for a query in an embedding is the best rank among all correct matches for that query, based on the similarity ranking we get with that embedding. In a perfect recognition system, the HRCM rank would be 1 for all queries. Figs. 6.5, 6.6, 6.7, and 6.8 show the median ENN

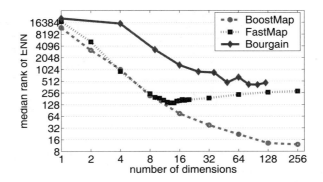

Figure 6.5 Median rank of ENN, vs. number of dimensions, in approximate similarity rankings obtained using three different methods, for 703 queries to the hand database.

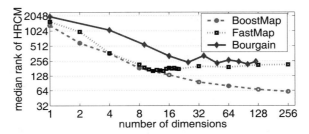

Figure 6.6 Median rank of HRCM, vs. number of dimensions, in approximate similarity rankings obtained using three different methods, for 703 queries to the hand database. For comparison, the median HRCM rank for the exact distance was 21.

ranks and median HRCM ranks for each data set, for different dimensions of BoostMap, FastMap and Bourgain embeddings. For the hand database, BoostMap gives significantly better results than the other two methods, for 16 or more dimensions. In the ASL database, BoostMap does either as well as FastMap or better than FastMap, in all dimensions. In both data sets, Bourgain embeddings overall do worse than BoostMap and FastMap.

With respect to Bourgain embeddings, we should mention that they are not quite appropriate for online queries, because they require evaluating too many distances in order to produce the embedding of a query. SparseMap [11] was formulated as a heuristic approximation of Bourgain embeddings that is appropriate for online queries. We have not implemented SparseMap but, based on its formulation, it would be a surprising result if SparseMap achieved higher accuracy than Bourgain embeddings.

6.6.1 Filter-and-refine Experiments

As described in subsection 6.3.3, we can use an embedding to perform filter-and-refine retrieval of nearest neighbors. The usefulness of an embedding in

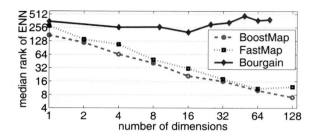

Figure 6.7 Median rank of ENN, vs. number of dimensions, in approximate similarity rankings obtained using three different methods, for 180 queries to the ASL database.

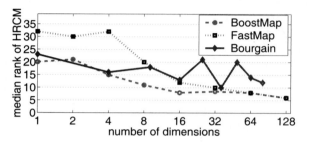

Figure 6.8 Median rank of HRCM, vs. number of dimensions, in approximate similarity rankings obtained using three different methods, for 180 queries to the ASL database. For comparison, the median HRCM rank for the exact distance was 3.

filter-and-refine retrieval depends on two questions: how often we successfully identify the nearest neighbors of a query, and how much the overall retrieval time is.

For both BoostMap and FastMap, we found the optimal combination of d (dimensionality of the embedding) and p (the number of candidate matches retained after the filter step) that would allow 1-NN retrieval to be correct 95% or 100% of the time, while minimizing retrieval time. Table 6.1 shows the optimal values of p and d, and the associated computational savings over standard nearest-neighbor retrieval, in which we evaluate the exact distance between the query and each database object. In both data sets, the bulk of retrieval time is spent computing exact distances in the original space. The time spent in computing distances in the Euclidean space is negligible, even for a 256D embedding. For the hand database, BoostMap leads to significantly faster retrieval, because we need to compute far fewer exact distances in the refine step, while achieving the same error rate as FastMap.

Table 6.1 Comparison of BoostMap, FastMap, and using brute-force search, for the purpose of retrieving the exact nearest neighbors successfully for 95% or 100% of the queries, using filter-and-refine retrieval. The letter d is the dimensionality of the embedding. The letter p stands for the number of top matches that we keep from the filter step (i.e., using the embeddings). D_X # per query is the total number of D_X computations needed per query, in order to embed the query and rank the top p candidates. The exact D_X column shows the results for brute-force search, in which we do not use a filter step, and we simply evaluate D_X distances between the query and all database images.

ENN retrieval accuracy and efficiency for hand database					
Method	BoostMap		FastMap		Exact D_X
ENN-accuracy	95%	100%	95%	100%	100%
Best d	256	256	13	10	N/A
Best p	406	3850	3838	17498	N/A
D_X # per query	823	4267	3864	17518	107328
seconds per query	2.3	10.6	9.4	42.4	260

ENN retrieval accuracy and efficiency for ASL database					
Method	BoostMap		FastMap		Exact D_X
ENN-accuracy	95%	100%	95%	100%	100%
Best d	64	64	64	32	N/A
Best p	129	255	141	334	N/A
D_X # per query	249	375	269	398	880
seconds per query	103	155	111	164	363

6.7   Discussion and Future Work

With respect to existing embedding methods, the main advantage of Boost-Map is that it is formulated as a classifier-combination problem that can take advantage of powerful machine learning techniques to assemble a high-accuracy embedding from many simple, 1D embeddings. The main disadvantage of our method, at least in the current implementation, is the running time of the training algorithm. However, in many applications, trading training time for embedding accuracy would be a desirable tradeoff. At the same time, we are interested in exploring ways to improve training time.

A possible extension of BoostMap is to use it to approximate not the actual distance between objects, but a hidden state space distance. For example, in our hand image data set, what we are really interested in is not retrieving images that are similar with respect to the chamfer distance, but images that actually have the same hand pose. We can modify the training labels Y provided to the training algorithm, so that instead of describing proximity with respect to the chamfer distance, they describe proximity with respect to actual hand pose. The resulting similarity rankings may be worse approximations of the chamfer distance rankings, but they may be better approximations of the actual pose-based rankings. A similar idea is described in Chapter 7, although in the context of a different approximate nearest-neighbor framework.

Acknowledgments

This research was funded in part by the U.S. National Science Foundation, under grants IIS-0208876, IIS-0308213, IIS-0329009, and CNS-0202067, and the U.S. Office of Naval Research, under grant N00014-03-1-0108.

References

1. V. Athitsos and S. Sclaroff. Estimating hand pose from a cluttered image. In *IEEE Conference on Computer Vision and Pattern Recognition*, volume 2, pages 432–439, 2003.

2. H.G. Barrow, J.M. Tenenbaum, R.C. Bolles, and H.C. Wolf. Parametric correspondence and chamfer matching: Two new techniques for image matching. In *International Joint Conference on Artificial Intelligence*, pages 659–663, 1977.

3. J. Bourgain. On Lipschitz embeddings of finite metric spaces in Hilbert space. *Israel Journal of Mathematics*, 52:46–52, 1985.

4. K. Chakrabarti and S. Mehrotra. Local dimensionality reduction: A new approach to indexing high dimensional spaces. In *International Conference on Very Large Data Bases*, pages 89–100, 2000.

5. T.J. Darrell, I.A. Essa, and A.P. Pentland. Task-specific gesture analysis in real-time using interpolated views. *IEEE Transactions on Pattern Analysis and Machine Intelligence*, 18(12), 1996.

6. A.A. Efros, A.C. Berg, G. Mori, and J. Malik. Recognizing action at a distance. In *IEEE International Conference on Computer Vision*, pages 726–733, 2003.

7. Ö. Egecioglu and H. Ferhatosmanoglu. Dimensionality reduction and similarity distance computation by inner product approximations. In *International Conference on Information and Knowledge Management*, pages 219–226, 2000.

8. C. Faloutsos and K.I. Lin. FastMap: A fast algorithm for indexing, data-mining and visualization of traditional and multimedia datasets. In *ACM SIGMOD International Conference on Management of Data*, pages 163–174, 1995.

9. A. Gionis, P. Indyk, and R. Motwani. Similarity search in high dimensions via hashing. In *International Conference on Very Large Databases*, pages 518–529, 1999.

10. G.R. Hjaltason and H. Samet. Properties of embedding methods for similarity searching in metric spaces. *IEEE Transactions on Pattern Analysis and Machine Intelligence*, 25(5):530–549, 2003.

11. G. Hristescu and M. Farach-Colton. Cluster-preserving embedding of proteins. Technical Report 99-50, CS Department, Rutgers University, 1999.

12. P. Indyk. *High-dimensional Computational Geometry*. PhD thesis, Stanford University, 2000.

13. K. V. R. Kanth, D. Agrawal, and A. Singh. Dimensionality reduction for similarity searching in dynamic databases. In *ACM SIGMOD International Conference on Management of Data*, pages 166–176, 1998.

14. Eamonn Keogh. Exact indexing of dynamic time warping. In *International Conference on Very Large Data Bases*, pages 406–417, 2002.

15. N. Koudas, B. C. Ooi, H. T. Shen, and A. K. H. Tung. Ldc: Enabling search by partial distance in a hyper-dimensional space. In *IEEE International Conference on Data Engineearing*, pages 6–17, 2004.

16. C. Li, E. Chang, H. Garcia-Molina, and G. Wiederhold. Clustering for approximate similarity search in high-dimensional spaces. *IEEE Transactions on Knowledge and Data Engineering*, 14(4):792–808, 2002.

17. N. Linial, E. London, and Y. Rabinovich. The geometry of graphs and some of its algorithmic applications. In *IEEE Symposium on Foundations of Computer Science*, pages 577–591, 1994.

18. S.T. Roweis and L.K. Saul. Nonlinear dimensionality reduction by locally linear embedding. *Science*, 290:2323–2326, 2000.

19. Y. Sakurai, M. Yoshikawa, S. Uemura, and H. Kojima. The a-tree: An index structure for high-dimensional spaces using relative approximation. In *International Conference on Very Large Data Bases*, pages 516–526, 2000.

20. R.E. Schapire and Y. Singer. Improved boosting algorithms using confidence-rated predictions. *Machine Learning*, 37(3):297–336, 1999.

21. G. Shakhnarovich, P. Viola, and T. Darrell. Fast pose estimation with parameter-sensitive hashing. In *IEEE International Conference on Computer Vision*, pages 750–757, 2003.

22. J.B. Tenenbaum, V. de Silva, and J.C. Langford. A global geometric framework for nonlinear dimensionality reduction. *Science*, 290:2319–2323, 2000.

23. E. Tuncel, H. Ferhatosmanoglu, and K. Rose. Vq-index: An index structure for similarity searching in multimedia databases. In *Proc. of ACM Multimedia*, pages 543–552, 2002.

24. P. Viola and M. Jones. Rapid object detection using a boosted cascade of simple features. In *IEEE Conference on Computer Vision and Pattern Recognition*, volume 1, pages 511–518, 2001.

25. M. Vlachos, M. Hadjieleftheriou, D. Gunopulos, and E.J. Keogh. Indexing multi-dimensional time-series with support for multiple

distance measures. In *ACM SIGKDD International Conference on Knowledge Discovery and Data Mining*, pages 216–225, 2003.

26. X. Wang, J.T.L. Wang, K.I. Lin, D. Shasha, B.A. Shapiro, and K. Zhang. An index structure for data mining and clustering. *Knowledge and Information Systems*, 2(2):161–184, 2000.

27. R. Weber and K. Bohm. Trading quality for time with nearest-neighbor search. In *International Conference on Extending Database Technology: Advances in Database Technology*, pages 21–35, 2000.

28. R. Weber, H.-J. Schek, and S. Blott. A quantitative analysis and performance study for similarity-search methods in high-dimensional spaces. In *International Conference on Very Large Data Bases*, pages 194–205, 1998.

29. D.A. White and R. Jain. Similarity indexing: Algorithms and performance. In *Storage and Retrieval for Image and Video Databases (SPIE)*, pages 62–73, 1996.

30. B.-K. Yi, H. V. Jagadish, and C. Faloutsos. Efficient retrieval of similar time sequences under time warping. In *IEEE International Conference on Data Engineering*, pages 201–208, 1998.

31. F.W. Young and R.M. Hamer. *Multidimensional Scaling: History, Theory and Applications*. Lawrence Erlbaum Associates, Hillsdale, New Jersey, 1987.

32. P. Zezula, P. Savino, G. Amato, and F. Rabitti. Approximate similarity retrieval with m-trees. *International Journal on Very Large Data Bases*, 4:275–293, 1998.

III APPLICATIONS: VISION

7   Parameter-Sensitive Hashing for Fast Pose Estimation

Gregory Shakhnarovich, Paul Viola, and Trevor Darrell

Example-based methods are most effective for parameter estimation problems when a large number of labeled examples is availabe, and a similarity measure appropriate for the domain at hand is defined. However, this is precisely the scenario in which the computational complexity of similarity search often makes example-based estimation prohibitively expensive. This is further complicated for high-dimensional domains, such as the articulated human pose. We introduce an approach to learning an embedding of the data into a space where a simple metric distance reflects the desired similarity notion. As a result we can apply locality-sensitive hashing in the embedding space to produce

7.1   Introduction

Many problems in computer vision can be naturally formulated as parameter estimation problems: given an image or a video sequence $\mathbf{x}$, we estimate the parameters θ of a model describing the scene or the object of interest. Here we focus on perhaps the most common problem of this type–the estimation of the configuration of an articulated body. Other examples of such tasks include estimating the contraction of muscles in the face, or the orientation of a rigid object.

Model-based approaches to estimation rely on fitting a model to the input-parameter relationship, which is typically parametric. In contrast, example-based methods capitalize on the availability of a large set of examples for which the parameter values are known: they infer the parameter values for the input from the known values in similar examples. This does not require modeling the global structure of the input-parameter relationship, which is only assumed to be sufficiently smooth to make such inference meaningful. Nearest-neighbor regression 1 and loclaly-weighted regression 5 are well-known instances of this family. However, the computational complexity of similarity search used by these methods in high-dimensional spaces and on very large data sets has made them infeasible for many vision problems. A feasible solution is to resort to approximate similarity search, and apply methods such as LSH. However, this limits the similarity measure to a metric, which may not be expressive or efficient enough.

In this chapter we describe a new example-based algorithm for fast parameter estimation using local models, which are dynamically built for each new input image. We overcome the problem of computational complexity with a recently developed algorithm for fast approximate similarity search, locality-sensitive hashing (LSH) [11]. The training examples are indexed by a number of hash tables, such that the probability of collision is large for examples similar in their parameters and small for dissimilar ones. For practical problems, such as pose estimation, good results can be achieved with a speedup factor of 10^3 to 10^4 over an exhaustive search in a database as large as 10^6 examples.

Our approach is motivated by the following intuitition: What one really wants is to base the estimate on examples similar to the input *in their parameter values*. In other words, we would like to find in the database examples poses that are close to the underlying pose in the input image. Of course we can not measure such similarity directly since this pose in the input image is precisely what we need to estimate! Instead, we will use a *proxy* similarity, measured in a space where distances are closely related to this target pose similarity. In order to

Consequently, we will have to change the definition of lacolity-snsitive functions on p. 1.5 to the following definition of a *parameter-sensitive* family over the data space $\mathcal{X}$. Let p_1, p_2 be probability values and S be the similarity function, such that $S(\mathbf{x}_1, \mathbf{x}_2) = +1$ if the poses in $\mathbf{x}_1$ and $\mathbf{x}_2$ are similar and -1 otherwise. A family $\mathcal{H}$ of functions $h : \mathcal{X} \rightarrow \{0, 1\}$ is (p_1, p_2, S)-sensitive if, for any $h \in \mathcal{H}$,

$$\mathrm{P}_{\mathbf{x},\mathbf{y}\sim \ p(\mathcal{X})^2}(h(\mathbf{x}) = h(\mathbf{y}) \mid S(\mathbf{x}, \mathbf{y}) = +1) \ \geq \ p_1, \qquad (7.1)$$

$$\mathrm{P}_{\mathbf{x},\mathbf{y}\sim \ p(\mathcal{X})^2}(h(\mathbf{x}) = h(\mathbf{y}) \mid S(\mathbf{x}, \mathbf{y}) = -1) \ \leq \ p_2. \qquad (7.2)$$

Note that, in contrast to the definition in chapter 1, the probabilities here are over random choice of *data* rather than functions. This formulation leads to parameter-sensitive hashing (PSH), a modification of LSH in which the bits that form hash functions are sampled from this family $\mathcal{H}$. When $\mathcal{H}$ contains M functions, this is equivalent to *embedding* the data into an M-dimensional binary space, in which distance are measured with L_1, and applying the standard LSH.

The key problem in this approach is the construction of $\mathcal{H}$. In this chapter we describe a learning algorithm that selects the functions in $\mathcal{H}$ through a feature selection process, based on a set of examples of images with similar and dissimilar poses. A set of pose-labeled images is indexed using PSH bases on the so learned family of functions. The pose estimate for a new image is produced by *robust LWR* which uses the approximate neighbors

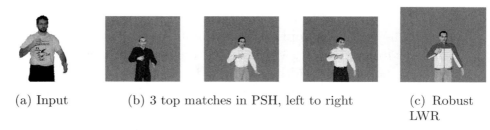

(a) Input   (b) 3 top matches in PSH, left to right   (c) Robust LWR

Figure 7.1 Pose estimation with parameter-sensitive hashing and local regression.

found by PSH to dynamically build a simple model of the neighborhood of the input. Our approach is schematically illustrated in figure 7.1.

The remainder of this chapter is organized as follows. Previous work is reviewed in section 7.2; it includes a brief overview of example-based estimation, a more detailed discussion of which was given in chapter 1. The PSH algorithm is presented in section 7.3 (the algorithm for constructing efficient hash functions is described in 7.3.1). We evaluate our framework on an articulated pose estimation problem: estimating the pose of a human upper body from a single image. The details of the task and our experiments are described in Section 7.4. We conclude and discuss some open questions in section 7.5.

7.2 Background and Previous Work

The body of literature on object parameter estimation from a single image, and in particular on estimating the pose of articulated bodies, is very large, and space constraints force us to mention only work most related to our approach.

In [18] a three-dimensional pose is recovered from the 2D projections of a number of known feature points on an articulated body. Other efficient algorithms for matching articulated patterns are given in [9, 16]. These approaches assume that detectors are available for specific feature locations, and that a global model of the articulation is available. In [15] a "shape context" feature vector is used to represent general contour shape. In [17], the mapping of a silhouette to a 3D pose is learned using multiview training data. These techniques were successful, but they were restricted to contour features and generally unable to use appearance within a silhouette.

Finally, in [1] a hand image is matched to a large database of rendered forms, using a sophisticated similarity measure on image features. This work is most similar to ours and in part inspired our approach. However, the complexity of nearest-neighbor search makes this approach difficult to apply to the very large numbers of examples needed for general articulated pose estimation with image-based distance metrics. Our goal is to alleviate this by employing the fast approximate search mechanism of PSH.

7.2.1   Example-Based Estimation

The task of example-based parameter estimation in vision can be formulated as follows. Input, which consists of image features (e.g., edge map, vector of responses of a filter set, or edge direction histograms) computed on the original image, is assumed to be generated by an unknown parametric process $\mathbf{x} = f(\theta)$. In our context of articulated pose, θ is a vector of joint angles. A training set of labeled examples $(\mathbf{x}_1, \theta_1), \dots, (\mathbf{x}_N, \theta_N)$ is provided. One must estimate θ_0 as the inverse of f for a novel input $\mathbf{x}_0$. The objective is to minimize the residual in terms of the distance (similarity measure) d_θ in the parameter space. Thus, we are facing a regression problem.

Methods based on nearest neighbors are among the oldest techniques for such estimation. The *k-NN estimate* [7] is obtained by averaging the values for the k training examples most similar to the input:

$$\hat{\theta}_{NN} = \frac{1}{k} \sum_{\mathbf{x}_i \in \text{neighborhood}} \theta_i \,, \qquad (7.3)$$

i.e., the target function is approximated by a constant in each neighborhood defined by k. This estimate is known to be consistent, and to asymptotically achieve Bayes-optimal risk under many loss functions [7]. Note that similarity (neighborhood) is defined in terms of the distance d_X in the input space.

A natural extension to k-NN, in which the neighbors are weighted according to their similarity to the query point, leads to *locally weighted regression* (LWR) [5, 2]: the target function is approximated locally (within any small region) by a function from a particular model class $g(\mathbf{x}; \vec{\beta})$. The parameters $\vec{\beta}$ are chosen to optimize the weighted learning criterion in the test input $\mathbf{x}_0$,

$$\vec{\beta}^* = \underset{\vec{\beta}}{\text{argmin}} \sum_{\mathbf{x}_i \in \text{neighborhood}} d_\theta \left(g(\mathbf{x}_i; \vec{\beta}), \theta_i \right) K \left(d_X(\mathbf{x}_i, \mathbf{x}_0) \right), \qquad (7.4)$$

where K is the *kernel* function that determines the weight falloff with increasing distance from the query point.

In *robust* LWR [4], the influence of outliers is diminished through a short iterative process. In each iteration after the model is fit, the neighborhood points are reweighted so that points with higher residual with respect to the fitted values become less influential.

There are two major problems with the straightforward application of example-based methods to parameter estimation in vision. The first is the computational complexity of the existing nearest-neighbor search algorithms, particularly in the high-dimensional spaces often encountered in vision tasks. Using fast approximate algorithms may overcome this obstacle. The idea of using approximate nearest-neighbor has been mentioned in previous work for object or texture classification [3, 10], and for some estimation tasks [14, 1]. However to our knowledge, no experiments using recent algorithms for estimation tasks have been conducted.

The second problem, not immediately solved by adopting an efficient similarity search algorithm, is the reliance of the search on the input space metric d_X, without explicitly taking into account d_θ. We will show how to explicitly select a feature subspace in which d_X approximates d_θ, without an explicit global model of this relationship. The data, training examples as well as new test examples, are embedded into this space. The approximate near neighbors with respect to L_1 distance in this space are of much higher relevance that neighbors retrieved using metric distance in the original data space.

7.3 Estimation with Parameter-Sensitive Hashing

Let $(\mathbf{x}_1, \theta_1), \ldots, (\mathbf{x}_N, \theta_N)$ be the training examples with their associated parameter values. An example is represented by a feature vector $\mathbf{x} = [x^1, \ldots, x^D]$, where x^j is computed by a scalar-valued function ϕ_j on the input image, such as a filter response at a certain location or a bin count in an edge direction histogram in a certain region. We assume the following:

1. A distance function d_θ is given which measures similarity between parameter vectors, and a radius R in the parameter space is given such that θ_1, θ_2 are considered *similar* if and only if $d_\theta(\theta_1, \theta_2) < R$.

2. The training examples are representative of the problem space, i.e., for a randomly drawn example there exists, with high probability, an example with similar parameter values.

3. The process that generates the examples is unbiased, or it is possible to correct for such bias.

The distance function and the similarity threshold are dependent on the particular task, and often reflect perceptual similarities between the scenes or objects.

The second assumption may appear a bit vague, and in fact its precise meaning depends on the nature of the problem. If we control the example generation process, we can attempt to "fill" the space, storing an example in every node on an R-grid in parameter space. This becomes infeasible very quickly as the dimension of θ increases. Alternatively, it has been often observed or conjectured [13, 19] that images of many real-world phenomena do not fill the space uniformly, but rather belong to an intrinsically low-dimensional manifold, and densely covering that manifold is enough to ensure this property.

The last assumption implies that there are no significant sources of variation in the examples besides the variation in the parameters, or that the contribution of such sources can be accounted for. While perhaps limiting, this is possible to comply with in many vision problems, either explicitly, by normalizing the examples, or implicitly, e.g., by using features invariant with respect to the "nuisance" parameters.

7.3.1   Parameter-Sensitive Hash Functions

Consider a two-bin hash table based on a binary-valued hashing function h. Let $p_1(h)$ and $p_2(h)$ be the probabilities of collision for similar or different examples, respectively: Recall from chapter 3 that a family of hash functions $\mathcal{H}$ is useful when, averaged over $h \in \mathcal{H}$, $p_2(h)$ is low and $p_1(h)$ is high. In [11] quantities like p_1 and p_2, that characterize the entire family, are derived for the task of finding neighbors in the input space. In our modified definitions, these quantities characterize each given hash function. For the parameter estimation task, where the goal is to find neighbors in the unknown parameter space, analytic derivation of $p_1(h)$ and $p_2(h)$ is infeasible since h is a measurement in the input (not parameter) domain. Instead, we will estimate these from data.

We can show that $p_1(h)$ and $p_2(h)$ have an intuitive interpretation in the context of the following classification problem. Let us assign to each possible pair of examples $(\mathbf{x}_i, \mathbf{x}_j)$ the label

$$y_{ij} = \begin{cases} +1 \text{ if } d_\theta(\theta_i, \theta_j) < r, \\ -1 \text{ if } d_\theta(\theta_i, \theta_j) > R, \\ \text{not defined otherwise,} \end{cases} \qquad (7.5)$$

where $r = R/(1 + \epsilon)$. Note that we do not define the label for the "gray area" of similarity between r and R, in order to conform to the definition of locality sensitive fuctions.

We can now formulate a classification task related to these labels. A binary hash function h either has a collision $h(\mathbf{x}_i) = h(\mathbf{x}_j)$ or not; we say that h predicts the label

$$\hat{y}_h(\mathbf{x}_i, \mathbf{x}_j) = \begin{cases} +1 \text{ if } h(\mathbf{x}_i) = h(\mathbf{x}_j) \quad \text{(collision)}, \\ -1 \text{ otherwise.} \end{cases} \qquad (7.6)$$

Thus, when h is interpreted as a classifier, $p_2(h)$ is the probability of a false positive $P(\hat{y}_{ij} = +1 | y_{ij} = -1)$. Similarly, $p_1(h)$ is the probability of a true negative. Such a *paired problem* set can be built from our training set of images labeled with poses, since we know d_θ, r, R.

Our goal, in learning a distance on images "faithful" to the pose similarity, is to find h's that are similarity sensitive in terms of (7.1). A reasonable objective that achieves this goal is to maximize the *gap* between the true positive and the false positive rate of h as a classifier on this paired classification problem; we have thus reduced our task to a feature selection task standard in machine learning.

One should be careful about two things when constructing the paired problem. First, one must not include pairs with similarity within the "gray area" between r and R, in order to allow for more efficient learning. Second, we should take into account the asymmetry of the classification task: there are many more negative examples among possible pairs than there are positive. Consequently, in order to represent the negative examples appropriately, we may need to include many more of them in the paired problem.

An alternative approach to dealing with this asymmety has been recently proposed [12]: under the assumptions that similar pairs are very rare (affirmed by our experiments in the pose domain, as described below), and that the expected rate of examples similar to any given example is roughly uniform, one can forgo sampling the negative examples alltogether. Instead, the expected false positive rate can be estimated in the following way. For a given feature ϕ and a threshold T, let π be the estimated probability of the event $\phi(\mathbf{x}) \leq T$. For a single (unpaired) data point $\mathbf{x}_i$, suppose, without loss of generality, that $\phi(\mathbf{x}_i) \leq T$. Now consider a pair formed by randomly selecting another example $\mathbf{x}_j$ and joining it with $\mathbf{x}_i$. With probability $P_{\phi,T} = \pi^2 + (1-\pi)^2$, this pair will be classified as positive by the function h parametrized by ϕ and T. Under the assumptions stated above, this random pair (and any random pair!) is with very high probability negative, i.e., dissimilar. Thus, the probability $P_{\phi,T}$ is a reasonable estimate of the false positive rate of h. This estimate of the probability mass over a one dimensional variable $\phi(\mathbf{x})$ is easily obtained as long as some unlabeled data points are available. In the experiments below, we have compared this approach to explicitly sampling large amounts of negative examples, and found that the results obtained with the two approaches are essentially identical, while the latter sampling-based estimation is significantly more time consuming.

The exact nature of the hash functions h will of course affect the feature selection algorithm. Here we consider h which are decision stumps:

$$h_{\phi,T}(\mathbf{x}) = \begin{cases} +1 \text{ if } \phi(\mathbf{x}) \geq T, \\ -1 \text{ otherwise,} \end{cases} \tag{7.7}$$

where $\phi(\mathbf{x})$ is a real-valued image function and T is a threshold. Algorithm 7.1 is the procedure that for a given ϕ finds the optimal T in two passes over the paired training set. Intuitively, it tries all possible distinct thresholds and counts the number of negative examples that are assigned the same hash value, as well as the number of positive examples that are assigned the same value. The former serves as an (unnormalized) estimate of the false positive rate $p_2(h)$; the latter, of the true positive rate p_1. Since examples are sorted by the feature value, these quantities can be updated with little work. The threshold T_{best} is the one that minimizes the gap between the two.

```
Require:  Feature φ;
Require:  Set of pairs X̃ = (x_{i_n}, x_{j_n}, y_n)_{n=1}^N, where y_n ∈ {±1} is the
   similarity label.
   Start with an empty array A.
   N_p := number of positive pairs;
   N_n := number of negative pairs (N_n + N_p = N).
   for n = 1 to N do
      v_1 := φ(x_{i_n}), v_2 = φ(x_{j_n})
      l_1 := 1 if v_{i_n} > v_{j_n}, 0 otherwise
      l_2 := -l_1
      A := A ∪ {< v_1, l_1, n >, < v_2, l_2, n >}
   end for
   /*At this point A has 2N elements. Each paired example is
   represented twice. /*
   Sort A by the values of v
   S_p := S_n := 0
   /*g is the best gap p̂_1 - p̂_2 for φ */
   g_best := 0
   for k = 1 to 2N do
     Let < v, l, n >= A[k]
     if y_n = +1 then
        S_p := S_p - l
     else if y_n = -1 then
        S_n := S_n - l
     end if
     g := (N_p - S_p) - (N_n - S_n)
     if g > g_best then
        g_best := g; T_best := v
     end if
   end for
```

Algorithm 7.1   Algorithm for evaluating potential hash functions based on axis-parallel decision stumps (see 7.3). The algorithm returns the threshold T_{best} that attains the maximal gap between the estimated true positive rate and the estimated false positive rate.

The family $\mathcal{H}$ of parameter-sensitive hash functions can now be constructed by selecting only $h_{\phi,T}$ for which $p_1(h_{\phi,T})$ and $p_2(h_{\phi,T})$ evaluated on the paired problem satisfy the desired thresholds.

7.3.2   Similarity Search

After $\mathcal{H}$ is selected, we project the data on only those feature dimensions ϕ for which $h_{\phi,T} \in \mathcal{H}$, obtain binary representation for our data by applying (7.7) and select k and l. We then build the l hash tables. For an unlabeled input, LSH is used to query the database rapidly, and finds the union of the l hash buckets, $X' = \bigcup_{j=1}^{l} g_j(\mathbf{x}_0)$. Let M be the number of distinct points in X'; with high probability $M \ll N$ (if $M = 0$ the algorithm terminates in failure mode). X' is exhaustively searched to produce the K (r, ϵ)-NN $\mathbf{x}'_1, \ldots, \mathbf{x}'_K$, ordered by increasing $d_X(\mathbf{x}'_i, \mathbf{x}_0)$, with parameters $\theta'_1, \ldots, \theta'_K$. The estimate is based on these points, which, with high probability, belong to an approximate neighborhood of $\mathbf{x}_0$ both in the parameter and in the input spaces.

7.3.3 Local Regression

The simplest way to proceed is by the (single) nearest-neighbor rule, that is, to return θ'_1 as the answer. There are two problems with this. First θ'_1 can be up to R away from the true parameter of the input, θ_0. Often, the R for which it is feasible to satisfy the representativeness property mentioned above is too large to make this an acceptable solution (see figure 7.4 for examples). The second problem is caused by our inability to directly measure $d_\theta(\theta_0, \theta)$; the search relies on the properties of LSHF, and on the monotonicity of d_X with respect to d_θ, which are usually not perfect. We need a robust estimate based on the approximate neighborhood found by PSH.

A possible way of achieving this is by using the k-NN estimate as a starting point of a gradient descent search [1]. Alternatively, active learning can be used to refine the "map" of the neighborhood [6]. Both approaches, however, require an explicit generative model of $p(\mathbf{x}|\theta)$, or an "oracle," which for a given value of θ generates an example to be matched to $\mathbf{x}_0$. While in some cases it is possible (e.g., with animation software which would render objects with a given pose), we would like to avoid such a limitation.

Instead, we use robust LWR to avoid overfitting; since we expect the number of neighbors to be small, we consider constant or linear model, which can be easily fit with weighted least squares. The model order and the kernel bandwidth, as well as the number of iterations of reweighting, can be chosen based on validation set.

7.4 Pose Estimation with PSH

We applied our algorithm to the problem of recovering the articulated pose of a human upper body. The model has 13 degrees of freedom (DOF): one DOF for orientation, namely the rotation angle of the torso around the vertical axis, and 12 DOFs in rotational joints (2 in each clavicle, 3 in each shoulder, and 1 in each elbow). We do not assume constant illumination or fixed poses for other body parts in the upper body (head and hands), and therefore need to represent the variation in these and other nuisance parameters, such as clothing and hairstyle, in our training set.

For this application, it is important to separate the problem of object detection from that of pose estimation. Given simple backgrounds and a stationary camera, body detection and localization are not difficult. In the

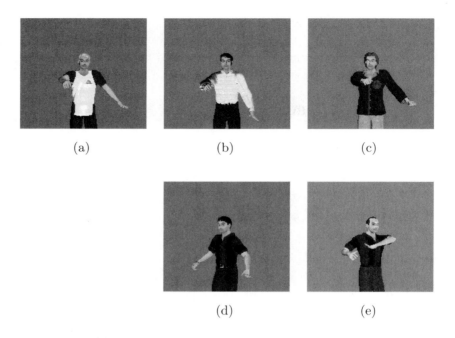

Figure 7.2 Positive and negative paired examples. For each image in (b)–(e), the ±1 label of the pair formed with (a) is based on the distance d_θ to the underlying parameters of (a), with similarity threshold $r = 0.25$.

experiments reported here, it is assumed that the body has been segmented from the background, scaled, and centered in the image. For more difficult scenarios, a more complex object detection system may be required.

Input images are represented in our experiments by *multi-scale edge direction histograms*. Edges are detected using the Sobel operator and each edge pixel is classified into one of four direction bins: $\pi/8, 3\pi/8, 5\pi/8, 7\pi/8$. Then, the histograms of direction bins are computed within sliding square windows of varying sizes (8, 16, 32 pixels) placed at multiple locations in the image. The feature space consists of the concatenated values of all of the histograms. We chose this representation, often used in image analysis and retrieval, because it is largely invariant to some of the nuisance parameters with respect to pose, such as illumination and color.

The training set consisted of 500,000 images rendered from a humanoid model using POSER [8], with parameter values sampled independently and uniformly within anatomically feasible ranges; the torso orientation is constrained to the range $[-90^o, 90^o]$. Each training image is 180×200 pixels. In our model, all angles are constrained to $[-\pi, \pi]$, so as a similarity measure we use

$$d_\theta(\theta_1, \theta_2) = \sum_{i=1}^{m} 1 - \cos(\theta_1^i - \theta_2^i) \qquad (7.8)$$

where m is the dimension of the parameter space (number of joint angles), and θ_j^i is the i-th component of θ_j. We found that this distance function, while not perfect, usually reflects our perception of pose similarity (see figure 7.2 for examples).

After examining large numbers of images corresponding to poses with various distances, we set $r = 0.25$ and $\epsilon = 1$. An LSH query is therefore considered successful if it returns examples within $R = 0.5$ of the input, using (7.8) as a distance between poses. Analysis of the distribution of d_θ over pairs of training examples reveals that only about 0.05% of the pairs constitute a positive example by this criterion (the distribution appears to be roughly log-normal). Figure 7.2 shows four of 1,775,000 paired examples used to select hash functions; out of 11,270 features, 219 hash functions were selected for which the gap between $p_1(h)$ and $p_2(h)$ is at least 0.25. Based on validation set performance, PSH was implemented with 80 hash tables using 19-bit hash functions.

Model	$k = 7$	$k = 12$	$k = 50$
k-NN	0.882 (0.39)	0.844 (0.36)	0.814 (0.31)
Linear	0.957 (0.47)	0.968 (0.49)	1.284 (0.69)
Const LWR	0.882 (0.39)	0.843 (0.36)	0.810 (0.31)
Linear LWR	0.885 (0.40)	0.843 (0.36)	0.808 (0.31)
Robust const LWR	0.930 (0.49)	0.825 (0.41)	0.755 (0.32)
robust linear LWR	1.029 (0.56)	0.883 (0.46)	0.738 (0.33)

Table 7.1 Mean estimation error for synthetic test data, over 1000 examples. Standard deviation shown in parentheses. Not shown are the baseline error of 1-NN, 1.614 (0.88), and of the exact 1-NN based on the input distance, 1.659.

To quantitatively evaluate the algorithm's performance, we tested it on 1000 synthetic images, generated from the same model. Table 7.1 summarized the results with different methods of fitting a local model; "linear" refers to a non-weighted linear model fit to the neighborhood, "constant" refers to a zeroth order model (weighted average). On average PSH searched 5100 candidates, about 3.4% of the data, per input example; in almost all cases, the true nearest neighbors under d_X were also the top PSH candidates.

The results confirm some intuitive expectations. As the number of approximate neighbors used to construct the local model increases, the non-weighted model suffers from outliers, while the LWR model improves; the gain is especially high for the robust LWR. Since higher-order models require more examples for a good fit, the order-1 LWR only becomes better for large neighborhood sizes. Although the differences between models that rely on multiple neighbors were not statistically significant, there is a clear trend that reflects consistent superiority of LWR models. In particular, note

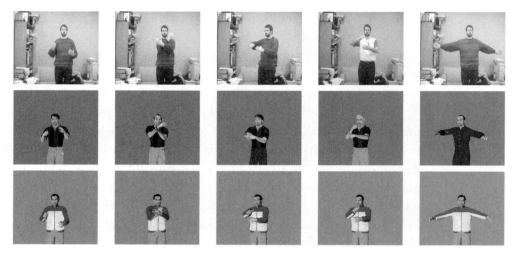

Figure 7.3 Examples of upper body pose estimation (see section 7.4). Top row: input images. Middle row: top PSH match. Bottom row: robust constant LWR estimate based on 12 NN. Note that the images in the bottom row are not in the training database - these are rendered only to illustrate the pose estimate obtained by LWR.

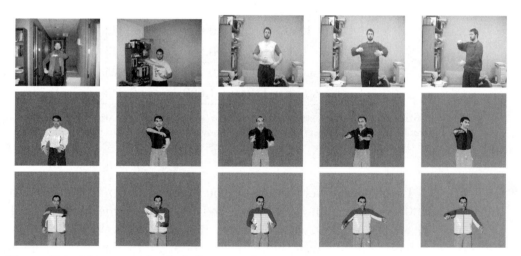

Figure 7.4 More examples, including typical "errors". In the leftmost column, the gross error in the top match is corrected by LWR. The rightmost two columns show various degrees of error in estimation.

that the robust linear LWR with 50-NN is on average more than twice better than the baseline 1-NN estimator.

We also tested the algorithm on 800 images of a real person; images were processed by a simple segmentation and alignment program. Figure 7.3 shows a few examples of pose estimation on real images. Note that the results in the bottom row are not images from the database, but a visualization of the pose estimated with robust linear LWR on 12-NN found by PSH; we used a Gaussian kernel with the bandwidth set to the median distance to the neighbors. In some cases (e.g., leftmost column in figure 7.4), there is a dramatic improvement vs. the estimate based on the single NN.

The number of candidates examined by PSH was, as expected, significantly lower than for the synthetic images–about 2000, or 1.3% of the database. It takes an unoptimized Matlab program less than 2 seconds to produce the pose estimate. This is a dramatic improvement over searching the entire database for the exact nearest-neighbor, which takes more than 2 minutes per query, and in most cases produces the same top matches as the PSH.

Lacking ground truth for these images, we rely on visual inspection of the pose for evaluation. For most of the examples the pose estimate was accurate; on some examples it failed to various extents. Figures 7.3 and 7.4 show a number of examples, including two definite failures. Note that in some cases the approximate nearest neighbor is a poor pose estimate, while robust LWR yields a good fit. We believe that there are three main sources of failure: significant mismatch between d_θ and d_X; imperfect segmentation and alignment; and the limitations of the training set, in terms of coverage and representativeness of the problem domain.

7.5 Summary and Conclusions

We present an algorithm that uses new hashing-based search techniques to rapidly find relevant examples in a large database of image data, and estimates the parameters for the input using a local model learned from those examples. Experiments show that our estimation method, based on PSH and robust LWR, is successful on the task of articulated pose estimation from static input. These experiments also demonstrate the usefulness of synthetically created data for learning and estimation.

In addition to the use of local regression to refine the estimate, our work differs from that of others, e.g., [1, 14], in that it allows accurate estimation when examining only a fraction of a data set. The running time of our algorithm is sublinear; in our experiments we observed a speedup of almost two orders of magnitude relative to the exhaustive exact nearest-neighbor search, reducing the time to estimate pose from an image from minutes to under two seconds without adversely affecting the accuracy. We expect an optimized version of the system to run at real-time speed. This has the potential of making previously infeasible example-based estimation paradigms attractive for such tasks.

There are many interesting questions that remain open. The learning algorithm, presented in 7.3.1, implicitly assumes independence between the features; we are exploring more sophisticated feature selection methods that would account for possible dependencies. Moreover, it should be pointed out that there exist fast algorithms for approximate similarity search other than LSH. It remains an open question whether those algorithms can be modified for parameter sensitivity and become useful for estimation tasks in vision, replacing LSH in our framework.

Finally, as we mentioned earlier, the presented framework is not specific to pose; we intend to investigate its use in other parameter estimation tasks.

Acknowledgments

This work were carried out in MIT Visual Interfaces Group, supported in part by DARPA, Project Oxygen, NTT, Ford, CMI, and ITRI, and in Mitsubishi Electric Research Laboratories.

References

1. V. Athitsos and S. Sclaroff. Estimating 3D Hand Pose from a Cluttered Image. In *IEEE Conf. on Computer Vision and Pattern Recognition*, pages 432–439, Madison, WI, June 2003.

2. C. G. Atkeson, A. W. Moore, and S. Schaal. Locally weighted learning. *Artificial Intelligence Review*, 11(1-5):11–73, 1997.

3. J. S. Beis and D. G. Lowe. Shape indexing using approximate nearest-neighbour search in high-dimensional space. In *IEEE Conf. on Computer Vision and Pattern Recognition*, pages 1000–1006, San Juan, PR, June 1997.

4. W. S. Cleveland. Robust locally weighted regression and smoothing scatter plots. *Journal of American Statistical Association*, 74(368):829–836, 1979.

5. W. S. Cleveland and S. J. Delvin. Locally weighted regression: an approach to regression analysis by local fitting. *Journal of American Statistical Association*, 83(403):596–610, 1988.

6. D. A. Cohn, Z. Ghahramani, and M. I. Jordan. Active learning with statistical models. *J. Artificial Intelligence Research*, 4:129–145, 1996.

7. T. M. Cover. Estimation by the nearest neighbor rule. *IEEE Transactions on Information Theory*, 14:21–27, January 1968.

8. Curious Labs, Inc., Santa Cruz, CA. *Poser 5 - Reference Manual*, 2002.

9. P. Felzenszwalb and D. Huttenlocher. Efficient matching of pictorial structures. In *IEEE Conf. on Computer Vision and Pattern Recognition*, pages 66–75, Los Alamitos, June 13–15 2000. IEEE.

10. B. Georgescu, I. Shimshoni, and P. Meer. Mean shift based clustering in high dimnensions: A texture classification example. In *International Conference on Computer Vision*, 2003.

11. A. Gionis, P. Indyk, and R. Motwani. Similarity search in high dimensions via hashing. In *Proceedings of the 25th International Conference on Very Large Data Bases (VLDB '99)*, pages 518–529, San Francisco, September 1999. Morgan Kaufmann.

12. Y. Ke, D. Hoiem, and R. Sukthankar. Computer vision for music identification. In *IEEE Conf. on Computer Vision and Pattern Recognition*, San Diego, CA, June 2005.

13. B. Moghaddam and A. Pentland. Probabilistic visual learning for object representation. *IEEE Transactions on Pattern Analysis and Machine Intelligence*, 19(7):696–710, 1997.

14. G. Mori, S. Belongie, and J. Malik. Shape contexts enable efficient retrieval of similar shapes. In *IEEE Conf. on Computer Vision and Pattern Recognition*, pages 723–730, Lihue, HI, 2001.

15. G. Mori and J. Malik. Estimating Human Body Configurations using Shape Context Matching. In *European Conference on Computer Vision*, pages 666–680, 2002.

16. R. Ronfard, C. Schmid, and B. Triggs. Learning to parse pictures of people. In *European Conference on Computer Vision*, Copenhagen, Denmark, 2002.

17. R. Rosales and S. Sclaroff. Specialized mappings and the estimation of body pose from a single image. In *IEEE Human Motion Workshop*, pages 19–24, Austin, TX, 2000.

18. C. J. Taylor. Reconstruction of articulated objects from point correspondences in a single uncalibrated image. *Computer Vision and Image Understanding*, 80(3):349–363, December 2000.

19. Y. Wu, J. Y. Lin, and T. S. Huang. Capturing natural hand articulation. In *International Conference on Computer Vision*, pages 426–432, Vancouver, BC, 2001.

8   Contour Matching Using Approximate Earth Mover's Distance

Kristen Grauman and Trevor Darrell

A shape may be represented by a set of local features, and the correspondences produced by the minimum cost matching between the two discrete feature distributions often reveal how similar the underlying shapes are. However, due to the complexity of computing the exact minimum cost matching, previous correspondence-based algorithms could only run efficiently with a limited number of features per example, and could not scale to perform retrievals from large databases. We present a matching algorithm that quickly computes a minimal cost correspondence field between sets of descriptive local contour features using a recently introduced low-distortion embedding of the Earth Mover's Distance (EMD) into a normed space. Given a novel embedded shape, the approximate nearest neighbors in a database of embedded examples are retrieved in time sublinear in the number of examples via Locality-Sensitive Hashing (LSH). We demonstrate our method on large databases of human figure contours and images of handwritten digits.

8.1   Introduction

The ability to measure the similarity between shapes has wide application in tasks such as object recognition, content-based image retrieval, and automatic video analysis. A shape may be represented by a set (or bag) of local features, such as a set of local histograms collected from its contour or edge points. The minimum cost of matching the local image features of one object to the features of another often reveals how similar the two objects are. The cost of matching two features may be defined as how dissimilar they are in spatial location, appearance, curvature, or orientation; the minimal weight matching is the correspondence field between the two sets of features that requires the least summed cost. A number of successful shape matching algorithms and distance measures require the computation of minimal cost correspondences between sets of features on two shapes (see [2, 19, 9, 7, 3]).

Unfortunately, computing the optimal matching for a single comparison has a complexity that is cubic in the number of features. The complexity is of course magnified when one wishes to search for similar examples ("neighbors") in a large database: a linear scan of the database would require computing a comparison of cubic complexity for each database member against the query. Hierarchical search methods, pruning, or the triangle inequality may be employed, yet query times are still linear in the size of the database in the worst case, and individual comparisons maintain their high complexity regardless.

To address the computational complexity of current correspondence-based matching algorithms, we propose a contour matching algorithm that incorporates recently developed approximation techniques and enables fast shape-based similarity retrieval from large databases. We treat contour matching as a graph matching problem, and use the Earth Mover's Distance (EMD)—the minimum cost that is necessary to transform one weighted point set into another—as a metric of similarity. We embed the minimum weight matching of contour features into L_1 via an EMD embedding, and then employ approximate nearest-neighbor search to retrieve the shapes that are most similar to a novel query. The embedding step alone reduces the complexity of computing a low-cost correspondence field to $O(nd \log \Delta)$, where n is the number of features, d is their dimension, and Δ is the diameter of the feature space (i.e., the greatest inter-feature distance).

For further efficiency, we introduce a low-dimensional shape descriptor subspace based on the shape context feature of [2], and successfully use it within the proposed approximate EMD shape matching method. Using many examples of high-dimensional local edge point histograms taken from shapes in a database, we construct a subspace that captures much of the descriptive power of the rich features, yet allows us to represent them compactly.

We demonstrate our contour matching method on databases of 136,500 human figure images (real and synthetic examples) and 60,000 handwritten digits. We report on the relative complexities (query time and space requirements) of approximate versus exact EMD. In addition, we study empirically how much retrieval quality for our approximate method differs from its exact-solution counterpart, optimal graph matching. Shape matching quality is quantified based on its performance as a k-nearest-neighbor (k-NN) classifier for 3D pose or digit classification. With our method it is feasible to quickly retrieve similar shapes from large databases—an ability which has applications in various example-based vision systems. Unlike other methods which must perform vector quantization in the feature space in order to do efficient online retrievals, our technique can efficiently match raw feature distributions, and it eliminates the constraint on input feature set size from which other matching techniques suffer.

8.2   Related Work

In this section we briefly review relevant related work on shape matching techniques requiring optimal correspondences between features, the use of EMD as a similarity measure, and an embedding of EMD into a normed space and fast approximate similarity search.

A number of shape matching techniques require optimal correspondences between feature sets at some stage. The authors of [2] obtain least cost correspondences with an augmenting path algorithm in order to estimate an aligning transform between two shapes. They achieve impressive shape matching results with their method, but they note that the run-time does not scale well with the representation size due to the cubic complexity of solving correspondences. The authors of [3] characterize local shape topologies with points and tangent lines and use a combinatorial geometric hashing method to compute correspondence between these "order structures" of two shapes. In [9], a graduated assignment graph matching method is developed for matching image boundary features; it operates in time polynomial in the size of the feature sets. For additional information about various distance metrics for shape matching and their computational complexities, please refer to [20].

In recent work, AdaBoost is used to learn an embedding that maps the Chamfer distance into Euclidean space, and it is applied to edge images of hands to retrieve 3D hand poses from large databases [1]. However, while [1] requires that a large number of exact (potentially expensive) distance computations be performed during training, our method requires no exact EMD computations; our "training" cost is only the $O(Nnd \log \Delta)$ cost of embedding N database members. Additionally, while in [1] retrievals are based on a linear scan of the database, our method's online query time is sublinear in the size of the database.

The concept of using an EMD-like distance to measure perceptual similarity between images was first explored in [17] for the purpose of comparing intensity images. More recently EMD has been utilized for color- or texture-based similarity in [18] and [12], and extended to allow unpenalized distribution transformations in [5]. Exact EMD is computed via a linear programming solution, and its complexity is exponential in the number of points per point set in the worst case. In [15] exact EMD is applied to a database of 1620 silhouettes whose shock graphs are embedded into a normed space; the method does not use an embedding to approximate the EMD computation itself, and thus may not scale well with input or database size. In [7], a pseudo-metric derived from EMD that respects the triangle inequality and positivity property is given and applied to measure shape similarity on edges.

Our goal is to achieve robust, perceptually meaningful matching results, but in a way that scales more reasonably with an arbitrary representation size and allows real-time retrieval from larger databases. To that end, in this work we show how EMD and Locality-Sensitive Hashing (LSH) can be used for contour-based shape retrievals. An embedding of EMD into L_1 and the use of LSH for approximate nearest neighbors was shown for the purpose of image retrieval using global color histograms in [14]. To our knowledge, this work is the first to use an EMD embedding or employ LSH for local feature-based matching, and it is the first to develop a compact shape context subspace feature.

8.3 Fast Similarity Search with EMD

In this section, for the reader's convenience, we briefly summarize the EMD metric and the randomized algorithms we use in our shape matching method: the approximate similarity search algorithm LSH [8], and the embedding of EMD into a normed space given in [14].

EMD is named for a physical analogy that may be drawn between the process of transforming one weighted point set into another and the process of moving piles of dirt spread around one set of locations to another set of holes in the same space. The points are locations, their weights are the size of the dirt piles and holes, and the ground metric between a pile and a hole is the amount of work needed to move a unit of dirt. To use this transformation as a distance measure, i.e., a measure of dissimilarity, one seeks the least cost transformation—the movement of dirt that requires the least amount of work.

When the total weights in the two point sets are equal, the solution is a complete one-to-one correspondence, and it is equivalent to the problem of bipartite graph matching. That is, for a metric space (X,D) and two n-element sets $\mathbf{A}, \mathbf{B} \subset X$, the distance is the minimum cost of a perfect matching π between $\mathbf{A}$ and $\mathbf{B}$:

$$EMD(\mathbf{A}, \mathbf{B}) = \min_{\pi:\mathbf{A} \to \mathbf{B}} \sum_{\mathbf{a} \in \mathbf{A}} D(\mathbf{a}, \pi(\mathbf{a})). \tag{8.1}$$

LSH indexes a database of examples residing in a normed space by a number of hash tables, such that the probability of collision is high for similar examples and low for dissimilar ones. In particular, LSH guarantees that if for a query point $\mathbf{q}$ there exists a point in the database $\mathbf{p}$ such that $D(\mathbf{p}, \mathbf{q}) \leq r$, then (with high probability) a point $\mathbf{p}'$ is returned such that $D(\mathbf{p}', \mathbf{q}) \leq (1 + \epsilon)r$. Otherwise, the absence of such a point is reported. The query time for a database of N d-dimensional examples is bounded by $O(dN^{(1/(1+\epsilon))})$. See [8] for details.

The low-distortion embedding of EMD given in [14] provides a way to map weighted point sets $\mathbf{A}$ and $\mathbf{B}$ from the metric space into the normed space L_1, such that the L_1 distance between the resulting embedded vectors is comparable to the EMD distance between **A** and **B** themselves. It is required that **A** and **B** have equal total weights. Working in a normed space is desirable since it allows the use of fast approximate nearest-neighbor search techniques such as LSH. The general idea of the embedding is to compute and concatenate several weighted histograms of decreasing resolution for a given point set.

Formally, given two point sets **A** and **B**, each of cardinality n, and each containing points in $\Re^d$: impose grids G_i, $-1 \leq i \leq \log(\Delta)$, on the space $\Re^d$, with grid G_i having side length 2^i, and Δ equal to the diameter of $\mathbf{A} \cup \mathbf{B}$. Each grid is translated by a vector chosen randomly from $[0, \Delta]^d$. To embed a point set **A**, a vector $\mathbf{v}_i$ is created for each G_i with one coordinate per grid cell, where each coordinate counts the number of points in the corresponding cell, i.e., each $\mathbf{v}_i$ forms a histogram of **A**. The embedding of **A** is then the concatenated vector of the $\mathbf{v}_i$'s, scaled by the side lengths:

$$f(\mathbf{A}) = \left[\frac{1}{2}\mathbf{v}_{-1}(\mathbf{A}), \mathbf{v}_0(\mathbf{A}), 2\mathbf{v}_1(\mathbf{A}), \ldots, 2^i\mathbf{v}_i(\mathbf{A}), \ldots \right]. \qquad (8.2)$$

The distortion C of a metric embedding f describes how much information loss the embedding induces:

$$\frac{1}{C}EMD(\mathbf{A}, \mathbf{B}) \leq ||f(\mathbf{A}) - f(\mathbf{B})||_{L_1} \leq EMD(\mathbf{A}, \mathbf{B}). \qquad (8.3)$$

The distortion of the embedding used in this work has an upper bound of $O(\log \Delta)$ [14].

The intuition behind how this embedding captures EMD's minimum cost correspondence is as follows: each increasingly coarse level of the hierarchy of histogram grids serves to "match" the yet unmatched points from one point set to another within a particular grid cell. Points not matched at a given level result in entries in the L_1 vectors with different indices, which will add a value proportional to that level's grid cell side length to the L_1 distance between the two point sets' embeddings.

8.4 Matching Contours and Shape Context Subspaces

In this work we develop an efficient contour matching method that exploits the approximate EMD embedding and nearest neighbor search algorithms described above, and a rich but compact contour descriptor subspace that is amenable to approximate EMD.

EMD provides an effective way for us to compare shapes based on their distributions of local features. To compare shapes with EMD is essentially to measure how much effort would be required to transform one shape into another. The measure of this "effort" is based on establishing the correspondence between two shapes' unordered set of descriptive local

Given: N weighted point sets $\mathbf{B}_1, \ldots, \mathbf{B}_N$, where $\mathbf{B}_i = \{(\mathbf{s}_1, w_1) \ldots, (\mathbf{s}_{m_i}, w_{m_i})\}$ is a weighted
point set composed of m_i features, $\mathbf{S}^i = \{\mathbf{s}_1, \ldots, \mathbf{s}_{m_i}\}$, $\mathbf{s}_j \in \Re^d$, with feature vector $\mathbf{s}_j$
associated with scalar weight w_j, and where Δ is the diameter of $\cup_{i=1}^N \mathbf{S}^i$,
1:   **for all** $i = 1, \ldots, N$ **do**
2:       $\mathbf{B}_i \leftarrow \{(\mathbf{s}_1, w_1/T), \ldots, (\mathbf{s}_{m_i}, w_{m_i}/T)\}$, where $T = \sum_{j=1}^{m_i} w_j$.
3:   **end for**
4:   Let $L = \lceil \log \Delta \rceil$.
5:   For $1 \leq l \leq L$, let each $\mathbf{t}^l = [t_1^l, \ldots, t_d^l]$ be a random vector from $[0, 2^l]^d$.
6:   **for all** $\mathbf{B}_i$, $1 \leq i \leq N$ **do**
7:       **for all** $(\mathbf{s}_j = [s_1^j, \ldots, s_d^j], w_j) \in \mathbf{B}_i$ **do**
8:           **for all** $\mathbf{t}^l$, $1 \leq l \leq L$ **do**
9:               $\mathbf{x}_l^j = [c(t_1^l, s_1^j), \ldots, c(t_d^l, s_d^j)]$,
                where $c(t_k^h, s) = trunc((s - t_k^h)/2^h)$
10:              $\mathbf{v}_l^j = w_j \times 2^l$
11:          **end for**
12:          $\mathbf{p}_j^i = [(\mathbf{x}_1^j, v_1^j), \ldots, (\mathbf{x}_L^j, v_L^j)]$
13:      **end for**
14:      $embed(\mathbf{B}_i) = tally(sort([\mathbf{p}_1^i, \ldots, \mathbf{p}_{m_i}^i]))$,
        where pairs $(\mathbf{x}, v)$ represent nonzero sparse vector entries with index $\mathbf{x}$ and value v, $sort()$
        returns $[(\mathbf{x}_{o_1}, v_{o_1}), \ldots, (\mathbf{x}_{o_n}, v_{o_n})]$ such that $\mathbf{x}_{o_i} \leq_{LEX} \mathbf{x}_{o_{i+1}}$ (lexicographic ordering of
        concatenated vector elements) and $tally()$ sums values of sparse vector entries with equal
        indices.
15: **end for**

Algorithm 8.1 L_1 embedding for sets of local features.

features that results overall in the lowest possible matching cost, where
matching cost is defined by a ground distance between two local features
(e.g., the L_2 norm). Our goal is to compare local feature sets in this manner,
but in an efficient way that will scale well with feature set cardinality and
database size.

To overcome the computational burden of the conventional methods
described above, we embed the problem of correspondence between sets
of local features into L_1, and use the approximate solution to match the
shapes or images. By mapping the computation of EMD over unordered
feature sets into a normed space, a complex correspondence-based distance
is reduced to a simple, efficiently computable norm over very sparse vectors.

Our method proceeds as follows: features are extracted from a database of
images, and each image's features are treated as a uniformly weighted point
set. Using the L_1 embedding of EMD over the point sets, one sparse vector is
produced for each input example. Next, a set of random LSH hash functions
are generated, and all of the embedded database vectors are entered into
the hash tables. Both the database embedding and hash table construction
are performed offline. Then, given a novel example, the embedding for its
features is computed using the same random grid translations used for
the database embedding. Finally, examples similar to the novel query are
retrieved from the database by computing the L_1 distance between the
query's embedding and only those vectors in the union of the hash buckets
that are indexed by the query's embedding. Pseudo-code for the EMD local
feature matching embedding is given in Algorithm 8.1.

The embedded vector resulting from an input point set is high-dimensional but very sparse; only $O(n \log \Delta)$ entries are nonzero. The time required to embed one point set is $O(nd \log \Delta)$. L_1 distances are computed in time proportional to the number of nonzero entries in the sparse vectors as follows: a sparse vector data structure is composed of a vector of nonzero indices plus a vector of values at those indices. At the time of embedding, the vectors are sorted according to their indices (an offline computational cost). Then computing the L_1 distance is a matter of running two pointers through the vectors to sum the absolute value of the difference of their values where they have the same index, or add the absolute value of one vector where the index is not shared.

Thus the computational cost of obtaining the near-optimal feature correspondences for our matching method will be $O(nd \log \Delta) + O(n \log \Delta) = O(nd \log \Delta)$, the cost of embedding two point sets, plus an L_1 distance on the sparse vectors. In comparison, the exact methods typically used in shape matching to solve for correspondences (such as the Hungarian method for bipartite graph matching or the transportation simplex algorithm for linear programming) require time cubic or exponential in n.

Once a database of example shapes or images is embedded into a normed space, we do fast (time sublinear in the database size) retrievals for a novel embedded query via LSH. In addition to the complexity savings for a single match described above, the time required for retrieving similar shapes or images is reduced to $O(sN^{(1/(1+\epsilon))})$, where N is the number of examples in the database, ϵ is the LSH parameter relating the amount of approximation of the normed distance between neighbors, and s is the dimension of the sparse embedded contour vectors, s having a space requirement of $O(n \log \Delta)$. Results showing the quality of the approximate nearest neighbor contours we retrieve with LSH are reported in section 8.5.

Probably the most direct application of EMD for 2D contour matching is to compose point sets from the literal points on the two contours (or some subsets of them) and use the Euclidean distance between two contour points' image coordinates as the ground distance D in (8.1). For this simple positional feature, examples must be translated and scaled to be on par with some reference shape. To embed a set of 2D contour points, we impose a hierarchy of grids on the image coordinates themselves, starting with a grid resolution where each image coordinate receives its own cell, and ending with a single cell grid the size of the largest image, $G_{\log \Delta}$ (see figure 8.1).

There are drawbacks to using the simple positional feature for shape matching with approximate EMD. Though straightforward to embed, it can be a brittle feature. In order to achieve scale or translation invariance this feature demands a pre-processing stage on all shapes (which requires some a priori knowledge about the shapes, and can itself be brittle). In addition, under EMD the positional feature is too weak to enforce consistent, meaningful correspondences; since it encodes nothing about the

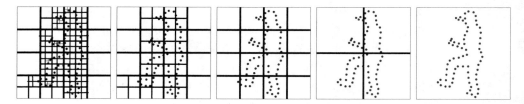

Figure 8.1   Imposing a hierarchy of grids on a set of 2D contour points to get its embedding.

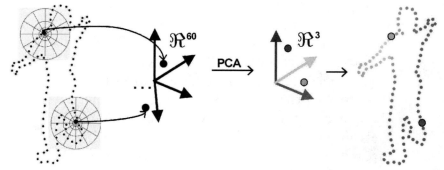

Figure 8.2   Projecting histograms of contour points onto the shape context subspace.

local shape appearance of the object, it will be greedily matched to points that are simply nearby on the other object.

To overcome these issues, we use a richer shape descriptor with the approximate EMD distance, as we expect to achieve more robust matchings and more meaningful correspondence fields from descriptive feature representations that encode the local shape in the neighborhood of each point. We employ the shape context descriptor of [2]. The shape context feature at a single contour point is a log-polar histogram of the coordinates of the rest of the point set, measured using the reference point as the origin. It is inherently translation invariant, and scale and rotation invariance may be added [2].

While matching with the full shape context feature is possible with our method, a low-dimensional feature descriptor is desirable since any change in point dimensions changes the constant distortion factor C in the embedding, and also changes the d factor in the complexity of computing the embedding itself. Thus we find a low-dimensional feature subspace based on a large sample of the shape context histograms, and then perform the embedding step in the domain of this subspace. The subspace is constructed from a large sample of features drawn from the database of contours on which we wish to apply our method. All contour features (from the database items and novel queries alike) are then projected onto the subspace, and the approximate EMD embedding is performed in the domain of a small number of their subspace coordinates (see figure 8.2). We use principal components analysis (PCA) to determine the set of bases that define this "shape context subspace."

We found that a very low-dimensional subspace was able to capture much of the local contour variation in our data sets. Figure 8.3 gives examples of the shape context subspace for human figures and handwritten digits. In section 8.5 we report results using the shape context subspace representation and discuss how to determine the most effective subspace dimension to use.

8.5   Results

In this section, we first describe each of the data sets we use in our experiments, as well as the feature representations and parameter settings that are used for each. Then we report on the matching performance of our method, followed by a discussion regarding its efficiency.

8.5.1   Data Sets and Representation

We have tested the proposed contour matching method on databases of human figures and handwritten digits. The human figure database contains 136,500 images of synthetic human figure contours in random poses that were generated with a computer graphics package called Poser [4]. We query this database with a separate test set of 7000 synthetic human figure images, and a test set of 1000 real images from a single human subject in various poses. The digit database we use is a publicly available benchmark data set, the MNIST database [16], which has been used to test many different pattern recognition algorithms. It contains 60,000 training images and 10,000 test images of digits written by about 250 different people. For the human figure images, we uniformly sampled 200 points from each silhouette contour, and for the digits we sampled 100 edge points per example.

We describe each contour with a set of shape context subspace features (see subsection 8.4). We construct shape context subspaces from 5×12 log-polar histograms extracted from the training sets; we used samples of 855,600 and 816,665 histograms from the human figure and handwritten digit data sets, respectively. The representation of a novel contour is determined by projecting its shape context histograms onto the low-dimensional subspace. This representation is translation invariant, and the scale of the shape context histograms initially extracted from the data is determined from the mean inter-point distance per shape. Because the coefficients are real-valued, they must be appropriately scaled and discretized before the embedding grids can be imposed. We remap the projection coefficients to positive integers by subtracting the minimum projection value from all examples, then scaling by 10^2.

There are several tradeoffs that must be considered when selecting d, the number of subspace dimensions to use for the shape context subspace features. The larger d is, the more exactly the projection coordinates will

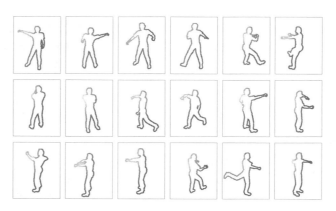

(a) Human figure database

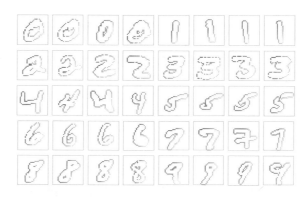

(b) Handwritten digits database

Figure 8.3 Visualization of feature subspace constructed from shape context histograms for two different data sets. The RGB channels of each point on the contours are colored according to its histogram's 3D PCA coefficient values. Matching with EMD in this feature space means that contour points of similar color have a low matching cost (require little "work"), while highly contrasting colors incur a high matching cost.

capture the original histogram feature extracted from the image (i.e., the smaller the PCA reconstruction error will be). However, larger d values will increase both the distortion over EMD that is induced by the embedding, as well as the complexity of computing the embedding. The dimension of the embedded vectors—and thus the time required to compute an L_1 distance on the embedded vectors—are also directly impacted by d. Moreover, higher-dimensional subspace projections, though strictly capturing the original data more faithfully, will not necessarily provide the most meaningful representation of the feature; one purpose of reducing the features' dimensionality with PCA is to distill the most significant modes of variation within the high-dimensional feature and use only those most discriminating dimensions as the descriptor. In fact, since we have a quantitative task by which retrievals may be judged (k-NN classification performance), it is more ap-

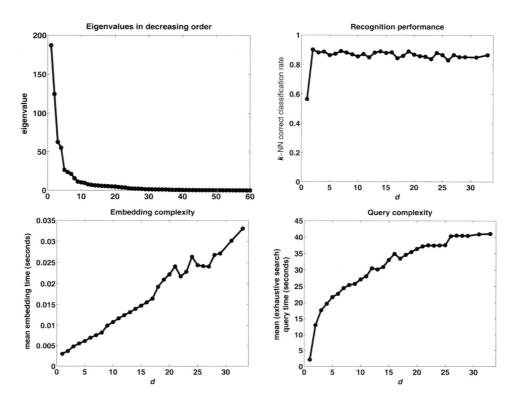

Figure 8.4 Example of using recognition performance to select the feature subspace dimension (d). These data are from the MNIST digits data set. A reserved portion (500 examples) of the training set was used to query the remaining 50,500 in order to optimize d for testing on the true test set. The top left graph shows the magnitudes of the eigenvalues for the PCA subspace over the shape context feature. The top right graph shows the k-NN classification performance that results when the 500 reserved training examples are used as queries, for projection dimensions varying from 1 to 34 ($k = 3$). The bottom left graph shows the corresponding mean embedding times for the same queries, and the bottom right graph shows the mean query times. Note that even though a number of principal components past the first two dimensions have eigenvalues of significant magnitude, the top right plot reveals that these dimensions are superfluous in terms of recognition performance. The data indicate that the choice of $d = 2$ is optimal for this data set, since there is an excellent balance between recognition performance and embedding/query efficiency at this point.

propriate to choose d with this objective than to select it solely on the number of eigenvalues with the highest magnitude (a standard approach).

Ultimately, the optimal setting of d—the setting that preserves both descriptiveness and efficiency—will depend on the data set. Thus in our experiments we determine the best setting by looking directly at the relationships between d and both recognition performance and retrieval efficiency. Using a reserved portion of the training set to query the remaining training examples, we record the correct k-NN classification rate, embedding times, and query times achieved with each increasing value of d. While seeking the optimal d in this way, we measure relative query times in terms of an exhaustive L_1 search on embedded vectors (i.e., without LSH). This ensures both that the best possible classification performance is observed, and that the query times are fairly uniform across examples for the same d, so as not to be influenced by outlier cases that may occur with LSH. Plotting the recognition rates, embedding times, and query times then reveals the tradeoffs between complexity and classification performance and allows us to choose an appropriate value of d to be applied for the actual test examples (see figure 8.4). Using this process, we found that for the human figure and MNIST digit data sets, a 2D projection adequately captured the descriptive power of the shape context feature and produced good contour matches, yet also yielded very efficient embedding and query complexities.

We constructed a separate set of hash functions for each image data set in order to perform LSH approximate nearest-neighbor retrievals. We determined the LSH parameters (number of hash tables and number of bits per hash value) based on the proof in [13] which shows how to select parameters for the case of the Hamming space over a non-binary alphabet, such that the desired level of approximation versus speed tradeoff is achieved. The radius r denotes the distance from a query point where similar points (its "r-neighbors") are believed to lie. The probability of collision of similar examples (examples within distance r), p_1, is set to $1 - \frac{r}{d'}$, where $d' = Zd$, d is the dimension of the embedded vectors, and Z is the largest coordinate value in any of the embeddings. The probability of collision for dissimilar examples (examples farther than $(1 + \epsilon)r$ from each other), p_2, is set to $1 - \frac{r(1+\epsilon)}{d'}$. Then the number of bits k and the number of hash tables l are set as follows:

$$ k = \log_{1/p_2}\left(\frac{N}{B}\right), \qquad l = \left(\frac{N}{B}\right)^{\frac{\log 1/p_1}{\log 1/p_2}}, \qquad (8.4) $$

where N is the total number of examples in the database, and B is the maximum number of examples we wish to search exhaustively after hashing. For the complete data set of 136,500 human figure examples, this meant using eight tables and 120-bit functions. For the MNIST digit data set, we used five tables and 96-bit functions. The radius r is determined for each data set by examining the distances and class labels corresponding to the nearest neighbors of an embedded point set under L_1. For all experiments ϵ is set to 1, which means the upper bound on the query time is $O(dN^{\frac{1}{2}})$.

8.5.2   Retrieval Quality

To quantitatively measure the quality of the database retrievals our contour matching method yields, we pose a k-NN classification task for each data set. A k-NN query selects the nearest k examples among a database of training examples, and then labels the test point by a majority vote of these samples. Though a simple method, the k-NN approach to classification is powerful since its error rate reaches the optimal Bayes rate when k and N go to infinity [6].

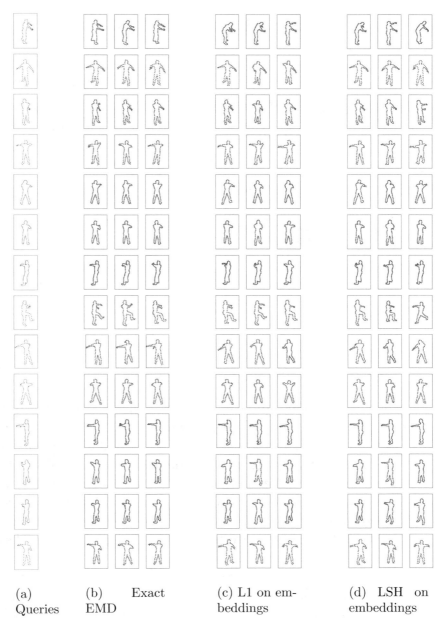

(a)　(b)　　Exact　　(c) L1 on em-　　(d) LSH on
Queries　EMD　　　　　beddings　　　embeddings

Figure 8.5 Approximate EMD retrieves shapes very similar to those retrieved by the optimal matching. This figure shows examples of the three nearest neighbors (left to right in rank order) retrieved with embedded EMD contour matching (c) and embedded EMD contour matching with LSH (d), compared to the nearest neighbors under exact EMD contour matching (b). Examples shown were chosen randomly from 7000 test set results, and nearest neighbors were retrieved from a database of 136,500 examples. Columns (c) and (d) use the embedded 2D shape context subspace feature; column (b) uses exact EMD applied to full 60D shape context features. Note that the embedded match results are qualitatively similar, yet are several orders of magnitude faster to compute.

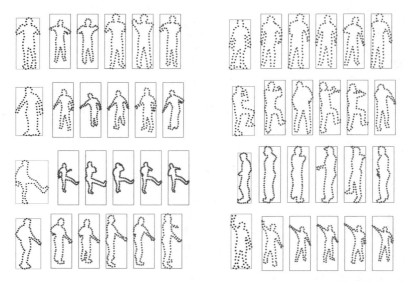

Figure 8.6 Real image queries: examples of query contours from a real person (left image in each group) and the five nearest-neighbor contours retrieved from a synthetic database of 136,500 images using L_1 on EMD embeddings of 2D shape context subspace features. The example results shown here are a random sample of the 1000 real queries that were performed.

8.5.2.1 Human Figures Data Set

For the human figures data set, we measure retrieval quality by comparing the 3D pose of each query example with the pose of the k most similar examples that are retrieved from the database. When the synthetic human figure database is generated, the 3D pose (a set of 19 3D joint positions) is recorded for each example. If the joint positions corresponding to a retrieved shape are on average within some threshold of distance from the known joint positions of the query example, we consider the retrieved shape a good match. We chose a threshold of 10 cm, since this is a distance at which the 3D poses are perceptually similar.

Figure 8.5 shows some example retrievals using our approximate EMD method with synthetic query images. Examples of the synthetic nearest neighbors that were retrieved for the images from a real person are shown in figure 8.6. These real image queries contain a single subject performing various actions against a static background. Background subtraction was done automatically using standard frame differencing followed by morphological operations.

Figure 8.7 (a) quantitatively compares the quality of results obtained with our approximate method with those obtained from exact EMD for a database of 10,000 images. Due to the complexity of exact EMD, the exact comparisons were necessarily computed with a parallel implementation. In this figure the optimal results were obtained by running the transportation simplex algorithm to compute EMD on full 60D shape context features,

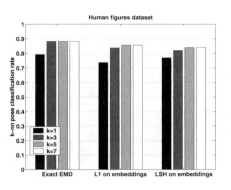
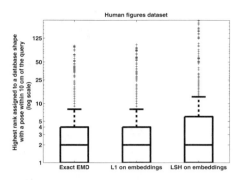

(a) Accuracy of approximate vs. exact method

(b) Matching performance

Figure 8.7 (a) Comparison of the quality of contour matching retrievals from the exact versus approximate methods for the human figures data set. Quality is measured via a k-NN classification task. The test set and training set are composed of 1000 and 10,000 examples, respectively. For this problem, our method achieves a speedup of four orders of magnitude over the exact method, at the cost of only a 4% reduction in accuracy. (b) Distributions of the highest rank of a correct match for human figure retrievals. Lines in center of boxes denote median value; the top and bottom of boxes denote upper and lower quartile values, respectively. The dashed lines show extent of rest of the data, and the pluses denote outliers. See text for details.

whereas results for the two approximations (the embedding and LSH) were obtained using only 2D shape context subspace features. There is a slight decrease in classification performance at each approximation level; however, we found that the practical bound on the distortion introduced by the EMD embedding is significantly (about one order of magnitude) lower than the theoretical upper bound. Moreover, the bar graph in figure 8.7 (a) demonstrates that our method shows only a 4% reduction in accuracy over the exact method, and as we discuss in subsection 8.5.3, this small error increase allows us a substantial speedup of four orders of magnitude.

Figure 8.7 (b) shows how well our contour matching method serves as a means of estimating 3D pose from a set of 2D occluding contour points. The boxplot shows the distributions of the highest rank that is assigned by our method to an example in the database with a very similar (within 10 cm) pose to a query. In most cases, the second nearest neighbor is a "correct" match, meaning it correctly identifies the pose of the query. We note that there are of course ambiguities in the task of inferring 3D pose from a single frame silhouette view; due to self-occlusions or ambiguities about the orientation of the person, the information provided by the outer contour may be an insufficient indicator of 3D pose. Nevertheless, we are encouraged by the fact that the correct matches in pose are generally among the highest ranked examples according to our method. In recent work we have also investigated how these example-based pose estimates may be integrated and improved by considering sequences of silhouette frames [11].

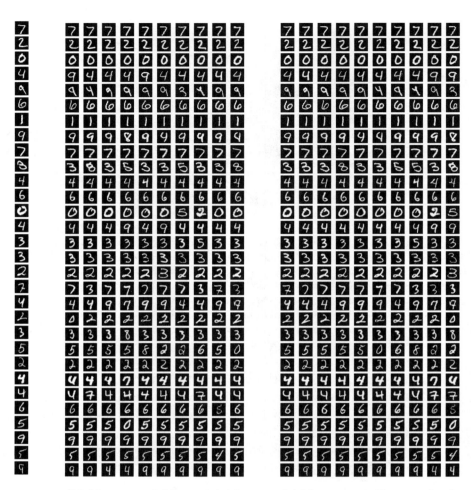

(a)   (b) Nearest neighbors: initial   (c) Nearest neighbors: refined
Queries   rankings   rankings

Figure 8.8 Example retrieval results for the MNIST handwritten digits database. Approximate EMD efficiently filters through the N-item database to find an initial set of w examples whose edge point histograms have minimal cost correspondences with the query's histograms. Then, in order to refine the initial rankings, a more expensive shape matching method (such as shape context matching [2]) can be applied to only the w examples that were retrieved with approximate EMD. Classification is then done using only the first k re-ranked examples ($k < w$). Each row shows one example. (a) shows some query digits from the MNIST test set. (b) shows the first $w = 10$ nearest neighbors for these queries under approximate EMD with L_1 (in rank order). (c) shows the same 10 nearest neighbors after they are re-ranked by the shape context distance. The first $k = 3$ refined nearest neighbors are used to classify the query digit.

8.5.2.2 Handwritten Digits Data Set

In a practical system, classification rates can be improved by adding a refining step: some number of the best matches retrieved by the fast approximate method may be fed as input to a more elaborate (and presumably more expensive) matching algorithm for re-ranking prior to k-NN classification. For the MNIST handwritten digits data set, we took this refinement approach. The goal is to correctly label the identity of a query handwritten digit based on the majority vote of its k-NN in the training set of 60,000 examples. First, we use our approximate EMD shape matching method with shape context subspace features to retrieve an initial set of w nearest neighbors for a query. Then we compute the exact shape context distance [2] between this initial nearest neighbor set and the query example, which yields a re-ranking of the neighbors.[1] The k closest neighbors in this re-ranked or refined set are then used to do the classification. Figure 8.8 shows some example matching results for the handwritten digits and illustrates the impact of the refinement stage.

Figure 8.9 shows classification performance for the handwritten digits data set. Since the MNIST digit database is a publicly available benchmark data set, we are able to compare our algorithm's performance against that of many other researchers. (See [16] for a summary of different algorithms' results.) At this writing, the best published classification performance was achieved by the shape context matching method of [2], which correctly classifies 99.37% of the 10,000-item test set. By combining our approximate EMD contour matching with shape context matching as described above, we are able to correctly classify 99.35% of the test set. Note that while the technique in [2] compares query shapes against every database item, with the refinement framework we need only evaluate the shape context distance between the query and a fraction of the database; so with $w = 6000$, our method misclassifies only 65 of the 10,000 test digits, but classification is an order of magnitude more efficient than doing a linear scan of the database.

Even with a much shorter refinement step that evaluates only 50 exact shape context distances, our method correctly classifies 97.42% of the test set. With only 100 exact shape context distances, it correctly classifies 98.08%. In comparison, the authors of [21] report a correct classification rate of 97.0% on the same data using their discriminative classifier, when allowing the same computational cost of 100 exact shape context distances against selected prototypes. In addition, our method's training stage is substantially more efficient and more easily updatable than that given in [21]. Since the method in [21] relies on k-medoids to determine prototypes from the training set (an $O(NdkT)$ operation for T iterations), it is not clear that it will be able to accommodate new training examples without an expensive re-training step. In contrast, since the "training" of our method consists only of embedding available training examples, additional examples

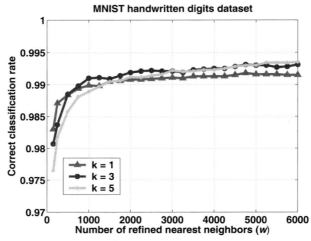

Figure 8.9   Contour matching-based classification of the MNIST handwritten digit test set. Given a query image, approximate EMD is used to obtain an initial set of nearest neighbors in the training set, and then shape context matching is used to refine the ranks of this set of neighbors. Classification is based on the refined rankings.

may be incorporated simply by embedding the new examples and entering them into the LSH hash tables.

8.5.3   Empirical Measure of Complexity

As discussed in section 8.4, the theoretical computational complexity of retrieving the approximate minimum cost feature correspondences with our method for feature sets of cardinality n and dimension d residing in a space of diameter Δ is $O(nd \log \Delta)$. The diameters of the spaces in which our point sets reside are on the order of 10^3 up to 10^5, depending on the representation; with n on the order of 10^2, $d = 2$, theoretically this means that a single embedding and L_1 distance cost requires on the order of 10^3 operations. This is the cost of embedding two point sets, plus performing an L_1 distance on the very sparse vectors.

  In practice, with $d = 2$ and $n = 200$, an unoptimized C implementation of our method takes about 0.005 second to perform a single matching between the human figure images with exact L_1 (less than 0.005 second to compute the two embeddings, plus 7.9×10^{-5} second to compute the L_1 distance). In comparison, to compute a single exact EMD distance using a C implementation of the simplex algorithm required on average 0.9 second for data of the same dimensions. In accordance with the upper bound on the embedding's space requirements, the number of nonzero entries in the sparse embedded vectors was on average 350 for the human figure contours with the shape context subspace representation. For the MNIST digits data, with $d = 2$ and $n = 100$, the average time needed to compute an embedding was 0.003 second, and each L_1 distance required 1.7×10^{-4} second.

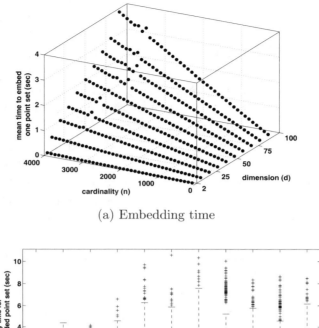

(a) Embedding time

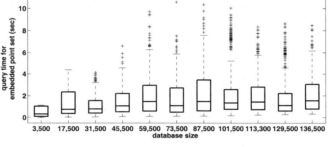

(b) Query time

Figure 8.10 (a) Mean embedding time per point set for 500 point sets with varying dimensions and cardinalities. (b) Query time distributions for embedded point sets for increasing database sizes. The test set is composed of 1000 examples from the human figure database, $d = 2$, $n = 200$. The lines in center of boxes denote median value; the top and bottom of boxes denote upper and lower quartile values, respectively. The dashed lines show extent of rest of the data, and the pluses denote outliers. The median query time for the 136,500 item database is only 1.56 seconds; exact EMD could require over a day to perform the same query.

Figure 8.10 (a) gives a summary of the empirical run-time behavior of the embedding. Our experiments confirm that the run-time for embedding point sets increases only linearly with the size of the input's dimension or cardinality. This means that our method scales well to handle inputs with large representation sizes.

The larger payoff for using the approximate embedding, however, comes when we use LSH to query a large database with an embedded point set. With ϵ set to 1, the upper bound on the query time is $O(dN^{\frac{1}{2}})$. The input must be compared against only a small fraction of the database's embedded vectors—those in the union of the hash buckets that are indexed by the query's embedding.

On average, in our experiments LSH needed to compute only 1915 L_1 distances per query for the human figures database, (less than 2% of the database). The median query time for the complete 136,500-item Poser database was only 1.56 seconds. In comparison, a single query with the exact EMD method would require 34 hours (performing a worst-case linear scan of the database). Figure 8.10 (b) shows how query time for the human figure data set varies with the database size.

For the MNIST digits data set, the median query time using LSH (and no refinement step) was 0.14 second, and on average a query's embedding was compared to 94 training examples, less than 1% of the database. When the refinement step described in subsection 8.5.2.2 is included, the query time increases by $w \times g$, where w is the number of rankings that are refined and g is the time needed to perform one shape context distance. (The implementation of the shape context distance that we are using requires $g = 0.07$ second.)

8.6   Conclusions

We have presented a new contour matching algorithm that utilizes an approximation to EMD to judge similarity between sets of local descriptors. Our technique enables fast (sublinear in the size of the database) local feature-based similarity retrievals from large databases, and its run-time is only linearly dependent on the number of features used to represent an object. We have also constructed a rich but compact contour feature subspace based on shape contexts that is appropriate for approximate EMD. We have demonstrated the application of our method for inferring pose from contours of human figures and classifying handwritten digits. We have also shown that our method is able to more efficiently produce matching results that are competitive with the best reported results on the MNIST digits data set.

In the future we intend to experiment with different shape representations under approximate EMD. Thus far we have applied our shape matching method to 2D inputs, i.e., contours. However, our method may also be applied to 3D data (e.g., visual hull data or stereo maps); the only necessary adjustment is to provide an appropriate 3D shape descriptor as the feature type in the point sets. We will also explore alternative means of compactly representing inherently continuous features within the discrete embedding framework, such as vector quantization or multi-dimensional scaling. We are also interested in investigating ways to improve the efficacy of the nearest neighbors hashing process in this context.

Acknowledgments

We would like to thank Piotr Indyk and Gregory Shakhnarovich for various helpful discussions, and Vassilis Athitsos for sharing his implementation of shape context matching. This work was supported in part by a Department of Energy Computational Science Graduate Fellowship.

Notes

[1] Note that the exact shape context distance is different from exact EMD. It first solves the optimal assignment problem, and then given those correspondences, it estimates the thin-plate spline transformation that best aligns the two shapes. The scalar measure of dissimilarity is then the sum of the matching errors between the corresponding points, plus the magnitude of the aligning transform [2].

References

1. V. Athitsos, J. Alon, S. Sclaroff, and G. Kollios. BoostMap: A method for efficient approximate similarity rankings. In *Proceedings of IEEE Conference on Computer Vision and Pattern Recognition*, Washington, DC, July 2004.

2. S. Belongie, J. Malik, and J. Puzicha. Shape matching and object recognition using shape contexts. *IEEE Transactions on Pattern Analysis and Machine Intelligence*, 24(24):509–522, April 2002.

3. S. Carlsson. Order structure, correspondence and shape based categories. In *International Workshop on Shape Contour and Grouping*, Palermo, Sicily, May 1998.

4. Curious Labs Egisys Co., Santa Cruz, CA. Poser 5 : The Ultimate 3D Character Solution, 2002.

5. S. Cohen and L. Guibas. The earth mover's distance under transformation sets. In *Proceedings of IEEE International Conference on Computer Vision*, Corfu, Greece, Sept 1999.

6. R. Duda, P. Hart, and D. Stork. *Pattern Classification*, pages 182–184. John Wiley & Sons, Inc., Hoboken, NJ, 2001.

7. P. Giannopoulos and R. Veltkamp. A pseudo-metric for weighted point sets. In *Proceedings of European Conference on Computer Vision*, Copenhagen, Denmark, May 2002.

8. A. Gionis, P. Indyk, and R. Motwani. Similarity search in high dimensions via hashing. In *Proceedings of the 25th International Conference on Very Large Data Bases*, 1999.

9. S. Gold and A. Rangarajan. A graduated assignment algorithm for graph matching. *IEEE Transactions on Pattern Analysis and Machine Intelligence*, 18(4):377–388, April 1996.

10. K. Grauman and T. Darrell. Fast contour matching using approximate earth mover's distance. In *Proceedings of IEEE*

Conference on Computer Vision and Pattern Recognition, Washington DC, June 2004.

11.   K. Grauman, G. Shakhnarovich, and T. Darrell. Virtual visual hulls: example-based 3D shape inference from silhouettes. In *Proceedings of the 2nd Workshop on Statistical Methods in Video Processing, in conjunction with ECCV*, Prague, Czech Republic, May 2004.

12.   H. Greenspan, G. Dvir, and Y. Rubner. Region correspondence for image matching via EMD flow. In *IEEE Workshop on Content-Based Access of Image and Video Libraries*, June 2000.

13.   P. Indyk. *High-Dimensional Computational Geometry*. PhD thesis, Stanford University, Stanford, CA, 2000.

14.   P. Indyk and N. Thaper. Fast image retrieval via embeddings. In *3rd International Workshop on Statistical and Computational Theories of Vision*, Nice, France, October 2003.

15.   Y. Keselman, A. Shokoufandeh, M. F. Demirci, and S. Dickinson. Many-to-many graph matching via metric embedding. In *Proceedings of IEEE Conference on Computer Vision and Pattern Recognition*, Madison, WI, June 2003.

16.   MNIST handwritten digits data set. *http://yann.lecun.com/exdb/mnist*.

17.   S. Peleg, M. Werman, and H. Rom. A unified approach to the change of resolution: space and gray-level. *IEEE Transactions on Pattern Analysis and Machine Intelligence*, 11(7):739–742, July 1989.

18.   Y. Rubner, C. Tomasi, and L. Guibas. The earth mover's distance as a metric for image retrieval. *International Journal of Computer Vision*, 40(2):99–121, 2000.

19.   T. Sebastian, P. Klein, and B. Kimia. Recognition of shapes by editing shock graphs. In *Proceedings of IEEE International Conference on Computer Vision*, Vancouver, Canada, December 2001.

20.   R. Veltkamp and M. Hagedoorn. State-of-the-Art in Shape Matching. *Technical Report UU-CS-1999-27*, Utrecht University, Utrecht, Netherlands, 1999.

21.   H. Zhang and J. Malik. Learning a discriminative classifier using shape context distances. In *Proceedings of IEEE Conference on Computer Vision and Pattern Recognition*, Madison, WI, June 2003.

9 Adaptive Mean Shift Based Clustering in High Dimensions

Ilan Shimshoni, Bogdan Georgescu, and Peter Meer

Feature space analysis is the main module in many computer vision tasks. The most popular technique, k-means clustering, however, has two inherent limitations: the clusters are constrained to be spherically symmetric and their number has to be known a priori. In nonparametric clustering methods, like the one based on mean shift, these limitations are eliminated but the amount of computation becomes prohibitively large as the dimension of the space increases. We exploit a recently proposed approximation technique, locality-sensitive hashing (LSH), to reduce the computational complexity of adaptive mean shift. In our implementation of LSH the optimal parameters of the data structure are determined by a pilot learning procedure, and the partitions are data driven. The algorithm is tested on two applications. In the first, the performance of mode and k-means-based textons are compared in a texture classification study. In the second, multispectral images are segmented. Again, our method is compared to k-means clustering.

9.1 Introduction

Representation of visual information through feature space analysis has received renewed interest in recent years, motivated by content-based image retrieval applications. The increase in the available computational power allows today the handling of feature spaces which are high-dimensional and contain millions of data points.

The structure of high-dimensional spaces, however, defies our three-dimensional(3D) geometric intuition. Such spaces are extremely sparse with the data points far away from each other [17, subsection 4.5.1]. Thus, when inferring about the local structure of the space when only a small number of data points may be available can yield erroneous results. The phenomenon is known in the statistical literature as the "curse of dimensionality", and its effect increases exponentially with the dimension. The curse of dimensionality can be avoided only by imposing a fully parametric model over the data [6, p.203], an approach which is not feasible for a high-dimensional feature space with a complex structure.

The goal of feature space analysis is to reduce the data to a few significant features through a procedure known under many different names, clustering, unsupervised learning, or vector quantization. Most often different variants of *k-means clustering* are employed, in which the feature space is represented as a mixture of normal distributions [6, subsection 10.4.3]. The number of mixture components k is usually set by the user.

The popularity of the k-means algorithm is due to its low computational complexity of $O(nkNd)$, where n is the number of data points, d the dimension of the space, and N the number of iterations which is always small relative to n. However, since it imposes a rigid delineation over the feature space and requires a reasonable guess for the number of clusters present, the k-means clustering can return erroneous results when the embedded assumptions are not satisfied. Moreover, the k-means algorithm is not robust; points which do not belong to any of the k clusters can move the estimated means away from the densest regions.

A robust clustering technique which does not require prior knowledge of the number of clusters, and does not constrain the shape of the clusters, is the *mean shift*-based clustering. This is also an iterative technique, but instead of the means, it estimates the modes of the multivariate distribution underlying the feature space. The number of clusters is obtained automatically by finding the centers of the densest regions in the space (the modes). See [1] for details. Under its original implementation the mean shift-based clustering cannot be used in high dimensional spaces. Already for $d = 7$, in a video sequence segmentation application, a fine-to-coarse hierarchical approach had to be introduced [5].

The most expensive operation of the mean shift method is finding the closest neighbors of a point in the space. The problem is known in computational geometry as *multidimensional range-searching* [4, chap.5]. The goal of the range-searching algorithms is to represent the data in a structure in which proximity relations can be determined in less than $O(n)$ time. One of the most popular structures, the kD-tree, is built in $O(n \log n)$ operations, where the proportionality constant increases with the dimension of the space. A query selects the points within a rectangular region delimited by an interval on each coordinate axis, and the query time for kD-trees has complexity bounded by $O\left(n^{\frac{d-1}{d}} + m\right)$, where m is the number of points found. Thus, for high dimensions the complexity of a query is practically linear, yielding the *computational curse of dimensionality*. Recently, several probabilistic algorithms have been proposed for approximate nearest-neighbor search. The algorithms yield sublinear complexity with a speedup which depends on the desired accuracy [7, 10, 11].

In this chapter we have adapted the algorithm in [7] for mean shift-based clustering in high dimensions. Working with data in high dimensions also required that we extend the adaptive mean shift procedure introduced in [2]. All computer vision applications of mean shift until now, such as image segmentation, object recognition, and tracking, were in relatively low-dimensional spaces. Our implementation opens the door to use mean shift in tasks based on high-dimensional features.

In section 9.2 we present a short review of the adaptive mean shift technique. Locality-sensitive hashing(LSH), the technique for approximate nearest-neighbor search, is described in section 9.3, where we have also introduced refinements to handle data with complex structure. In section 9.4 the performance of adaptive mean shift (AMS) in high dimensions is investigated, and in section 9.5 AMS is used for texture classification based on textons and for segmentation of multispectral images. We conclude in section 9.6.

9.2   Adaptive Mean Shift

Here we only review some of the results described in [2] which should be consulted for the details.

Assume that each data point $\mathbf{x}_i \in \mathcal{R}^d$, $i = 1, \ldots, n$ is associated with a bandwidth value $h_i > 0$. The *sample point* estimator

$$\hat{f}_K(\mathbf{x}) = \frac{1}{n} \sum_{i=1}^{n} \frac{1}{h_i^d} k \left(\left\| \frac{\mathbf{x} - \mathbf{x}_i}{h_i} \right\|^2 \right) \tag{9.1}$$

based on a spherically symmetric kernel K with bounded support satisfying

$$K(\mathbf{x}) = c_{k,d} k(\|\mathbf{x}\|^2) > 0 \qquad \|\mathbf{x}\| \le 1 \tag{9.2}$$

is an adaptive nonparametric estimator of the density at location $\mathbf{x}$ in the feature space. The function $k(x)$, $0 \le x \le 1$, is called the *profile* of the kernel, and the normalization constant $c_{k,d}$ assures that $K(\mathbf{x})$ integrates to one. The function $g(x) = -k'(x)$ can always be defined when the derivative of the kernel profile $k(x)$ exists. Using $g(x)$ as the profile, the kernel $G(\mathbf{x})$ is defined as $G(\mathbf{x}) = c_{g,d} g(\|\mathbf{x}\|^2)$.

By taking the gradient of (9.1) the following property can be proven

$$\mathbf{m}_G(\mathbf{x}) = C \frac{\hat{\nabla} f_K(\mathbf{x})}{\hat{f}_G(\mathbf{x})}, \tag{9.3}$$

where C is a positive constant and

$$\mathbf{m}_G(\mathbf{x}) = \frac{\sum_{i=1}^{n} \frac{1}{h_i^{d+2}} \mathbf{x}_i \, g \left(\left\| \frac{\mathbf{x} - \mathbf{x}_i}{h_i} \right\|^2 \right)}{\sum_{i=1}^{n} \frac{1}{h_i^{d+2}} g \left(\left\| \frac{\mathbf{x} - \mathbf{x}_i}{h_i} \right\|^2 \right)} - \mathbf{x} \tag{9.4}$$

is called the *mean shift vector*. The expression (9.3) shows that at location $\mathbf{x}$ the weighted mean of the data points selected with kernel G is proportional to the normalized density gradient estimate obtained with kernel K. The mean shift vector thus points toward the direction of maximum increase in the density. The implication of the mean shift property is that the iterative procedure

$$\mathbf{y}_{j+1} = \frac{\sum_{i=1}^{n} \frac{\mathbf{x}_i}{h_i^{d+2}} g\left(\left\| \frac{\mathbf{y}_j - \mathbf{x}_i}{h_i} \right\|^2 \right)}{\sum_{i=1}^{n} \frac{1}{h_i^{d+2}} g\left(\left\| \frac{\mathbf{y}_j - \mathbf{x}_i}{h_i} \right\|^2 \right)} \qquad j = 1, 2, \ldots \qquad (9.5)$$

is a hill-climbing technique to the nearest stationary point of the density, i.e., a point in which the density gradient vanishes. The initial position of the kernel, the starting point of the procedure $\mathbf{y}_1$, can be chosen as one of the data points $\mathbf{x}_i$. Most often the points of convergence of the iterative procedure are the modes (local maxima) of the density.

There are numerous methods described in the statistical literature to define h_i, the bandwidth values associated with the data points, most of which use a pilot density estimate [17, subsection 5.3.1]. The simplest way to obtain the pilot density estimate is by nearest neighbors [6, section 4.5]. Let $\mathbf{x}_{i,k}$ be the k-nearest neighbor(k-NN) of the point $\mathbf{x}_i$. Then, we take

$$h_i = \|\mathbf{x}_i - \mathbf{x}_{i,k}\|_1, \qquad (9.6)$$

where L_1 norm is used since it is the most suitable for the data structure to be introduced in the next section. The choice of the norm does not have a major effect on the performance. The number of neighbors k should be chosen large enough to assure that there is an increase in density within the support of most kernels having bandwidths h_i. While the value of k should increase with d the dimension of the feature space, the dependence is not critical for the performance of the mean shift procedure, as will be seen in section 9.4. When all $h_i = h$, i.e., a single global bandwidth value is used, the AMS procedure becomes the fixed bandwidth mean shift discussed in [1].

A robust nonparametric clustering of the data is achieved by applying the mean shift procedure to a representative subset of the data points. After convergence, the detected modes are the cluster centers, and the shape of the clusters is determined by their basins of attraction. See [1] for details.

9.3   Locality-Sensitive Hashing

The bottleneck of mean shift in high dimensions is the need for a fast algorithm to perform neighborhood queries when computing (9.5). The problem has been addressed before in the vision community by sorting the data according to each of the d coordinates [13], but a significant speedup was achieved only when the data are close to a low-dimensional manifold.

Recently, new algorithms using tools from probabilistic approximation theory were suggested for performing approximate nearest neighbor search in high dimensions for general data sets [10, 11] and for clustering data [9, 14]. We use the approximate nearest neighbor algorithm based on *locality-sensitive hashing* [7] and adapted it to handle the complex data met in computer vision applications. In a task of estimating the pose of articulated objects [16], the LSH technique was extended to accommodate distances in the parameter space.

9.3.1 High-Dimensional Neighborhood Queries

Given n points in $\mathcal{R}^d$ the mean shift iterations (9.5) require a neighborhood query around the current location $\mathbf{y}_j$. The naive method is to scan the whole data set and test whether the kernel of the point $\mathbf{x}_i$ covers $\mathbf{y}_j$. Thus, for each mean computation the complexity is $O(nd)$. Assuming that for every point in the data set this operation is performed N times (a value which depends on the h_i's and the distribution of the data), the complexity of the mean shift algorithm is $O(n^2 dN)$.

To improve the efficiency of the neighborhood queries the following data structure is constructed. The data is tessellated L times with random partitions, each defined by K inequalities (fig. 9.1). In each partition K pairs of random numbers, d_k and v_k, are used. First, d_k, an integer between 1 and d, is chosen, followed by v_k, a value within the range of the data along the d_kth coordinate.

The pair (d_k, v_k) partitions the data according to the inequality

$$x_{i,d_k} \leq v_k \qquad i = 1, \ldots, n, \tag{9.7}$$

where x_{i,d_k} is the selected coordinate for the data point $\mathbf{x}_i$. Thus, for each point $\mathbf{x}_i$ each partition yields a K-dimensional Boolean vector (inequality true/false). Points which have the same vector lie in the same cell of the partition. Using a hash function, all the points belonging to the same cell are placed in the same bucket of a hash table. As we have L such partitions, each point belongs simultaneously to L cells (hash table buckets).

To find the neighborhood of radius h around a query point $\vec{q}$, L Boolean vectors are computed using (9.7). These vectors index L cells C_l, $l = 1, \ldots, L$ in the hash table. The points in their union $C_\cup = \bigcup_{l=1}^{L} C_l$ are the ones returned by the query (fig. 9.1). Note that any $\vec{q}$ in the intersection $C_\cap = \bigcap_{l=1}^{L} C_l$ will return the same result. Thus $C_\cap$ determines the resolution of the data structure, whereas $C_\cup$ determines the set of the points returned by the query. The described technique is called *locality-sensitive hashing* and was introduced in [10].

Points close in $\mathcal{R}^d$ have a higher probability for collision in the hash table. Since $C_\cap$ lies close to the center of $C_\cup$, the query will return most of the nearest neighbors of $\vec{q}$. The example in fig. 9.1 illustrates the approximate nature of the query. Parts of an L_1 neighborhood centered on $\vec{q}$ are not covered by $C_\cup$, which has a different shape. The approximation errors can be reduced by building data structures with larger $C_\cup$'s; however, this will increase the running time of a query.

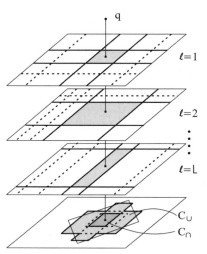

Figure 9.1   The LSH data structure. For the query point $\vec{q}$ the overlap of L cells yields the region $C_\cup$, which approximates the desired neighborhood.

9.3.2   Optimal Selection of K and L

The values for K and L determine the expected volumes of $C_\cap$ and $C_\cup$. The average number of inequalities used for each coordinate is K/d, partitioning the data into $K/d+1$ regions. Qualitatively, the larger the value for K, the number of cuts in a partition, the smaller the average volume of the cells C_l. Conversely, as the number of partitions L increases, the volume of $C_\cap$ decreases and of $C_\cup$ increases. For a given K, only values of L below a certain bound are of interest. Indeed, once L exceeds this bound all the neighborhood of radius h around $\vec{q}$ has been already covered by $C_\cup$. Thus, larger values of L will only increase the query time with no improvement in the quality of the results.

The optimal values of K and L can be derived from the data. A subset of data points $\mathbf{x}_j, j = 1, \cdots, m \ll n$, is selected by random sampling. For each of these data points, the L_1 distance h_j (9.6) to its k-NN is determined accurately by the traditional linear algorithm.

In the approximate nearest-neighbor algorithm based on LSH, for any pair of K and L, we define for each of the m points $h_j^{(K,L)}$, the distance to the k-NN returned by the query. When the query does not return the correct

k-NNs $h_j^{(K,L)} > h_j$. The total running time of the m queries is $t(K,L)$. The optimal (K,L) is then chosen such that

$$(K,L) = \arg\min_{K,L} t(K,L) \qquad \text{subject to:} \qquad \frac{1}{m}\sum_{j=1}^{m} \frac{h_j^{(K,L)}}{h_j} \leq (1+\epsilon),$$

where ϵ is the LSH approximation threshold set by the user.

The optimization is performed as a numerical search procedure. For a given K we compute, as a function of L, the approximation error of the m queries. This is shown in fig. 9.2(a) for a 13D real data set. By thresholding the family of graphs at $\epsilon = 0.05$, the function $L(K)$ is obtained (fig. 9.2(b)). The running time can now be expressed as $t[K, L(K)]$, i.e., a 1D function in K, the number of employed cuts (fig. 9.2(c)). Its minimum is K_{min} which together with $L(K_{min})$, are the optimal parameters of the LSH data structure.

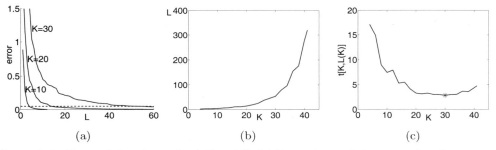

| (a) | (b) | (c) |

Figure 9.2 Determining the optimal K and L. (a) Dependence of the approximation error on L for $K = 10, 20, 30$. The curves are thresholded at $\epsilon = 0.05$ (dashed line). (b) Dependence of L on K for $\epsilon = 0.05$. (c) The running time $t[K, L(K))]$. The minimum is marked $*$.

The family of error curves can be efficiently generated. The number of partitions L is bounded by the available computer memory. Let L_{max} be that bound. Similarly, we can set a maximum on the number of cuts, K_{max}. Next, the LSH data structure is built with (K_{max}, L_{max}). As the result of a query is the union of the results on all the L_{max} partitions, the approximation error can be computed incrementally for $L = 1, \cdots, L_{max}$ by adding one partition at a time, yielding the approximate error for all values of L. This yields $L(K_{max})$ which is subsequently used as L_{max} for $K_{max} - 1$, etc.

9.3.3 Data-Driven Partitions

The strategy of generating the L random tessellations has an important influence on the performance of LSH. In [7] the coordinates d_k have equal chance to be selected and the values v_k are uniformly distributed over the range of the corresponding coordinate. Under this assumption and when given a distance r, probabilities p_1 and p_2, and an uncertainty value ϵ, an LSH data structure can be built using appropriate values of K and L to satisfy the following requirements. Given a query point q and a data point p, then if the distance between them is less than r, then the probability that the query will return p is greater than p_1. On the other hand, if the distance between them is greater than $(1 + \epsilon)r$, then the probability that the query will return p is less than p_2. This partitioning strategy works well only when the density of the data is approximately uniform in the entire space (i.e., the distance to the required neighbors is less than r). However, feature spaces associated with vision applications are often multimodal and with large differences in the density. In [10, 11] the problem of nonuniformly distributed data was dealt with by building several data structures associated with different values of r which have different values of K and L to accommodate the different local densities. The query is performed first under the assumption of a high density (small value of r), and when it fails to find the required neighbors the process is repeated for larger values of r. The process terminates when the nearest neighbors are found.

Our approach is to sample according to the marginal distributions along each coordinate. We use K points $\mathbf{x}_i$ chosen at random from the data set. For each point one of its coordinates is selected at random to define a cut. Using more than one coordinate from a point would imply sampling from partial joint densities, but that does not seem to be more advantageous. Our adaptive, data driven strategy assures that in denser regions more cuts will be made yielding smaller cells, while in sparser regions there will be fewer cuts. On average all cells will contain a similar number of points.

The 2D data in fig. 9.3(a) and 9.3(b) comprised of four clusters and uniformly distributed background is used to demonstrate the two sampling strategies. In both cases the same number of cuts were used but the data driven method places most of the cuts over the clusters [see fig. 9.3(b)]. For a quantitative performance assessment a data set of ten normal distributions with arbitrary shapes (5000 points each) were defined in fifty dimensions. When the data-driven strategy is used, the distribution of the number of points in a cell is much more compact and their average value is much lower [fig. 9.3(c)]. As a consequence, the data driven strategy yields more efficient k-NN queries for complex data sets. For more uniformly distributed data sets the data-driven method converges to the original LSH method.

9.4 Mean Shift in High Dimensions

Given $\mathbf{y}_j$, the current location in the iterations, an LSH-based query retrieves the approximate set of neighbors needed to compute the next location (9.5). The resolution of the data analysis is controlled by the user. In the fixed bandwidth mean shift method the user provides the bandwidth parameter h. In the AMS method, the user sets the number of neighbors k

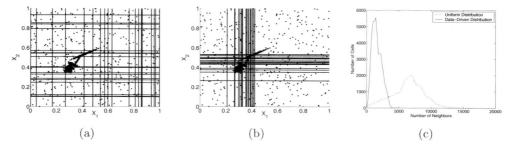

Figure 9.3 Uniform vs. data-driven partitions. Typical result for 2D data obtained with (a) uniform, (b) data-driven strategy. (c) Distribution of points per cell for a 50D data set.

used in the pilot density procedure. The parameters K and L of the LSH data structure are selected employing the technique discussed in subsection 9.3.2. The bandwidths h_i associated with the data points are obtained by performing n neighborhood queries. Once the bandwidths are set, the adaptive mean shift procedure runs at approximately the same cost as the fixed bandwidth mean shift. Thus, the difference between mean shift and AMS is only one additional query per point.

An ad hoc procedure provides further speedup. Since the resolution of the data structure is $C_\cap$, with high probability one can assume that all the points within $C_\cap$ will converge to the same mode. Thus, once any point from a $C_\cap$ is associated with a mode, the subsequent queries to $C_\cap$ automatically return this mode and the mean shift iterations stop. The modes are stored in a separate hash table whose keys are the L Boolean vectors associated with $C_\cap$.

9.4.1 Adaptive vs. Fixed Bandwidth Mean Shift

To illustrate the advantage of adaptive mean shift, a data set containing 125,000 points in a 50D cube was generated. From these 10×2500 points were generated from ten spherical normal distributions (clusters) whose means were positioned on a line through the origin. The standard deviation increases as the mean becomes more distant from the origin. For an adjacent pair of clusters, the ratio of the sum of standard deviations to the distance between the means was kept constant. The remaining 100,000 points were uniformly distributed in the 50D cube. Plotting the distances of the data points from the origin yields a graph very similar to the one in fig. 9.4(a). Note that the points farther from the origin have a larger spread.

The performance of the fixed bandwidth mean shift and the AMS procedures is compared for various parameter values in fig. 9.4. The experiments were performed for 500 points chosen at random from each cluster, a total of 5000 points. The location associated with each selected point *after* the mean shift procedure is the employed performance measure. Ideally this location should be near the center of the cluster to which the point belongs.

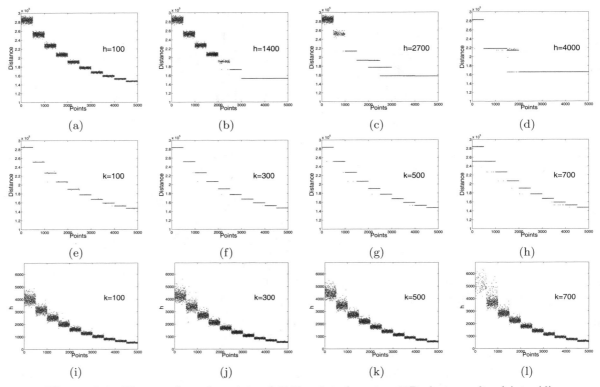

Figure 9.4 Distance from the origin of 5000 points from ten 50D clusters *after* (a) to (d): fixed bandwidth mean shift, and (e) to (h): AMS. The parameters: mean shift – bandwidth h; AMS – number of neighbors k. (i) to (l): the adaptive bandwidths for AMS data points.

In the mean shift strategy, when the bandwidth h is small due to the sparseness of the high-dimensional space, very few points have neighbors within distance h. The mean shift procedure does not detect any neighbors and the allocation of the points is to themselves [fig. 9.4(a)]. On the other hand, as h increases the windows become too large for some of the local structures and points may converge incorrectly to the center (mode) of an adjacent cluster [fig. 9.4(b) to (d)].

The pilot density estimation in the AMS strategy automatically adapts the bandwidth to the local structure. The parameter k, the number of neighbors used for the pilot estimation, does not have a strong influence. The data are processed correctly for $k = 100$ to 500, except for a few points [fig. 9.4(e) to (g)], and even for $k = 700$ only some of the points in the cluster with the largest spread converge to the adjacent mode [fig. 9.4(h)]. The superiority of the adaptive mean shift in high dimensions is clearly visible. In fig. 9.4(i) to (l) the bandwidth values for the AMS procedure are shown. Note the wide spread of values for the different points. This shows that the attempt to choose a single bandwidth for all the data points is futile. Due to the sparseness of the 50D space, the 100,000 points in the background did not interfere with the mean shift processes under either strategy, proving its robustness.

The use of the LSH data structure in the mean shift procedure assures a significant speedup. We have derived four different feature spaces from a texture image with the filter banks discussed in the next section. The spaces had dimension $d = 4, 8, 13$, and 48, and contained $n = 65,536$ points. An AMS procedure was run both with linear and approximate queries for 1638 points. The number of neighbors in the pilot density estimation was $k = 100$. The approximation error of the LSH was $\epsilon = 0.05$. The running times (in seconds) in table 9.1 show the achieved speedups.

Table 9.1 Running times of AMS implementations

d	Traditional	LSH	Speedup
4	1507	80	18.8
8	1888	206	9.2
13	2546	110	23.1
48	5877	276	21.3

The speedup will increase with the number of data points n, and will decrease with the number of neighbors k. Therefore in the mean shift procedure the speedup is not as high as in applications in which only a small number of neighbors are required.

9.5 Applications

The adaptive mean shift procedure in high dimensions has been implemented. This procedure has been used in two different applications: texture classification and multispectral image segmentation. In both cases the mean shift method is compared to k-means-based methods.

9.5.1 Texture Classification

Efficient methods exist for texture classification under varying illumination and viewing direction [3, 12, 15, 18]. In the state-of-the-art approaches a texture is characterized through *textons*, which are cluster centers in a feature space derived from the input. Following [12] this feature space is built from the output of a filter bank applied at every pixel. However, as was shown recently [19], neighborhood information in the spatial domain may also suffice.

The approaches differ in the employed filter bank.

– **LM**: A combination of forty eight anisotropic and isotropic filters was used by Leung and Malik [12] and Cula and Dana [3]. The filters are Gaussian masks, their first derivative, and Laplacian, defined at three scales. Because of the oriented filters, the representation is sensitive to texture rotations. The feature space is 48D.

– **S**: A set of thirteen circular symmetric filters was used by Schmid [15] to obtain a rotationally invariant feature set. The feature space is 13D.

– **M4**, **M8**: Both representations were proposed by Varma and Zissermann [18]. The first one (M4) is based on two rotationally symmetric and twelve oriented filters. The second set is an extension of the first one at three different scales. The feature vector is computed by retaining only the maximum response for the oriented filters (two out of twelve for M4 and six out of thirty six for M8), thus reducing the dependence on the global texture orientation. The feature space is 4D and 8D respectively.

To find the textons, usually the standard k-means clustering algorithm is used, which, as was discussed in section 9.1, has several limitations. The shape of the clusters is restricted to be spherical and their number has to be set prior to the processing.

The most significant textons are aggregated into the *texton library*. This serves as a dictionary of representative local structural features and must be general enough to characterize a large variety of texture classes. A texture is then modelled through its *texton histogram*. The histogram is computed by defining at every pixel a feature vector, replacing it with the closest texton from the library (vector quantization) and accumulating the results over the entire image.

Let two textures i and j be characterized by the histograms H_i and H_j built from T textons. As in [12] the χ^2 distance between these two texton distributions,

$$\chi^2(H_i, H_j) = \sum_{t=1}^{T} \frac{[H_i(t) - H_j(t)]^2}{H_i(t) + H_j(t)}, \tag{9.8}$$

is used to measure similarity, although note the absence of the factor $1/2$ to take into account that the comparison is between *two* histograms derived from data. In a texture classification task the training image with the smallest distance from the test image determines the class of the latter.

In our experiments we substituted the k-means based clustering module with the AMS-based robust nonparametric clustering. Thus, the textons instead of being *mean-based* are now *mode-based*, and the number of the significant ones is determined automatically.

The complete Brodatz database containing 112 textures with varying degrees of complexity was used in the experiments. Classification of the Brodatz database is challenging because it contains many nonhomogeneous textures. The 512×512 images were divided into four 256×256 subimages with half of the subimages being used for training (224 models) and the other half for testing (224 queries). The normalizations recommended in [18] (both in the image and filter domains) were also performed.

The number of significant textons detected with the AMS procedure depends on the texture. We have limited the number of mode textons extracted from a texture class to five. The same number was used for the mean textons. Thus, by adding the textons to the library, a texton histogram has at most $T = 560$ bins.

Table 9.2 Classification results for the Brodatz database

Filter	M4	M8	S	LM
Random	84.82%	88.39%	89.73%	92.41%
k-means	85.71%	94.64%	93.30%	97.32%
AMS	85.27%	93.75%	93.30%	98.66%

The classification results using the different filter banks are presented in table 9.2. The best result was obtained with the LM mode textons, an additional three correct classifications out of the six errors with the mean textons. However, there is no clear advantage in using the mode textons with the other filter banks.

The classification performance is close to its upper bound defined by the texture inhomogeneity, due to which the test and training images of a class can be very different. This observation is supported by the performance degradation obtained when the database images were divided into sixteen 128×128 subimages and the same half/half partition yielded 896 models and 896 queries. The recognition rate decreased for all the filter banks. The best result of 94%, was again obtained with the LM filters for both the mean and mode textons. In [8], with the same setup but employing a different texture representation, and using only 109 textures from the Brodatz database, the recognition rate was 80.4%.

A texture class is characterized by the histogram of the textons, an approximation of the feature space distribution. The histogram is constructed from a Voronoi diagram with T cells. The vertices of the diagram are the textons, and each histogram bin contains the number of feature points in a cell. Thus, variations in textons translate in approximating the distribution by a different diagram, but appear to have a weak influence on the classification performance. When by uniform sampling five random vectors were chosen as textons, the classification performance (RANDOM) decreased only between 1% and 6%. The reduction in performance is probably due to textons located in sparse areas of the distributions. But when they are located in more dense regions as a result of the mean shift or the k-means procedures the performance improves somewhat.

The k-means clustering imposes rigidly a given number of identical spherical clusters over the feature space. Thus, it is expected that when this structure is not adequate, the mode based textons will provide a more meaningful decomposition of the texture image. This is proven in the following two examples.

In fig. 9.5 the LM filter bank was applied to a regular texture. The AMS procedure extracted twenty one textons, the number also used in the k-means clustering. However, when ordered by size, the first few mode textons

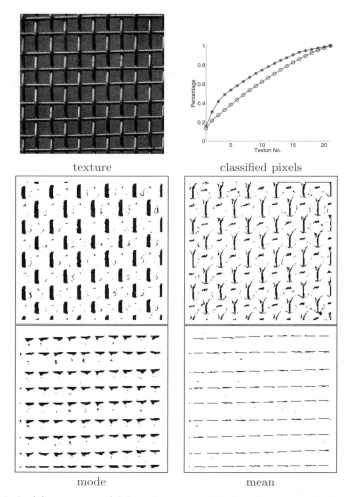

texture   classified pixels

mode   mean

Figure 9.5 Mode (∗)- vs. mean (∘)-based textons. The local structure is better captured by the mode textons. D001 texture, LM filter bank.

are associated with more pixels in the image than the mean textons, which always account for a similar number of pixels per texton. The difference between the mode and mean textons can be seen by marking the pixels associated with textons of the same local structure (fig. 9.5, bottom). The advantage of the mode-based representation is more evident for the irregular texture in fig. 9.6, where the cumulative distribution of the mode textons classified pixels has a sharper increase.

Since textons capture local spatial configurations, we believe that combining the mode textons with the representation proposed in [19] can offer more insight into why the texton approach is superior to previous techniques.

9.5.2   Multispectral Image Segmentation

In a second set of experiments we compared mean shift-based segmentation with k-means-based segmentation. The inputs were multispectral images. Each pixel consisted of thirty one bands in the visual spectrum. In the

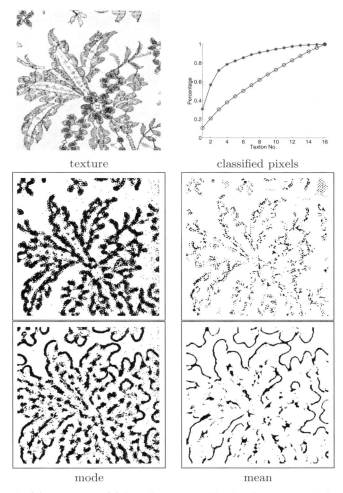

texture   classified pixels

mode   mean

Figure 9.6 Mode (∗)- vs. mean (○)-based textons. The local structure is better captured by the mode textons. D040 texture, S filter bank.

experiments only the photometric data were used. The x-y coordinates of the pixels were discarded. As in the previous experiments the number of clusters recovered by the mean shift clustering was used as the value of k for the k-means clustering. In the following two examples, shown in fig. 9.7, the differences between the two methods can be seen. In both examples the mean shift-based segmentation better segments the images. Consider the large leaf on the left side of the first image. The mean shift segmentation correctly segments the leaf into two segments whereas the k-means clustering method oversegments the light green part of the leaf. The reason for that is that the intensity of light falling on the leaf changes depending on the surface normal. This causes all the thirty one bands to change depending on the normal, creating an approximately 1D surface in $\Re^{31}$. Mean shift clustering can deal clusters of arbitrary shape as long as they are continuous. k-means clustering on the other hand assumes that the clusters are spherical and thus in this case oversegments the single natural cluster. The mean shift clustering is also able to detect other meaningful clusters, e.g., a segment of specular pixels.

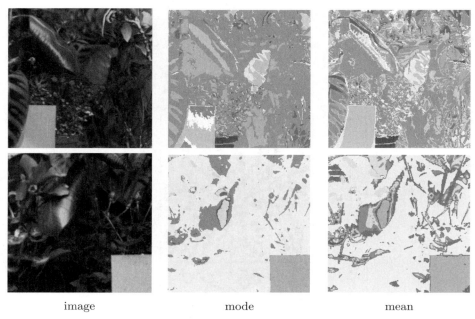

image   mode   mean

Figure 9.7   Multispectral image segmentation. Mode- vs. mean-based classification.

9.6   Conclusion

We have introduced a computationally efficient method that makes possible the detection of modes of distributions in high dimensional spaces. By employing a data structure based on LSH, a significant decrease in the running time was obtained while maintaining the quality of the results. The new implementation of the mean shift procedure opens the door to the development of vision algorithms exploiting feature space analysis - including learning techniques - in high dimensions. The C++ source code of this implementation of mean shift can be downloaded from http://www.caip.rutgers.edu/riul.

Acknowledgments

We thank Bogdan Matei of the Sarnoff Corporation, Princeton, NJ, for calling our attention to the LSH data structure. This work was done during the sabbatical of I.S. at Rutgers University. The support of the National Science Foundation under grant IRI 99-87695 is gratefully acknowledged.

References

1. D. Comaniciu and P. Meer. Mean shift: A robust approach toward feature space analysis. *IEEE Transactions on Pattern Analysis and Machine Intelligence*, 24(5):603–619, 2002.

2. D. Comaniciu, V. Ramesh, and P. Meer. The variable bandwidth mean shift and data-driven scale selection. In *Proceedings of the Eighth International Conference on Computer Vision*, Vancouver, Canada, volume I, pages 438–445, July 2001.

3. O. G. Cula and K. J. Dana. Compact representation of bidirectional texture functions. In *Proceedings of IEEE Conference on Computer Vision and Pattern Recognition*, Kauai, HI, volume 1, pages 1041–1047, 2001.

4. M. de Berg, M. van Kreveld, M. Overmars, and O. Schwartzkopf. *Computational Geometry. Algorithms and Applications*, Berlin, second edition, Springer-Verlag, 2000.

5. D. DeMenthon. Spatio-temporal segmentation of video by hierarchical mean shift analysis. In *Proceedings of Statistical Methods in Video Processing Workshop*, Copenhagen, 2002. Also CAR-TR-978 Center for Automatation Research, University of Maryland, College Park.

6. R.O. Duda, P.E. Hart, and D.G. Stork. *Pattern Classification.* second edition, Hoboken NJ, Wiley & Sons, 2001.

7. A. Gionis, P. Indyk, and R. Motwani. Similarity search in high dimensions via hashing. In *Proceedings of International Conference on Very Large Data Bases*, pages 518–529, 1999.

8. G. M. Haley and B. S. Manjunath. Rotation-invariant texture classification using a complete space-frequency model. *IEEE Transactions on Image Processing*, 8(2):255–269, 1999.

9. P. Indyk. A sublinear time approximation scheme for clustering in metric spaces. In *Proceedings of IEEE Symposium on Foundations of Computer Science*, pages 154–159, 1999.

10. P. Indyk and R. Motwani. Approximate nearest neighbors: towards removing the curse of dimensionality. In *Proceedings of Symposium on Theory of Computing*, pages 604–613, 1998.

11. E. Kushilevitz, R. Ostrovsky, and Y. Rabani. Efficient search for approximate nearest neighbor in high dimensional spaces. In *Proceedings of Symposium on Theory of Computing*, pages 614–623, 1998.

12. T. Leung and J. Malik. Representing and recognizing the visual appearance of materials using three-dimensional textons. *International Journal of Computer Vision*, 43(1):29–44, 2001.

13. S.A. Nene and S.K. Nayar. A simple algorithm for nearest-neighbor search in high dimensions. *IEEE Transactions on Pattern Analysis and Machine Intelligence*, 19(9):989–1003, 1997.

14. R. Ostrovsky and Y. Rabani. Polynomial time approximation schemes for geometric k-clustering. In *Proceedings of IEEE Symposium on Foundations of Computer Science*, pages 349–358, 2000.

15.   C. Schmid. Constructing models for content-based image retrieval. In *Proceedings of IEEE Conference on Computer Vision and Pattern Recognition,* Kauai, HI, volume 2, pages 39–45, 2001.

16.   G. Shakhnarovich, P. Viola, and T. Darrell. Fast pose estimation with parameter-sensitive hashing. In *Proceedings of the Ninth International Confernce on Computer Vision,* Nice, pages 750–757, 2003.

17.   B. W. Silverman. *Density Estimation for Statistics and Data Analysis.* London, Chapman & Hall, 1986.

18.   M. Varma and A. Zisserman. Classifying images of materials. In *Proceedings of the European Conferebce on Computer Vision,* Copenhagen , volume 3, pages 255–271, 2002.

19.   M. Varma and A. Zisserman. Texture classification: Are filter banks necessary? In *Proceedings of IEEE Conference on Computer Vision and Pattern Recognition,* Madison, WI, volume 2, pages 691–698, 2003.

10 Object Recognition using Locality Sensitive Hashing of Shape Contexts

Andrea Frome and Jitendra Malik

At the core of many computer vision algorithms lies the task of finding a correspondence between image features local to a part of an image. Once these features are calculated, matching is commonly performed using a nearest-neighbor algorithm. In this chapter, we focus on the topic of object recognition, and examine how the complexity of a basic feature-matching approach grows with the number of object classes. We use this as motivation for proposing approaches to feature-based object recognition that grow sublinearly with the number of object classes.

10.1 Regional Descriptor Approach

Our approach to object recognition relies on the matching of feature vectors (also referred to here as *features*) which characterize a region of a two-dimensional (2D) or 3D image, where by "3D image" we mean the point cloud resulting from a range scan. We use the term *descriptor* to refer to the method or "template" for calculating the feature vector. There are several lines of work which develop descriptors for use in object recognition. [15] introduced jet-based features; [12] introduced the scale- and rotation-invariant feature transform (SIFT) descriptor for recognition and matching in intensity images; [10] describes the *spin image* descriptor for recognizing objects by shape in 3D range scans; [3] describes a histogram-based descriptor for recognizing objects in 2D images by shape, called the *shape context*, which is extended to the *generalized shape context* in [14]; and [6] presents the *3D shape context*, an extension of the shape context to three dimensions, and experimentally evaluates its performance against the spin image descriptor in difficult range image recognition tasks.

The spin image and shape context descriptors share a *regional* approach to feature calculation; the features incorporate information within a *support region* of the image centered at a chosen *basis point*. The locality of these *regional descriptors* make them robust to clutter and occlusion, while at the same time each feature contains more information than purely local descriptors due to their extended support. In some recognition approaches the features are computed at particularly salient locations in the image determined by an *interest operator*, such as in [12]. In other approaches, including the cited works that make use of spin images and shape contexts, the basis points at which features are computed are chosen randomly and are not required to posses any distinguishing characteristics.

Object recognition algorithms typically work by calculating features from a query image and comparing those features to other features previously calculated from a set of *reference* images, and return a decision about which object or image from among the reference set best matches the query image. We consider *full object recognition* to be achieved when the algorithm returns the identity, location, and position of an object occurring in a query image. Our discussion in this chapter focuses on a relaxed version of the full recognition problem where the algorithm returns a *short list* of objects, at least one of which occurs *somewhere* in the image. An algorithm solving this relaxed recognition problem can be used to prune a large field of candidate objects for a more expensive algorithm which solves the full recognition problem. In a more complex system it could be used as an early stage in a cascade of object recognition algorithms which are increasingly more expensive and discriminating, similar in spirit to the cascade of classifiers made popular in the vision community by [16]. A pruning step or early cascade stage is effective when it reduces the total computation required for full recognition and does not reduce the recognition performance of the system. To this end, we want a short-list recognition algorithm which (1) minimizes the number of misses, that is, the fraction of queries where the short list does not include any objects present in the query image, and (2) minimizes its computational cost.

Object recognition algorithms based on features have been shown to achieve high recognition rates in the works cited above and many others, though often in a an easy or restricted recognition setting. We will demonstrate methods for speeding a simple matching algorithm while maintaining high recognition accuracy in a difficult recognition task, beginning with an approach which uses an exhaustive k-nearest-neighbor (k-NN) search to match the *query features* calculated from a query image to the *reference features* calculated from the set of reference images. Using the distances calculated between query and reference features, we generate a short list of objects which might be present in the query image.

It should be noted that the method we examine does not enforce relative geometric constraints between the basis points in the query and reference images, and that most feature-based recognition algorithms do use this additional information. For example, for reference features centered at basis points p_1 and p_2 and query features centered at basis points q_1 and q_2, if p_1 is found to be a match for q_1, p_2 a match for q_2, and we are considering rigid objects, then it should be the case that the distance in the image between p_1 and p_2 should be similar to the distance between q_1 and q_2. There are many methods for using these types of constraints, [8], RANSAC, and [5] to name a few. We choose not to use these constraints in order to demonstrate the power of matching feature vectors alone. A geometric-based pruning or verification method could follow the matching algorithms described in this chapter.

The drawback of an exhaustive search of stored reference features is that it is expensive, and for the method to be effective as a pruning stage, it needs to be fast. Many of the descriptors listed above are high-dimensional; in the works cited, the scale-invariant feature transform (SIFT) descriptor has 160 dimensions, the spin image has about 200, the 2D shape context has 60 (the generalized version has twice as many for the same number of bins), and the 3D shape context has almost 2000. The best algorithms for exact nearest-neighbor search in such high-dimensional spaces requires time linear in the number of reference features. In addition, the number of reference features is linear in the number of example objects the system is designed to recognize. If we aim to build systems that can recognize hundreds or thousands of example objects, then the system must be able to run in time sublinear in the number of objects.

The goal of this chapter is to present ways to maintain the recognition accuracy of this "short-list" algorithm while reducing its computational cost. Locality-sensitive hashing (LSH) plays a key role in a final approach that is both accurate and has complexity sublinear in the number of objects being recognized. In our experiments we will be evaluating variations on the basic matching method with the 3D shape context descriptor.

10.2 Shape Context Descriptors

We will focus on a type of descriptor called the *shape context*. In their original form, shape context features characterize shape in 2D images as histograms of edge pixels (see [2]). In [14] the authors use the same template as 2D shape contexts but capture more information about the shape by storing aggregate edge orientation for each bin. In [4], the authors developed the notion of *geometric blur* which is an analog to the 2D shape context for continuous-valued images. We extended the shape context to three dimensions in [6], where it characterizes shape by histogramming the position of points in a range scan. In the rest of this section, we describe the basics of the 2D and 3D shape context descriptors in more detail, and introduce the experimental framework used in the rest of the chapter.

10.2.1 Two-dimensional Shape Contexts

To calculate a 2D shape context feature from an image, first run your favorite edge detector on the image. Next, choose a coordinate in the edge map to be a basis point, and imagine a radar-like template like the one in figure 10.1 laid down over the image, centered at that point. The lines of this pattern divide the image into regions, each of which corresponds to one dimension of the feature vector. The value for the dimension is calculated as the number of edge pixels which fall into the region. This feature vector can be thought of as a histogram which summarizes the spatial distribution of edges in the image relative to the chosen basis point. Each region in the template corresponds to one bin in the histogram, and we use the term *bin* to refer to the region in the image as well as the dimension in the feature vector. Note that if the bins were small enough to each contain one pixel, then the histogram would be an exact description of the shape in the support region.

This template has a few advantageous properties. The bins farther from the center summarize a larger area of the image than those close to the center. The gives a foveal effect; the feature more accurately captures and weights more heavily information toward the center. To accentuate this property of shape context descriptors, we use equally spaced log-radius divisions. This causes bins to get "fuzzy" more quickly as you move from the center of the descriptor.

When comparing two shape context features, even if the shapes from which they are calculated are very similar, the following must also be similar in order to register the two features as a good match:

- orientation of the descriptor relative to the object
- scale of the object

To account for different scales, we can search over scale space, e.g., by calculating a Gaussian pyramid for our query image, calculating query features in each of the down- and upscaled images, and finding the best match at each scale. We could sidestep the issue of orientation by assuming that objects are in a canonical orientation in the images, and orient the template the same way for all basis points. Or, to make it robust to variation, we could orient the template to the edge gradient at the basis point or include in our training set images at different orientations.

10.2.2 Three-dimensional Shape Contexts

In order to apply the same idea to range images, we extended the template to three dimensions (see figure 10.1 for a visualization). We use a spherical support volume, and divide the sphere at regular angles along the elevation and azimuth dimensions. Again we use the log-radius division as with the

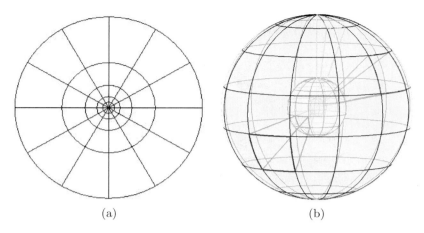

(a) (b)

Figure 10.1 Example templates for the shape contexts: (a) for 2D, (b) for 3D. The number of divisions shown are not the same as we used in our experiments.

2D shape contexts. The value for a bin is the count of the number of points in three dimensions from the raw range image that fall into its region.

When working with 3D range scans, we do not need to consider differences in scale since the scanner measurements in both the query and reference scans are reported in real-world dimensions. In three dimensions there are 2 degrees of freedom in the orientation of the template. We solve half of the problem by aligning the north pole with the surface normal calculated at the basis point. However, this still leaves a free rotation in the azimuth dimension. We account for that freedom with sampling; if we divide the azimuth into twelve sections, then we include in the reference set twelve discrete rotations of the feature vector. Since we are rotating the reference features, we do not need to rotate the query features. We could just as easily rotate the query features instead, but it should become clear why we rotate the reference features when we discuss our use of LSH later in the chapter.

Spin images, another descriptor used for 3D object recognition presented in [10], is very similar to the 3D shape context. It differs primarily in the shape of its support volume and its approach to the azimuth degree of freedom in the orientation: the spin image sums the counts over changes in azimuth. See [6] for a direct comparison between spin images and 3D shape contexts in similar experiments.

10.2.3 Experiments with Three-dimensional Shape Contexts

In this subsection, we introduce the data set that we use throughout the chapter to evaluate recognition with 3D shape contexts. The 3D shape contexts we calculate are the same as those used in [6]: they have twelve azimuth divisions, eleven elevation divisions, and fifteen radial divisions. These values were chosen after a small amount of experimentation with a similar data set.

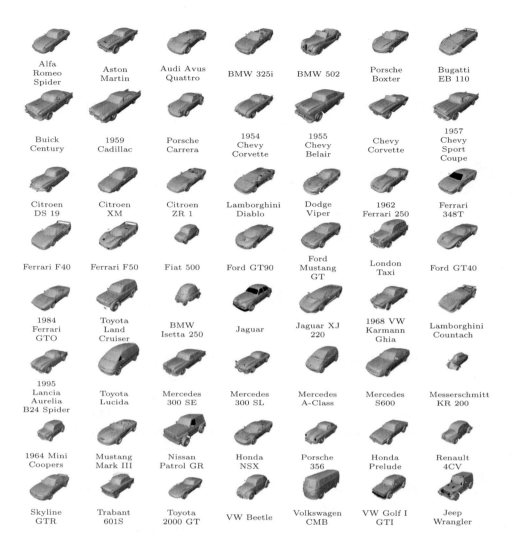

Figure 10.2   The fifty-six car models used in our experiments.

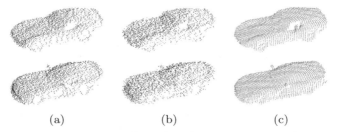

(a)   (b)   (c)

Figure 10.3 The *top row* shows scans from the 1962 Ferrari 250 model, and the *bottom* scans are from the Dodge Viper. The scans in column *(a)* are the query scans at 30 degrees elevation and 15 degrees azimuth with $\sigma = 5$ cm noise, and those in *(b)* are from the same angle but with $\sigma = 10$ cm noise. With 10 cm noise, it is difficult to differentiate the vehicles by looking at the 2D images of the point clouds. Column *(c)* shows the reference scans closest in viewing direction to the query scans (45 degrees azimuth and 45 degrees elevation).

The range scans from which we calculate the features are simulated from a set of fifty-six 3D car models, and are separated into reference scans (our training set) and query scans. The full models are shown in figure 10.2. The reference scans were generated from a viewpoint at 45 degrees elevation (measured from the horizon) and from four different azimuth positions, spaced 90 degrees apart around the car, starting from an angle halfway between the front and side views of the vehicle. The query scans were generated from a viewpoint at 30 degrees elevation and at one azimuth position 15 degrees different from the nearest reference scan. We also added Gaussian noise to the query scans along the viewing direction, with either a 5 cm or 10 cm standard deviation. This amount of noise is comparable to or greater than the noise one could expect from a quality scanner. An example of the noisy query scans next to the nearest reference scan for two of the car models is shown in figure 10.3.

From the reference scans, we calculated normals at the points, and calculated 3D shape context features at basis points sampled uniformly over the surface, an average of 373 features per scan. For each noisy query scan, we calculated the normals, then calculated features at 300 randomly chosen basis points. Now we can describe our first experiment.

10.3 Basic Matching Experiment

Experiment 1

Given a query scan, we want to return the best match from among the reference scans. Each of the 300 query features from the query scan casts a "vote" for one of the fifty-six car models, and the best match to the query scan as a whole is the model which received the most votes. We determine a query feature's vote by finding its nearest neighbor from among the reference features, and awarding the vote to the model that produced that reference feature. We could also give the n best matches by ordering the models by the number of votes received, and returning the top n from that list. We run this procedure for all fifty-six query scans and calculate the recognition rate as the percentage of the fifty-six query scans which were correctly identified.

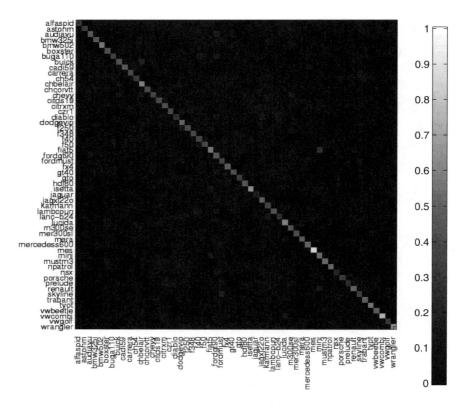

Figure 10.4 Confusion matrix for experiment 1 for 5 cm noise queries. Each row corresponds to one query and each column to one reference model. A square in the matrix represents the percentage of votes for the column's reference models by the row's query, where each row sums to 100%. The scale at the far right maps the colors to numbers. The strong diagonal means that most of the votes for each 5 cm noise query went to the correct corresponding model, giving us 100% recognition in the top choice.

The results we get are shown as confusion matrices in figure 10.4 for the 5 cm and figure 10.5 for 10 cm queries. Each row corresponds to the results for one query scan, and each column to one car model (four reference scans). Each square is a color corresponding to the number of votes that the query gave for the model. If every query feature voted for the correct model, then the matrix would have a dark red diagonal and otherwise be dark blue. Perfect recognition is achieved when the diagonal has the largest number from each row, which is the case here for the 5 cm noise data set. In the 10 cm experiment, we got fifty-two out of fifty-six queries correct, giving a recognition rate of 92.86%. The correct model is always in the top four matches, so if we are want a short list of depth four or greater, then our recognition is 100%.

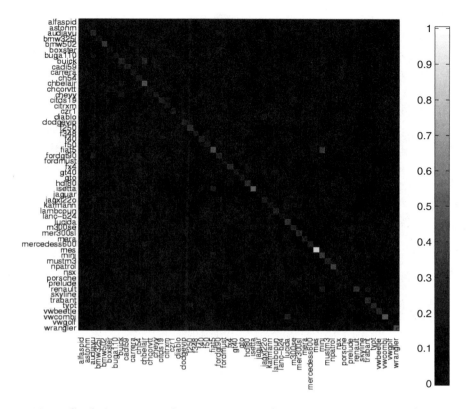

Figure 10.5 Confusion matrix for experiment 1 for 10 cm noise queries. See caption of figure 10.4 for legend. There was more confusion here than with 5 cm noise, with fifty-two of the fifty-six models correctly identified in the top choice, and 100% recognition within the top four choices.

10.3.1 Complexity and Computation Time

Take

- m to be the number of reference images (assume one object per reference image),
- n_r the number of features calculated per reference image,
- n_q the number of features calculated per query image,
- d the dimensionality of the features,
- p the number of pixels or points in the query scene, and
- s the number of scales over which we need to search.

Let us first look at the cost of computing each query feature. For the 2D shape context, we need to compute edge features at all the pixels that may lie in one of the descriptors' support, and then count the number of edge pixels in each bin. This gives us a preprocessing cost of $O(p)$ and a computation cost of $O(p)$ for each query feature, for a total of $O(p)+O(p{\cdot}n_q)$ for the query image as a whole.

For the 3D shape context, we do not need to preprocess all the points in the scan, just the neighborhood around the basis point to get the normal at that point. We still need to look through the points in the scene to calculate the bin contents, giving a cost of $O(p \cdot n_q)$.

Once we have the query features, we need to search through the $m \cdot n_r$ reference features. If we are performing an exact nearest-neighbor search as in experiment 1, we need to calculate the distance between each of those reference features and each of the query features. The cost for that is $O(m \cdot n_r \cdot n_q \cdot d)$. If we are working with 2D shape contexts, then we may also have to search over scale, increasing the cost to $O(m \cdot n_r \cdot n_q \cdot d \cdot s)$.

For the 3D shape contexts, this gives us a total cost of $O(p \cdot n_q) + O(m \cdot n_r \cdot n_q \cdot d)$. In experiment 1, $n_q = 300$, $m = 224$, $n_r = 4476$ (average of 373 features per reference scan times the twelve rotations through the azimuth for each), and $d = 1980$ ($11 \times 12 \times 15$), so the second term sums to 5.96×10^{11} pairs of floating point numbers we need to examine in our search. On a 1.3 GHz 64-bit Itanium 2 processor, the comparison of 300 query features to the full database of reference features takes an average of 3.3 hours, using some optimization and disk blocking. The high recognition rate we have seen comes at a high computational cost.

The rest of this chapter focuses on reducing the cost of computing these matches, first by reducing n_q using the *representative descriptor method* and then by reducing n_r using LSH. The voting results for $n_q = 300$ using exact nearest neighbor provides a baseline for performance, to which we will compare our results.

10.4   Reducing Running Time with Representative Descriptors

If we densely sample features from the reference scans (i.e., choose a large n_r), then we can sparsely sample basis points at which to calculate features from query scans. This is the case for a few reasons.

• Because the features are fuzzy, they are robust to small changes due to noise, clutter, and shift in the center point location. This makes it possible to match a feature from a reference object and a feature from a query scene even if they are centered at slightly different locations on the object or are oriented slightly differently. This also affects how densely we need to sample the reference object.

• Since regional descriptors describe a large part of the scene in fuzzy terms and a small part specifically, few are needed to describe a query scene well.

• Finally, these features can be very discriminative. Even with the data set we use below where we are distinguishing between several very similar objects, the features are descriptive enough that only a few are enough to tell apart very similar shapes.

We make use of these properties via the *representative descriptor* method. The method was originally introduced in [13] as *representative shape contexts* for the speeding search of 2D shape contexts, and were renamed in [6] to encompass the use of other descriptors such as spin images. Each of the few features calculated from the query scene is referred to as a *representative descriptor* or *RD*. What we refer to as the *representative descriptor method* really involves four aspects:

1. Using a reduced number of query points as centers for query features
2. A method for choosing which points to use as representative descriptors
3. A method for calculating a score between an RD and a reference object
4. A method for aggregating the scores for the RDs to give one score for the match between the query scene and the reference object

In our experiments, we try a range of values for the number of RDs and find that for simple matching tasks (e.g., low-noise queries), few are needed to achieve near-perfect performance. As the matching task becomes more difficult, the number required to get a good recognition rate increases.

We choose the basis points for the RDs uniformly at random from the 300 basis points from the query scans. This is probably the least sophisticated way to make the choice, and we do so to provide a baseline. Instead, we could use an interest operator such as those used with SIFT descriptors.

We take the score between one RD and a particular car model to be the smallest distance between the RD and a feature from one of the four reference scans for the model. To calculate the score between the query scene as a whole and the model, we sum the individual RD scores for that model. The model with the smallest summation is determined to be the best match. We have found this summation to be superior to the "voting" method where we take a maximum over the scores; the individual distances give a notion of the quality of the match, and summing makes use of that information, whereas taking a maximum discards it.

10.4.1 Experiment and Results

Experiment 2

Calculate n_q features from the query scan, which will be our RDs. Find the nearest neighbors to each of the RDs from each of the models, and calculate the scores. The model with the smallest score is the best match. Repeat for all queries and calculate the recognition rate as the percentage of query models that were correctly matched. Repeat the experiment several times with different randomly chosen sets of n_q features, and report the average recognition rate across these runs. Perform the experiment for different values of n_q.

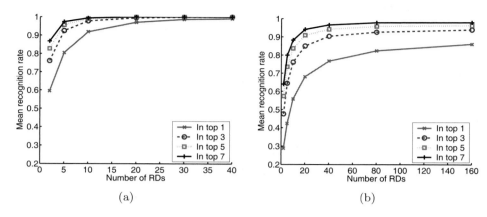

Figure 10.6 Results from experiment 2, shown as the number of RDs vs. mean recognition rate for the *(a)* 5 cm noise and *(b)* 10 cm noise queries. While our performance has dropped when considering only the top match, our recognition within a short list of matches is still very good, while we are performing a fraction of the feature comparisons. Note that the number of feature comparisons increases linearly with the number of RDs.

The graphs in figure 10.6 show the results. Note that the number of comparisons increases linearly with the number of RDs. For example, if the voting method with 300 query features required n comparisons, then using thirty RDs requires $n \times \frac{30}{300}$ comparisons. With the 5 cm queries, we achieve 100% recognition with thirty descriptors if we consider the top seven matches. If we use forty RDs, we achieve 99.9% in the top two matches and 100% in the top three. The performance on the 10 cm noise query degrades quickly with fewer RDs. Because of the noise, fewer of the original 300 query points are useful in matching, so we randomly choose more RDs in the hopes that we will get more of the distinctive query features. With the 10 cm queries, we achieve 97.8% mean recognition in the top seven results using eighty RDs. The mean recognition within the top seven with 160 RDs is 98%.

When we consider only our top match, our performance has dropped significantly with both query sets. However, we are primarily interested in getting a *short list* of candidates, and for the 5 cm queries we can reduce the number of computations required by 87% to 90% (depending on the length of our short list) by using the RD method over voting. And for almost all choices of the forty RDs, we find the correct match in the top five returned. With the 10 cm set, we can reduce our computation by 47% to 73%. Also keep in mind that these are recognition rates averaged across 100 different random selections of the RDs; for many choices of the RDs we are achieving perfect recognition.

10.5   Reducing Search Space with a Locality-Sensitive Hash

When comparing a query feature to the reference features, we could save computation by computing distances only to the reference features that are nearby. Call this the "1, 2, 3, many" philosophy: the few close ones play a large role in the recognition; the rest of the features have little meaning for the query. One way to achieve this is to use an algorithm for approximate k-NN search that returns a set of candidates that probably lie close to the query feature. The method we will look at is LSH, first introduced in [9].

We use a version of the simple LSH algorithm described in [7] (see chapter 3 for a more recent version). To create a hash, we first find the range of the data in each of the dimensions and sum them to get the total range. Then choose k values from that range. Each of those values now defines a cut in one of the dimensions, which can be visualized as a hyperplane parallel to that dimension's axis. These planes divide the feature space into hypercubes, and two features in the same hypercube hash to the same bucket in the table. We represent each hypercube by an array of integers, and refer to this array as the *first-level hash* or *locality-sensitive hash*. There are an exponential number of these hashes, so we use a standard second-level hash function on integer arrays to translate each to a single integer. This is the number of the bucket in the table, also called the *second-level hash* value. To decrease the probability that we will miss close neighbors, we create l tables, independently generating the k cuts in each. In most of our experiments in this section, we will use twenty tables. We will use the notation $b = h_i(\cdot)$ to refer to the hash function for the ith table which takes a feature vector and returns a second-level hash, or bucket, number. $T_i(b_i)$ will refer to the set of identifiers stored in bucket b_i in the ith table.

To populate the ith hash table, we calculate $b_i = h_i(f_j)$ for each feature f_j in the set of features calculated from the reference scans, and store the unique integer identifier j for the feature f_j in bucket b_i. Given a query feature q, we find matches in two stages. First, we retrieve the set of identifiers which are the union of the matches from the l tables: $\mathbb{F} = \bigcup_{i=1}^{l} T_i(h_i(q))$. Second, we retrieve from a database on disk the feature vectors for the identifiers, and calculate the distances $\mathrm{dist}(q, f_j)$ for all features f_j where $j \in \mathbb{F}$.

The first part is the LSH query overhead, and in our experiments this takes 0.01 to 0.03 second to retrieve and sort all the identifiers from twenty tables. This is small compared to the time required in the second step, which ranges from an average of 1.12 to 2.96 seconds per query feature, depending upon the number of matches returned. Because the overhead for LSH is negligible compared to the time to do the feature comparisons, we will compare the "speed" of our queries across methods using the number of feature comparisons performed. This avoids anomalies common in timing

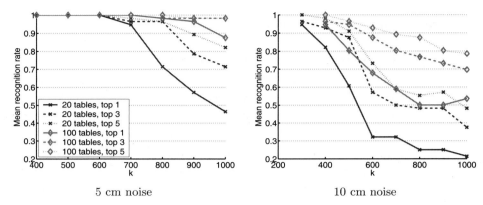

5 cm noise   10 cm noise

Figure 10.7 Results for experiment 3 using the voting method with 300 query features. The graph shows the recognition rate vs. the number of hash divisions (k) for 20 and 100 tables and for short lists of length one, three, and five (the legend applies to both graphs). The left and right graphs show results for the 5 cm and 10 cm noise queries, respectively. In general, as the number of hash divisions increases for a given number of tables, the performance degrades, and if the number of tables is increased, for a given value of k, performance increases. To see how the same factors affect the number of comparisons performed, see figure 10.8. To visualize the tradeoff between the number of comparisons and recognition rate, see section 10.9.

numbers due to network congestion, disk speed, caching, and interference from other processes.

As we mentioned earlier, we are storing in the hash tables the azimuth rotations of the reference features instead of performing the rotations on the query features. If LSH returns only the features that are most similar to a query q, it will effectively select for us the rotations to which we should compare, which saves us a linear search over rotations.

10.5.1   LSH with Voting Method

We first examine the performance of LSH using the voting method from subsection 10.2.3 to provide a comparison with the strong results achieved using exact nearest neighbor.

Experiment 3

Given the number of hash divisions k and the number of LSH tables l, perform LSH search with 300 features per query, and tabulate the best matches using the voting scheme, as we did in experiment 1. Perform for 5 cm and 10 cm noise queries.

We created 100 tables, and ran experiments using all 100 tables as well as subsets of 20, 40, 60, and 80 tables. In figure 10.7, we show how the recognition rate changes with variations in the number of hash divisions for the 5 cm and 10 cm queries. We show results for experiments with 20 and 100 tables, and show the recognition rate within the top choice, top three choices, and top five choices. In the 5 cm experiment, we maintain 100%

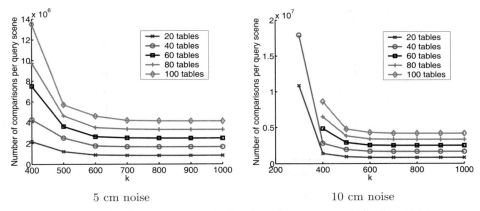

5 cm noise   10 cm noise

Figure 10.8 Results for experiment 3, showing the mean number of comparisons per query scene vs. the number of hash divisions (k), using 20, 40, 60, 80, or 100 tables. The left and right graphs show results for the 5 cm noise and 10 cm noise queries, respectively. The scale of the y-axis in the 10 cm graph is larger than in the 5 cm graph to accommodate the $k = 300$ results, though the number of comparisons required for each k and l combination is fewer with the 10 cm queries.

recognition with up to 600 hash divisions when using twenty tables, and up to 800 hash divisions if we use 100 tables and consider a short list of length five. Notice that when using twenty tables, recognition degrades quickly as k increases, whereas recognition is better maintained when using 100 tables.

In the 10 cm experiments, we only achieve 100% recognition looking at the top five and using 300 or 400 hash divisions, with recognition declining quickly for larger values of k. Also notice that recognition falls with increasing k more quickly in the 10 cm experiments. As the queries become more difficult, it is less likely we will randomly generate a table with many divisions that performs well for many of our query features.

The recognition rate is only one measure of the performance. In figure 10.8, we show the mean number of comparisons per query scene vs. the number of hash divisions. Here we show results for 20, 40, 60, 80, and 100 tables. In both the 5 cm and 10 cm queries, we see a decline in the number of comparisons with increasing k, though the decline quickly becomes asymptotic. We also see a linear increase in the number of computations with a linear increase in the number of tables used.

For the 10 cm query, we tried using 300 hash divisions, but for more than forty tables, the queries were computationally too expensive. The range on the y-axis is larger in the 10 cm graph than in the 5 cm graph due to the jump at $k = 300$, but the number of computations performed for all other combinations of k and l are fewer in the 10 cm experiments. This seems to indicate that in general, the 10 cm query features lie farther away from the reference features in feature space than the 5 cm query features.

We see that as k decreases or the number of tables increases, the recognition improves, but the number of comparisons increases. To evaluate the trade off between speed and accuracy, we show in figure 10.9 the number of

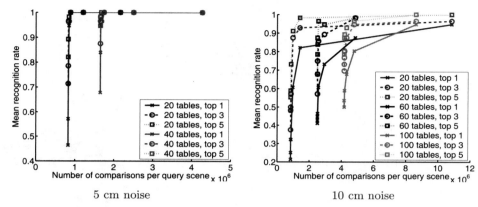

5 cm noise   10 cm noise

Figure 10.9   Results for experiment 3, where we vary the value of k along each line to show the tradeoff between the number of comparisons performed and the mean recognition rate. The ideal point is in the upper-left corner where the number of comparisons is low and recognition is perfect. Exact nearest neighbor is off the graph in the upper-right corner, and would lie at $(3.0 \times 10^8, 1)$ if it were plotted.

comparisons vs. the recognition rate, varying k along each line. The ideal point would be in the upper-left corner, where the recognition rate is high and the number of comparisons is low. Exact nearest neighbor gives us a point at $(3.0 \times 10^8, 1)$, off the graph in the far upper-right corner. In the 5 cm graph, the leftmost point still at 100% recognition is from the experiment with 600 divisions and twenty tables. We can see that there is little to gain in increasing the number of divisions or the number of tables. The rightmost points in the 10 cm graph correspond to the experiments with 300 divisions, showing that the high recognition comes at a high computational cost. The points closest to the upper-left corner are from experiments using twenty tables and either 400 or 500 hash divisions. Unless we require perfect recognition for all queries, it makes little sense to use fewer than 400 divisions or more than twenty tables.

Lastly, while we are still achieving 100% mean recognition with $k = 600$ on the 5 cm queries using the voting method, the confusion matrix in figure 10.10 shows that we are not as confident about the matches relative to the confusion matrix for exact nearest neighbor (see figures 10.4 and 10.5). The RD method depends upon having several distinguishing query features, so if we combine LSH with RD, we expect a decrease in the number of comparisons but also a further degradation in recognition performance.

10.5.2   Using RDs with LSH

Experiment 4

Perform LSH search with varying numbers of RDs, values of k, and numbers of tables. Using the model labels returned with each feature, tabulate scores as we did in experiment 2, with one exception: it is possible

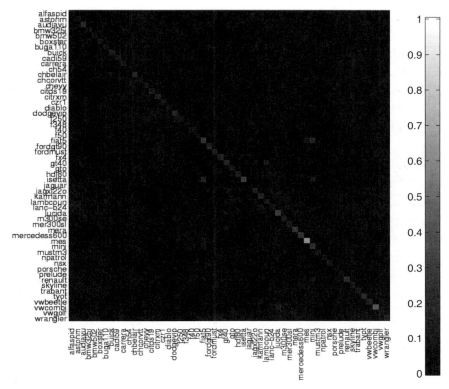

Figure 10.10 Confusion matrix showing the results for the 5 cm query for $k = 600$ from experiment 3. While we achieved 100% recognition with the top choice, comparing this matrix to the one from experiment 1 using exact nearest neighbor (see figures 10.4 and 10.5) shows that we are less certain of our choices.

that LSH does not return any matches corresponding to a particular model, and in that case, we substitute for the RD model score a number larger than any of the distances as a penalty.

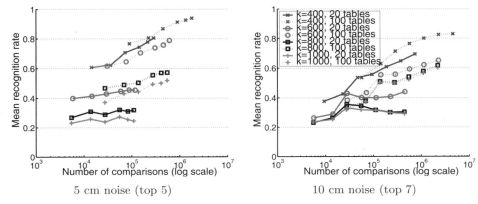

5 cm noise (top 5)   10 cm noise (top 7)

Figure 10.11 Results for experiment 4, showing number of comparisons vs. recognition rate with varying numbers of RDs along each line. We ran the experiment for different values of k and different numbers of tables. The legend applies to both graphs. In the left graph we show the recognition within the top five results for the 5 cm queries, and in the right graph we show recognition within the top seven results for the 10 cm queries.

The tradeoff for experiment 4 between number of comparisons and mean recognition rate is shown in figure 10.11. Along each line we varied the number of RDs, and show results for combinations of 400, 600, 800, and 1000 divisions and 20 and 100 tables. For the 5 cm experiment, we show recognition in a short list of five, and show results within the top seven for the 10 cm experiment. The mean recognition in the 5 cm experiment using 400 divisions and twenty tables reaches 80%, which is much worse than before. With $k = 600$ and twenty tables, which demonstrated a good tradeoff when we using the voting method with 300 query features, only a 45% mean recognition rate is achieved. We do see however, that increasing the number of tables has helped us; using $k = 400$ with 100 tables yields a mean recognition rate of 94%. We see similar degradation with the 10 cm experiments, achieving only 83% mean recognition withing the top seven results using 400 divisions and 100 tables.

Recognition performance is decreased when using LSH because LSH misses many of the nearest neighbors to the query points, resulting in a heavy penalty. We can improve performance by being more "forgiving" and including in the RD sum only the closest x percent of the RD model matches, hopefully discarding the large values that arise because LSH unluckily misses good matches. If we are using twenty RDs and we are summing the top 50%, then for a given model, we would search for the model's closest reference features to each of the twenty RDs, and include in the sum only the ten of those which are closest.

Experiment 5

We perform LSH search with varying numbers of RDs, values of k, and numbers of tables. We tally the RD scores by including in the sum the distances from only the best 50% of the RD model matches.

The results for experiment 5 in figure 10.12 show that this method improved performance significantly within the top five results for 5 cm and top seven for 10 cm. In the 5 cm experiments, our sweet spot appears to be forty RDs, 400 divisions, and twenty tables with a mean recognition rate of 99.8% within the top five matches (and 95.3% with the top match; 99.4% within the top three, not shown). In the 10 cm experiments we reach 96% mean recognition with 160 RDs, 400 divisions, and 100 tables within the top seven matches (and 93.6% in the top five, not shown). We reach 90% mean recognition with 160 RDs, 400 divisions, and twenty tables within the top seven matches, which requires less than one-sixth the number of comparisons as with the same settings except with 100 tables.

The key to further improving performance lies primarily with getting better results from our approximate nearest-neighbor algorithm. In the next section, we examine the quality of the LSH results relative to exact nearest

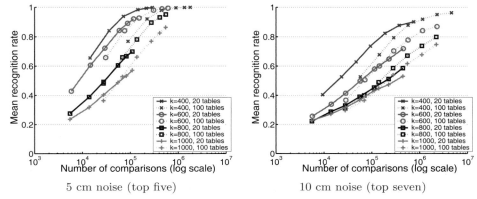

5 cm noise (top five)   10 cm noise (top seven)

Figure 10.12 Results from experiment 5, where we use the RD method but sum only the top half of the RD scores. The graphs show the number of comparisons vs. the mean recognition rate, with the number of RDs varying along each line. In the left graph we show the recognition within the top 5 results for the 5 cm queries, and in the right graph we show recognition with the top 7 results for the 10 cm queries. Note the logarithmic scale along the x-axis.

neighbor, and use this to motivate the need for algorithms that provide better nearest-neighbor performance.

10.6   Nearest-Neighbor Performance of LSH

In this section, we look at the performance of LSH as an approximate nearest-neighbor algorithm, independent of any recognition procedure. In most work on approximate nearest-neighbor algorithms, the performance is measured using the *effective distance error* or a similar measure [11, 7, 1], defined for the nth nearest neighbor as

$$E = \frac{1}{Q} \sum_{q \in Q} \left(\frac{d_{alg,n}}{d_n^*} - 1 \right), \tag{10.1}$$

where Q is the set of query features, d_n^* is the distance from the query q to the nth true nearest neighbor, and $d_{alg,n}$ is the distance from q to the nth best feature returned from the approximate algorithm. The effective distance error with increasing rank depth n is shown for the 5 cm and 10 cm queries in the first row of figure 10.13. Each line of the graphs represents one LSH query with a different number of hash divisions (k).

The effective distance error does not capture whether an approximate nearest-neighbor algorithm is returning the *correct* nearest neighbors, only how close it gets to them. In a recognition setting, the *identity* of the features returned is of primary interest, so we suggest a better measure would be *error by rank*. If we want the n nearest neighbors, the error by rank is the percentage of the true n nearest neighbors that were missing in the list of n returned by the approximate algorithm. The graphs in the second row of figure 10.13 show the error by rank with increasing n for the 5 cm and 10 cm queries.

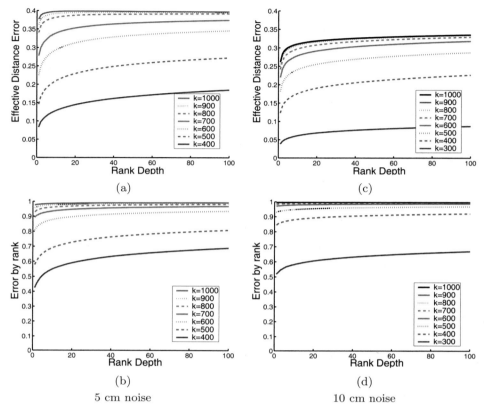

Figure 10.13 LSH performance, relative to exact nearest neighbor. The graphs in the first column show the performance on the 5 cm queries, using effective distance error in (a) and error by rank in (b). The second column shows results for the 10 cm query, with (c) showing effective distance error and (d) showing error by rank. All results are for twenty tables.

In the first column of figure 10.13 we see that for the 5 cm query, the effective distance error reaches a maximum at 40% for 800, 900, and 1000 hash divisions, but the same LSH results show almost 100% error by rank, meaning that almost never are any of the correct nearest neighbors returned. The second column of the figure shows results for the 10 cm queries. Notice that, relative to the 5 cm queries, the ceiling on the effective distance error is actually lower; the 900 and 1000 hash division LSH queries level off around 0.32, and all queries except LSH with 400 and 500 hash divisions are actually performing better by this measure than in the 5 cm query. However, we know from our recognition results that this should not be the case, that recognition results for the 10 cm queries were worse than the 5 cm queries for the same LSH settings. Indeed, we can see in the error-by-rank graph that the 10 cm queries are performing much worse than the 5 cm queries for all LSH settings.

As an aside, the lines on these graphs are monotonically increasing, which does not have to be the case in general. If an approximate nearest-neighbor algorithm misses the first nearest neighbor, but then correctly finds every nearest neighbor of deeper rank, than the error by rank would decrease with increasing rank depth, from 100% to 50% to 33%, etc. It is also true that the effective distance error need not increase with increasing rank depth. It is a feature of LSH that we get fewer correct results as we look further from the query, which means that we cannot expect to increase our recognition performance by considering a greater number of nearest neighbors.

In figure 10.14, we show the tradeoff for different numbers of tables and hash divisions (l and k). Each line corresponds to a fixed number of divisions, and we vary the number of tables along the line, with the largest number of tables at the rightmost point on each line. As expected, with a greater number of tables we see better performance but we also perform more comparisons.

In general, recognition performance should increase as error by rank decreases, though to what degree will depend upon the recognition algorithm and data set. Next we introduce a variant of LSH which will find the same or more of the nearest neighbors as LSH, but at a computational cost between LSH and exact nearest neighbor.

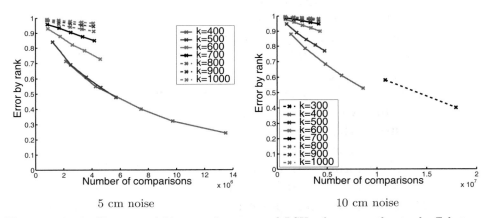

5 cm noise   10 cm noise

Figure 10.14 Nearest-neighbor performance of LSH, shown as the tradeoff between the number of comparisons and the error-by-rank for the 5 cm and 10 cm query sets. The lower-right corner of the graph is the ideal result, where the number of comparisons and the error by rank are low. The number of tables used is varied from 20 to 100 along each line. With 400 divisions, we drive down the error by rank, but also dramatically increase the number of comparisons required.

10.7   Associative LSH

In order to improve the error-by-rank and recognition performance, we introduce a variation which we will refer to as *associative LSH*. This

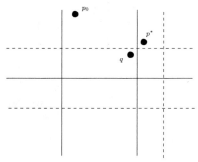

Figure 10.15 A 2D LSH example showing the space divided into bins by axis-parallel lines. The solid lines represent the divisions from one hash table, and the dashed lines represent divisions from another. Note that although p^* is the nearest neighbor to q, they do not occupy the same bin in either of the tables. It is the case, however, that p^* can be reached from q: q and p_0 are binmates in the solid-line table and p_0 and p^* are binmates in the dashed-line table.

algorithm begins with the results returned from LSH, and then uses the LSH tables to further explore the neighborhood around the query feature.

Consider the situation in figure 10.15 where we have a query q and the closest point to it, p^*, where for all tables i, $h_i(q) \neq h_i(p^*)$. It may be the case that there exists a point p_0 such that for two different tables i and j, $h_i(q) = h_i(p_0)$ and $h_j(p_0) = h_j(p^*)$. This suggests that we could use p_0 to find p^*.

First, a word about the data structures necessary. We will need the l LSH hash tables. To speed the algorithm we will also use precomputed l reverse hashes $b_i = R_i(j)$, which take an integer feature identifier and return the bucket in the ith table in which it is stored. Note that this is the reverse of the $T_i(b_i)$ function. Note that these reverse hashes are not necessary since we could retrieve the feature f_j from disk and calculate $h_i(f_i)$.

Results will be written to a structure $\mathcal{R}$ that for each match found so far stores the integer feature identifier j and the distance to the query, $\text{dist}(q, f_j)$, sorted by distance. This is the same structure we used for results when performing LSH queries. We will keep lists of the numbers of the buckets we have visited, one for each of the tables. Call the ith of these lists $\mathcal{B}_i$. We will also have a set of integer identifiers $\mathcal{A}$ which is initially empty.

The algorithm takes as input a rank depth r and a query feature q and outputs the results structure $\mathcal{R}$. Notice that the first three steps below are identical to the original LSH algorithm as described earlier, with the exception of the use of $\mathcal{B}_i$ for record-keeping.

1. For all i, calculate $b_i = h_i(q)$. Add b_i to $\mathcal{B}_i$ so that we do not visit the bucket b_i in the ith table again.

2. Calculate $\mathbb{F} = \bigcup_{i=1}^{l} T_i(b_i)$.

3. For all $j \in \mathbb{F}$, calculate $\text{dist}(q, f_j)$ and add to the results list R.

4. Find a feature identifier that is within the top r results in $\mathcal{R}$ and that is not in the set $\mathcal{A}$, call it a. If such a feature does not exist, then terminate.

5. Add a to the set $\mathcal{A}$. This, with the check above, ensures that we do not iterate using this feature again.

6. For all i, find $b_i = R_i(a)$, the bucket in which a is stored in the ith table.

7. For all i where $b_i \notin \mathcal{B}_i$ (i.e., we have not already looked in bucket b_i in table i), retrieve $\mathbb{F} = \bigcup_i T_i(b_i)$, the identifiers in the buckets in which a resides.

8. For all i, add b_i to $\mathcal{B}_i$.

9. For each identifier $j \in \mathbb{F}$ that is not already in $\mathcal{R}$, calculate $\text{dist}(q, f_j)$ and store the result in $\mathcal{R}$.

10. Go to step 4.

This algorithm requires only one parameter, r, that LSH does not require. In our experiments, we did not tune r, setting it only to two. Setting it higher would result in more comparisons and perhaps better results. The data structures for $R_i(\cdot)$ are l arrays, each with an element for each reference feature stored in the LSH tables. This roughly doubles the amount of memory required to hold the LSH tables, though it does not need to be stored on disk as it can quickly be generated when the tables are loaded from disk. Note that any variation on LSH that randomly generates the hash divisions can be used with this method as well.

The running time of the algorithm is dependent upon the number of associative iterations performed and the number of features retrieved on each iteration. The additional bookkeeping required for associative LSH over regular LSH adds a negligible amount of overhead. Step 4 requires a $O(r)$ search through the results list and comparison with the hashed set $\mathcal{A}$, but r will be set to a small constant (two in our experiments). Steps 8 and 9 require additional bookkeeping using the structure $\mathcal{B}_i$, but the complexity in both cases is $O(l)$ if we make $\mathcal{B}_i$ a hashed set.

In figure 10.16 we show the tradeoff between the number of comparisons performed and the error by rank for our associative LSH queries. We see a drop in the error by rank over regular LSH, especially when comparing results using the same number of hash divisions, but we see a corresponding increase in the number of comparisons.

In figure 10.16 we show the tradeoff between comparisons and error by rank using associative LSH. Comparing to the results for LSH in figure 10.14 we see that we achieve a better tradeoff. For example, in the 5 cm experiments using 400 divisions, associative LSH achieves a slightly lower error and about the same number of comparisons using twenty tables as LSH does using eighty tables. Similarly, using 600 divisions, associative LSH achieves 65% error in 5×10^6 comparisons using twenty tables, whereas LSH reaches only 72% error in the same number of comparisons using 100 tables. From these results we can see that our search using associative LSH is more focused; we are finding a comparable number of nearest neighbors

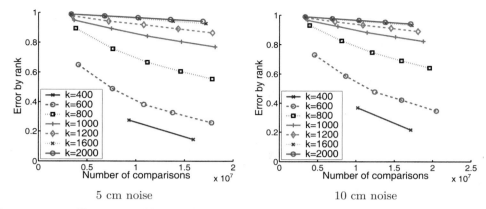

5 cm noise   10 cm noise

Figure 10.16   Nearest-neighbor performance of associative LSH, shown as the tradeoff between the number of comparisons and the error by rank for the 5 cm and 10 cm query sets. Compare these graphs to those in figure 10.14 showing nearest-neighbor performance of LSH. The number of tables used is varied from 20 to 100 along each line.

with associative LSH but with fewer comparisons. In the 10 cm experiments, this effect is more dramatic as associative LSH is able to achieve much lower error rates with a comparable number of comparisons.

Another important difference is that associative LSH is much less sensitive to the choices of k and the number of tables. With LSH, error changes dramatically with a change in the number of tables, and we see a quick degradation with an increase in the number of divisions.

10.8   Summary

In this chapter, we have performed an analysis of methods for performing object recognition on a particular data set, with a focus on the tradeoff between the speed of computation and the recognition performance of the methods. We made use of LSH for improving the speed of our queries, and demonstrated ways in which it could be made more robust.

In figure 10.17 we display as a scatterplot results from the different methods discussed earlier in the chapter on the 5 cm query data set. For each method, we show points for all the variations of number of RDs, number of hash divisions, and number of tables. In general, results for associative LSH using voting lie between LSH and exact nearest neighbor using voting, with the same true for all three methods using RDs. Looking at the left graph showing results using the top choice, the best associative LSH results using RDs is close both in recognition and speed to LSH results using voting. If we can accept finding the match in the top three results returned, all the methods presented can get us to 100% recognition, with LSH with RDs achieving the lowest number of comparisons by a small margin over LSH with voting and associative LSH with RDs. We note again that the range

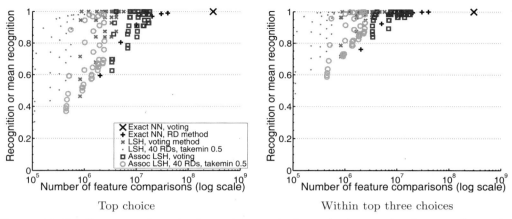

Top choice   Within top three choices

Figure 10.17 Summary of results for various methods on the 5 cm noise data set. For each method, we show points for all the variations of number of RDs, number of hash divisions, and number of tables discussed earlier in the chapter. The legend applies to both graphs.

of k using in the associative LSH experiments is much larger than in the LSH experiments, showing that we can achieve similar performance with less precise tuning of the parameters.

In figure 10.18 we give a scatterplot of the results for the various 10 cm noise experiments. Again we see that the associative LSH results lie between LSH and exact nearest neighbor, though as we see in the first plot, LSH using 300 divisions and the voting method shows a slightly higher recognition rate and lower comparisons than associative LSH. In general, however, associative LSH yields a higher recognition rate than LSH, though by performing more comparisons. We also note that when using the voting method, the results for associative LSH are more tightly packed than the LSH results, despite using a wider range of parameters for associative LSH in the experiments. This indicates that associative LSH can yield similar results on this data set with less tuning of the parameters.

In conclusion, we have found that LSH is an effective method for speeding nearest-neighbor search in a difficult object recognition task, but at the cost of some recognition performance. We have touched upon the connection between the reduction in recognition performance and the performance of LSH as a nearest-neighbor algorithm, and have presented a variation, associative LSH, which gives an improvement in nearest-neighbor performance on our data set. This increase in nearest-neighbor performance translates only roughly into recognition performance, showing small gains in recognition performance on this data set for an additional computational cost.

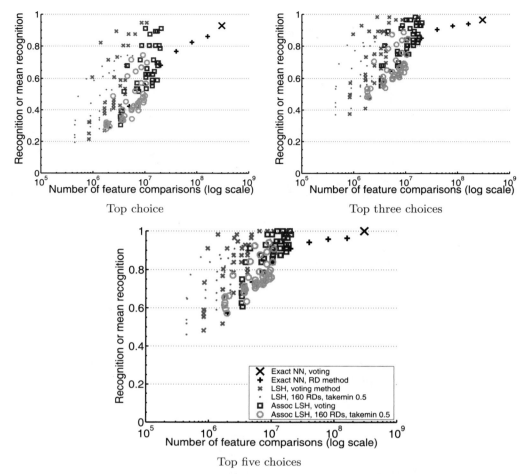

Top choice

Top three choices

Top five choices

Figure 10.18 Summary of results for various methods on the 10 cm noise data set, showing results for the top choice, top three, and top five choices. For each method, we show points for all the variations of number of RDs, number of hash divisions, and number of tables discussed earlier in the chapter. The legend in (c) applies to all three plots.

References

1. S. Arya, D.M. Mount, N.S. Netanyahu, R. Silverman, and A.Y. Wu. An optimal algorithm for approximate nearest neighbor searching fixed dimensions. *Journal of the ACM*, 45(6):891–923, November 1998.

2. S. Belongie, J. Malik, and J. Puzicha. Matching shapes. In *Eighth IEEE International Conference on Computer Vision*, volume 1, pages 454–461, July 2001.

3. S. Belongie, J. Malik, and J. Puzicha. Shape matching and object recognition using shape contexts. *IEEE Transactions on Pattern Analysis and Machine Intelligence*, 24(4):509–522, April 2002.

4. A. Berg and J. Malik. Geometric blur for template matching. In *Proceedings of IEEE Conference on Computer Vision and Pattern Recognition*, pages 607–614, 2001.

5. A.C. Berg, T.L. Berg, and J. Malik. Shape matching and object recognition using low distortion correspondence. Technical Report UCB//CSD-04-1366, University of California Berkeley, Computer Science Division, Berkeley, December 2004.

6. A. Frome, D. Huber, R. Kolluri, T. Bülow, and J. Malik. Recognizing objects in range data using regional point descriptors. In *Proceedings of the European Conference on Computer Vision*, volume 3, pages 224–237, May 2004.

7. A. Gionis, P. Indyk, and R. Motwani. Similarity search in high dimensions via hashing. In *Proceedings of Twenty-Fifth International Conference on Very Large Data Bases (VLDB)*, pages 518–529, 1999.

8. D.P. Huttenlocher and S. Ullman. Recognizing solid objects by alignment with an image. *International Journal of Computer Vision*, 5(2):195–212, November 1990.

9. P.Indyk and R.Motwani. Approximate nearest neighbor—towards removing the curse of dimensionality. In *Proceedings of the Thirtieth Symposium on Theory of Computing*, pages 604–613, 1998.

10. A.E. Johnson and M. Hebert. Using spin images for efficient object recognition in cluttered 3D scenes. *IEEE Transactions on Pattern Analysis and Machine Intelligence*, 21(5):433–449, 1999.

11. T. Liu, A.W. Moore, A. Gray, and K.Yang. An investigation of practical approximate nearest neighbor algorithms. In *Advances in Neural Information Processing Systems*, December 2004.

12. D.Lowe. Object recognition from local scale-invariant features. In *Proceedings of the International Conference on Computer Vision*, pages 1000–1015, September 1999.

13. G. Mori, S. Belongie, and J. Malik. Shape contexts enable efficient retrieval of similar shapes. In *Proceedings of IEEE Conference on Computer Vision and Pattern Recognition*, volume 1, pages 723–730, 2001.

14. G. Mori and J. Malik. Recognizing objects in adversarial clutter: Breaking a visual captcha. In *Proceedings of IEEE Conference on Computer Vision and Pattern Recognition*, 2003.

15. C.Schmid and R.Mohr. Combining greyvalue invariants with local constraints for object recognition. In *Proceedings of IEEE Conference on Computer Vision and Pattern Recognition*, pages 872–877, June 1996.

16. P. Viola and M.J. Jones. Robust real-time face detection. *International Journal of Computer Vision*, 57(2):137–154, May 2004.

Contributors

Jonathan Alon
Boston University
Boston, MA 02215
USA

Alexandr Andoni
MIT
Cambridge, MA 02139
USA

Vassilis Athitsos
Siemens Corporate Research
Princeton, NJ 08540
USA

Kenneth L. Clarkson
Bell Laboratories,
Lucent Technologies
Murray Hill, NJ 07974
USA

Trevor Darrell
MIT
Cambridge, MA 02139
USA

Mayur Datar
Google
Mountain View, CA 94043
USA

Aaron D'Souza
University of Southern California
Los Angeles, CA 90089
USA

Bogdan Georgescu
Siemens Corporate Research
Princeton, NJ 08540
USA

Kristen Grauman
MIT
Cambridge, MA 02139
USA

Alexander Gray
Georgia Institute of Technology
Atlanta, GA 30332
USA

Andrea Frome
University of California, Berkeley
Berkeley, CA 94720
USA

Nicole Immorlica
MIT
Cambridge, MA 02139
USA

Piotr Indyk
MIT
Cambridge, MA 02139
USA

George Kollios
Boston University
Boston, MA 02215
USA

Ting Liu
Carnegie-Mellon University
Pittsburgh, PA 15213
USA

Peter Meer
Rutgers University
Piscataway, NJ 08854
USA

Andrew W. Moore
Carnegie-Mellon University
Pittsburgh, PA 15213
USA

Stan Sclaroff
Boston University
Boston, MA 02215
USA

Ilan Shimshoni
Haifa University
Haifa 31905
Israel

Paul Viola
Microsoft Research
Redmond, WA 98052
USA

Jitendra Malik
University of California, Berkeley
Berkeley, CA 94720
USA

Vahab Mirrokni
MIT
Cambridge, MA 02139
USA

Stefan Schaal
University of Southern California
Los Angeles, CA 90089
USA

Gregory Shakhnarovich
Brown University
Providence, RI 02912
USA

Sethu Vijayakumar
University of Edinburgh
Edinburgh EH9 3EL
United Kingdom

Index